Urban Saniscapes

African History and Culture

SERIES EDITOR

Peter Alegi, *Michigan State University*

African History and Culture is a book series that builds upon and expands Michigan State University's commitment to the study of Africa. The series features books on African history, anthropology, sociology, and political science, as well as interdisciplinary studies, works on the African diaspora, and digital scholarship.

Urban Saniscapes

SLUMS, HOUSING, AND EVERYDAY SANITATION IN ACCRA AND NAIROBI, 1908–1963

Waseem-Ahmed Bin-Kasim

Michigan State University Press | *East Lansing*

Michigan State University Press
East Lansing, Michigan 48823-5245

Library of Congress Cataloging-in-Publication Data
Names: Bin-Kasim, Waseem-Ahmed author
Title: Urban saniscapes : slums, housing and everyday sanitation
in Accra and Nairobi, 1908–1963 / Waseem-Ahmed Bin-Kasim.
Description: East Lansing : Michigan State University Press, [2025] |
Series: African history and culture |
Includes bibliographical references and index.
Identifiers: LCCN 2025005060 | ISBN 9781611865493 paperback |
ISBN 9781609177942 | ISBN 9781628955576
Subjects: LCSH: Sanitation—Ghana—Accra—History—20th century |
Sanitation—Kenya—Nairobi—History—20th century |
Urbanization—Ghana—Accra—History—20th century |
Urbanization—Kenya—Nairobi—History—20th century |
Urban health—Ghana—Accra—History—20th century |
Urban health—Kenya—Nairobi—History—20th century
Classification: LCC RA545 .B556 2025
LC record available at https://lccn.loc.gov/2025005060

Cover photo: Aerial view of housing estates,
Nairobi, Kenya, 1961, The National Archives.

Visit Michigan State University Press at *www.msupress.org*

Contents

Preface

THIS BOOK COMPARES ENVIRONMENTAL SANITATION IN THE HISTORICAL DEVELOPment of Accra and Nairobi over the first half of the twentieth century. The cities were crucial capitals of British non-settler and settler colonies of the Gold Coast (now Ghana) in West Africa and Kenya (East African Protectorate until 1920) in East Africa. The cities served as the administrative centers where colonial officials ruled the Gold Coast and Kenya. Imperial planners and colonial officials chose to establish the capital of the Gold Coast in the already diverse and cosmopolitan city of Accra. In contrast, they conveniently built Nairobi from the ground up during railway construction. The broad histories of the territories these cities were in also shaped their historical evolution. In the early twentieth century, the Gold Coast increasingly gained popularity in West Africa for its cocoa economy, whereas Kenya became the main settler colony in East Africa. Unlike the Gold Coast, where Europeans controlled much of the trade but did not establish permanent homes and farms, Europeans in Kenya appropriated most of the best land, using it to dominate the colonial economy and society. Despite the differences in trade and settlement histories, imperial and official visions for Accra and Nairobi as projections of British power shaped diverse urban experiences of Africans. Acquisition of land by officials, professionals, and settlers for communication and transportation infrastructure, warehouse facilities, banks, trading facilities, security installations, residential buildings, and administrative structures was crucial in establishing Accra and Nairobi as seats of colonial and settler power. As the cities grew into commercial and administrative hubs, they became centers of urbanization. This urban growth, in turn, led to British colonial regulations emphasizing racial residential segregation and Western standards of sanitation infrastructure and orderly urbanization. The degree to which officials and municipal authorities could enforce these regulations depended on land tenure.

Sanitation as the Unit of Analysis

Sanitation was an essential aspect of the urban built environment, which I hope to disentangle in this book. The book looks at sanitation specifically as a European cultural tradition. Sanitation was a set of public health measures to prevent exposure to pathogenic microbes through material infrastructure, municipal regulations, and services. From its inception, it has been a Western concept that evolved to address the poor urban conditions that resulted from the Industrial Revolution.[1] The modern ways of achieving sanitation had their roots in Western Europe's public health movement in response to a series of cholera outbreaks in the nineteenth century. European physicians and social reformers, like Edwin Chadwick, John Snow, and John Simon, linked diseases to filth and urged state intervention through laws to clean cities. Chadwick provided a leading role in urban sanitation and public health reform; John Snow, a London surgeon, traced the cause of cholera to feces-infested water in Soho; and John Simon, London's chief medical officer, latched onto Snow's discovery to raise funds to build sanitation infrastructure in the city, including water and sewage systems, replacing cesspools and local pumps. Regular sanitation services to clean up Britain's cities strengthened as the reformers and physicians convinced the urban bourgeois of the connection between diseases and filth. In 1866, Britain's Sanitary Act set minimum standards for water and sewage systems for local governments. All these changes occurred when Louis Pasteur discovered that microorganisms or pathogens could cause diseases.[2]

The public health moment in Britain coincided with Haussmannization, which transformed the physical appearance of central Paris and helped resolve the cholera problem in the latter half of the nineteenth century. With vast powers bestowed on him by Emperor Louis Napoleon III, Georges-Eugène Haussmann oversaw an enormous public works scheme that demolished overcrowded neighborhoods and what were considered unhealthy areas and replaced them with parks, squares, gardens, and wide thoroughfares. The scheme also included the construction of new sewer networks.[3] In seeking to prevent cholera and other diseases, public health measures recognized the importance of constructing drainage and sewage systems; government regulations in urban areas; and regular services to remove filth from homes, streets, and roads and improve the water supply. Not only did the measures enhance the aesthetic appearances of the cities, but they also reshaped the built environment.

Thus, in this book I define sanitation as sets of constructed, regulated, and serviced public health infrastructures. Sanitation was crucial in Accra and Nairobi because it promised to secure the health and lives of European officials, traders, and settlers upon whom the political economies of the Gold Coast and Kenya hinged. In the minds of officials and imperialists, the health benefits would extend to African laborers after securing the health and lives of Europeans. The poor sanitation in cities across Britain, the ensuing sanitation reforms, and global outbreaks of sanitation-related diseases like cholera and plague, capable of severely disrupting transoceanic trade and colonial societies, had given rise to growing professions, like physicians and sanitation experts, with the power to reorder colonial cities along modern Western sanitation lines.[4] The health professionals, along with experts in urban planning, design, and development, increasingly assumed a technocratic role by making their knowledge indispensable to the strength and wealth of the empire. Since Accra and Nairobi were the seats of power and commercial centers, they became the early sites of experimenting with burgeoning health and urban planning expertise to enable European merchants, officials, and missionaries to live and work in the tropics while enjoying high mortality and morbidity. Land played a critical role in developing health infrastructures and urban plans. However, Africans also lived in the places where these metropolitan-inspired experimentations took place. The sanitation policies and practices impacted the lives and livelihoods of the African residents of Accra and Nairobi, and the strategies employed by the residents to cope with urbanization influenced colonial urban sanitation policies and practices. The ways British colonial officials imposed sanitation did not always align with the interests and aspirations of Africans. For that reason, dealing with sanitation sometimes yielded unexpected results.

Because of Accra's longstanding African settlement and urbanization history, African chiefs, lineage heads, and individuals controlled urban and suburban land.

The colonial state attempted to assert unbridled control of land through the 1876 Public Lands Ordinance to seize land for public purposes. It extended the power of land control using the 1892 Towns Ordinance, which helps explain the perceived sanitation importance of state-controlled land, among others.[5] Additionally, the Western-educated and elite Africans prevented a lands bill seeking to place urban and rural land under British Crown ownership.[6] Seen through colonial-driven sanitation schemes, officials failed to achieve complete land control.[7] The inability of officials to enforce its sanitation order through legislation partly explains a proverb in the Gold Coast that "laws are passed to throw dust in the eyes of the Colonial Office" in the metropole that the local colonial regime had their subjected communities under control.[8]

Unlike in Accra, European settlers dominated Nairobi's land. The settlers were determined to establish Kenya as a "white man's country" in Africa, placing land at the heart of the politics of racial hierarchy.[9] In 1903, the concept of the "white highland," championed by Charles Eliot, the newly appointed Kenya commissioner, had profound implications. It assured Europeans exclusive rights to vast, seemingly sparsely populated land between Machakos and Fort Ternan, a decision that would shape the colony's political future. The land was relatively fertile and the climate favorable. Eliot intended to reinforce the justification for laying the railway from Kenya to Uganda. He wanted to guarantee a means for paying for its construction through settler exploitation. The settlers had even greater control of Nairobi's land than the rest of the colony.[10] Despite having greater land control power than officials in Accra, settlers still faced significant challenges in making Nairobi a "white city" based on the logics of sanitation.

Brief Histories of Accra and Nairobi

Accra

Before becoming the British colonial capital city of the Gold Coast, Accra was the home of Ga communities since the end of the sixteenth century. Arriving in different groups at different times from the Gold Coast's eastern interior with diverse customs and traditions, the Ga settled among aboriginal Kpeshi in Accra. The area around the coastline settlement was characterized by an undulating plain, sparsely wooded and bordered by the Akwapim Mountains and the Shai Hills to the north and the Atlantic Ocean to the south. It provided the Ga with opportunities for farming and

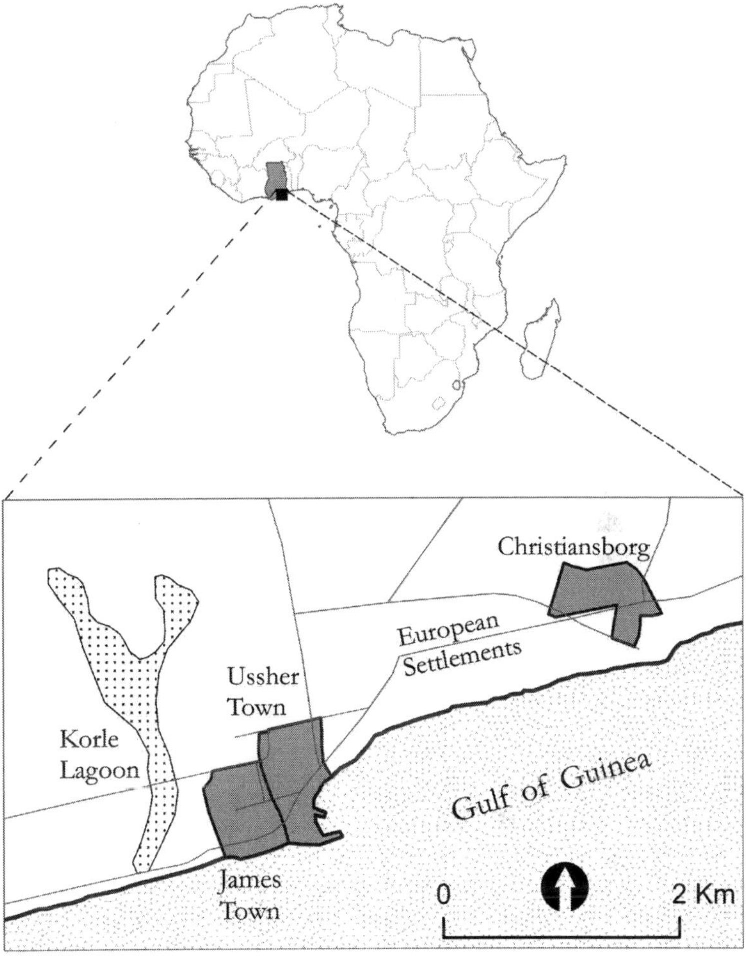

FIGURE 1. By 1903, the first European Victoriaborg took shape in Accra. The expansion of the Victoriaborg along the coastline of the Gulf of Guinea (Atlantic Ocean) threatened to displace the Ga people of Accra from their longstanding communities in James Town, Ussher Town, and Christiansborg. The Ga had built Accra since the seventeenth century as fishing communities and trading entrepôts serving Africans in the interior and the expanding Atlantic economy. The Ga communities established Accra as the center of their urbanism. By the interwar years, the city's built environment acquired the characteristics of a port city serving imperial capitalism. SOURCE: JOHN PARKER, *MAKING THE TOWN: GA STATE AND SOCIETY IN EARLY COLONIAL ACCRA* (PORTSMOUTH, NH: HEINEMANN, 2000), XVII–XIX.

fishing. Fishing and salt making became the main economic occupations. The Ga lived in close quarters along the coast for mutual defense from frequent conflicts and threats of aggression from neighboring African states.

About a century later, the presence of forts, lodges, and a castle on the coastline showed that Portuguese, Dutch, English, Danes, and Swedish merchants were vying to dominate trading with the Ga. Accra had become a busy southern terminus of trade in ivory, gold, and enslaved people from beyond its borders. The Ga occupied the crucial middle position between the land and sea trades. Their men and women negotiated the expanding trade between Europeans in the Atlantic system and Africans in the interior of the coast. Three of the Ga coastal settlements formed the nucleus of what would become Accra. They were the "seaside towns" (*nshonamajii*) of James Town (Nleshi), Ussher Town (Kinka), and Christiansborg (Osu), shown in figure 1. Each seaside town was composed of various quarters. James Town consisted of Alata, Sempe, and Akanmaji. Abola, Gbese, Otublohum, and Asere constituted Ussher Town. Christiansborg, to the east, had Kinkawe, Asante Blohum, Alata, and Anecho.[11] James Town adjoined Ussher Town between Korle Lagoon to the west and a little beyond Horse Road and Otoo Street to the northeast. The area of the two towns' was 0.6 square miles. Three miles east along the coast was Christiansborg.[12] The coastal towns were the Ga's religious, political, and economic center.

About four years before Accra became the capital of the Gold Coast in 1877, Henry Morton Stanley, a special correspondent for the *New York Herald,* traveled in West Africa and described the city's built environment. As an outsider without insights into the historical and social relationships that shaped Accra, Stanley portrayed a cosmopolitan urban setting as marked by whitewashed houses with wide verandas and open spaces belonging to wealthy merchants and Basel (Swiss and German) Christian missionaries, a port and lighthouse in the center, and a congestion of African and European houses. Stanley quickly linked poor sanitation to congestion, a connection that later colonial officials and experts would also perceive and instrumentalize in an attempt to reorder the city. Stanley contrasted the whitewashed wide-veranda houses and open spaces with overcrowded homes. The whitewashed houses with wide verandas and open spaces afforded wealthy residents fresh air, but the congested communities did not. Amid the more densely populated areas, there were thatch-roof houses constructed in a perceived-to-be disorderly pattern, resulting in narrow, crooked streets.[13] Accra's built environment became the subject of imperial and colonial correspondence and discussion when officials considered the city the Gold Coast's capital. They chose Accra despite the critiques of its sanitation. The city had some advantages that others in the colony lacked, including scarce swamps nearby, thriving commerce, and ample land for healthy living in the countryside. In March 1877, British officials transferred the capital of the Gold Coast to Accra.[14]

Accra became a focus of sanitation reform as the seat of the colonial power, a port city, and an economic hub. The congestion in James Town, Ussher Town, and Christiansborg took center stage in the colonial discourse about sanitation improvement. Officials thought of cleansing the city of filth and (re)ordering the arrangement of buildings, infrastructure, and open spaces, which, in their minds, would make it worthy of being a British capital city. To remake the city through sanitation, officials passed the Towns, Police, and Public Health Ordinance in 1878.[15] The ordinance was the first public health law intended to improve sanitation in the city. Under the ordinance, landowners could not build without the governor's permission. The ordinance required them to repair or demolish deteriorated property. The colonial administration reserved the power to impose fines for sanitation violations. The law also charged the colonial surveyor with making, cleaning, and draining streets. A year before the transfer of the capital city, officials promulgated the Public Lands Ordinance, which would provide the legal basis for compulsory land purchase to facilitate the remaking of Accra.[16] By 1894, visible changes in the cityscape included public cemeteries instead of home burials, streetlamps, toilets (latrines), and dustbins. Sanitation laborers regularly kept the main streets and European areas clean.[17] Bringing about sanitation in Accra provoked the construction, maintenance, and regulation of different elements of the urban landscape.

The Accra Town Council Ordinance of 1896 defined James Town, Ussher Town, and Christiansborg as the municipality and gave the colonial state new powers over sanitation. Its creation sparked protests and riots because of diverse and competing interests among officials, traditional African chiefs, and Western-educated African elites. While the colonial state wanted to relieve itself of municipal governance, the chiefs and elites wanted to exercise control. The sticking issue was the council's task of direct taxation through rates and license fees, a plan that instigated widespread urban protests. Because of the protests, most residents received a tax exemption due to poverty. However, a handful of affluent African residents agreed to pay. The council comprised an official European majority, an African minority elected by the wealthy residents, and a member of the European business community. The colonial state's policy of leaving sanitation in the hands of the council was a severe challenge to improving the city since it could not raise adequate revenue for that purpose. The council was unpopular, frequently criticized by the Gold Coast press, and needed help from the colonial state to keep up with the growing city's sanitation challenges. The colonial state supported it financially, but its assistance was inadequate.[18] Partly because of the insufficient funds, the municipality's sanitation services were uneven and inadequate, resulting in a noticeable disparity along racial lines in the cityscape. While the council maintained and improved European housing and residential areas, the "native town" of James Town, Ussher Town, and Christiansborg was a "standing menace to the health of the community at large."[19] This poor sanitation in the African communities fueled both official and unofficial discourse about slums, demolition of entire neighborhoods, housing Africans, and equal waste management across the city throughout the colonial period.

Nairobi

Unlike Accra, Nairobi did not develop on a preexisting African urban agglomeration. Instead, African communities, such as the Kikuyu and Maasai, had utilized the unbuilt area that became Nairobi for trading and cattle grazing. The name "Nairobi," for the new city, came from a Maasai description, "Enkari Nayrobi," meaning a place of cold waters. It was the area where the Nairobi River emerged from the swamp. The Maasai and Kikuyu were not interested in establishing their homes near the swampy area.[20] Nairobi's growth as a city began in 1899 when British engineers, whose influence would shape the city's future, constructed the railway line and set up camp on the site approximately three hundred miles from Mombasa. The Uganda Railway Committee at the Foreign Office in London granted significant power to the engineers, independent of the civil colonial officials in Kenya, allowing them to control the plain south of the swamp. The rapid urbanization of Nairobi caught the attention of colonial officials, leading to the transfer of the Ukamba provincial administration under Colonel John Ainsworth from Machakos to Nairobi in that very year. Ainsworth built his administration center north of the swamp so as not to infringe on the landed property of the railway administration.[21] The control of two different parts of Nairobi by the railway authority and Ainsworth presented a double competing vision for planning and managing the city that profoundly impacted sanitation. Meanwhile, the colonial state had to decide how to tap Kenya's highland forest and agricultural resources for the benefit of the British Empire and to pay the cost of the railway construction. Officials dismissed

Africans' ability to develop their natural resources and sought out others to provide the economic and technical skills required.[22] There were numerous transnational South Asian populations whose trading in and knowledge of the region stretched over centuries. They also provided the labor and resources for the construction of the railway. Charles Eliot sought European settlers from Britain and South Africa to invest in developing agricultural and forest resources. The initial target of successful capitalists in North America and Australia did not materialize as envisioned. Still, Kenya attracted European settlers from Britain and South Africa who had moved to Nairobi in waves.

Compared to Accra, sanitation played a pivotal role in establishing Nairobi as a European urban center and the capital of Kenya. When the chief engineer, George Whitehouse of the railway authority, camped at the site, thereby founding the nucleus of Nairobi, it was because the land was a large plain, allowing for trains to shunt. The plain had a limited water supply, enough for railway purposes. The railway authority developed workshops, stores, housing, and other property employing Europeans, South Asians, and Africans as physicians, accountants, police, magistrates, and laborers. The presence of the railway attracted ancillary populations who came to live in Nairobi outside the jurisdiction of the railway authority to benefit from the economic opportunities available. The influx of people, some of whom were South Asian and Arab from Mombasa and Zanzibar, came to settle in Nairobi to sell their wares and services to railway workers. Regulating the environmental sanitation of ancillary populations' locations was not the concern of the railway authority. It did not restrict the sprawl of the population and their locations, which lacked roads, drains, sewage, and other sanitation infrastructure. These unplanned developments, contrasting with the railway residential and official property, established Nairobi as a city divided from its foundation. Amid this growth, medical and sanitation discourse about Nairobi's (un)suitability for urbanization from a health perspective circulated widely. It intensified with an outbreak of a plague in 1902. While some medical officials condemned the site as unsuitable and advocated moving Nairobi to salubrious locations, others argued that sanitation infrastructures such as sewage and drainage would make the site habitable because of its healthy attitude. Further, recurring plague outbreaks and large areas in Nairobi suffering from malaria because of poor soil drainage made the argument for relocation more persuasive. Deciding to move or keep the current Nairobi location took over seven years of debate. While the discussion prolonged,

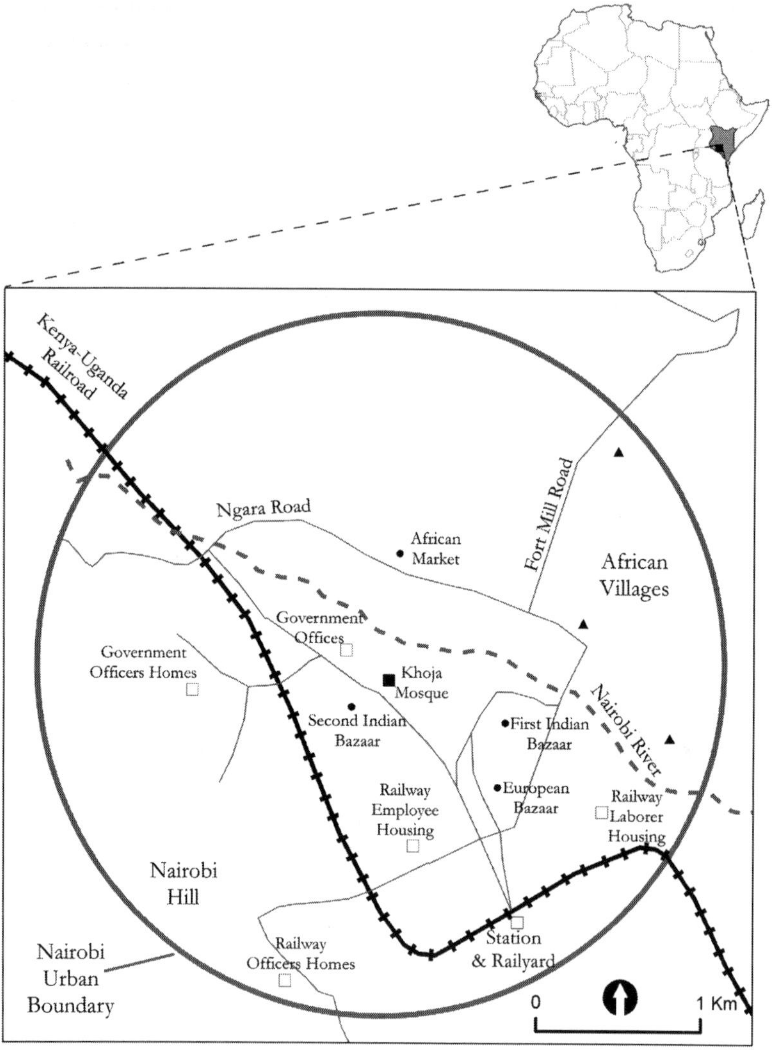

FIGURE 2. Map of Nairobi circa 1903. The British imperial system established the city from the foundation not because of a preexisting African settlement but a strategic importance. The system designated a town of about seven square miles. Nairobi performed primarily railway and administrative functions. While Africans established a commanding presence in Nairobi, they did not have an official residential location until after World War I. SOURCE: KENNETH GORDON MCVICAR, "TWILIGHT OF AN EAST AFRICAN SLUM: PUMWANI AND THE EVOLUTION OF AFRICAN SETTLEMENT IN NAIROBI" (PHD THESIS, UNIVERSITY OF CALIFORNIA LOS ANGELES, 1968), 12.

the development outside the railway section continued haphazardly. In 1905, when Nairobi became the capital city, it was too late to relocate. The politics against relocation rested on sustained investment and development in the area.[23]

As the municipal authority, the Nairobi Township Committee's work to improve sanitation was crucial. Two years before the plague outbreak, Nairobi published its first municipal regulations, which defined a boundary of one and a half square miles from the office of the Ukamba provincial subcommissioner. The city constituted a township committee and laid down the rules governing its duties to regulate urban growth and development, ensure Nairobi's cleanliness, and determine tax rates. In naming the township committee, Ainsworth aimed to resolve Nairobi's overlapping and competing management and its negative impact on sanitation.[24] The committee of two South Asians, two Europeans, and the provincial subcommission soon became divided over questions of sanitation that morphed into a complex interplay of European settler politics, the colonial state, and South Asian residents. As more Europeans arrived in Nairobi, further settler politics, which aimed for autonomy from the colonial metropole, added an intriguing layer to the city's history of sanitation administration. Early European settlers encouraged further white settlement to counter the significant presence of South Asians, whose demographic advantage and longstanding knowledge of and dealings in the region made Nairobi appear more like a city in India than a European one. White settler politics excluded South Asians from Kenya's highlands, reserved the best land in Nairobi for whites' exclusive use, and dominated crucial committees in the municipal authority responsible for sanitation and public health. Marginalization of the South Asian communities grew worse as more settlers from South Africa arrived during World War I. Settler hostilities toward Africans manifested in their refusal to admit them to municipal authority until the 1940s.[25] Thus, the municipal authority lost focus on one of its core mandates to ensure Nairobi's growth along Western sanitation lines because of racial politics.

The decisions made by the colonial state and the settler-dominated municipal authority regarding residential patterns had a profound and enduring impact on the urban health and Nairobi's physical development, shaping it well beyond the colonial period. To the high altitude north and west of the railway line, Europeans acquired volcanic red soil land that was well drained and unlikely to swamp during rains and harbor mosquitos (see figure 2). They built large, spacious buildings on the land. By the 1940s, each European resident took up over one acre of land compared to thirty South Asians and three hundred Africans who would typically occupy that area. The only Africans who lived in the European areas were domestic servants. The settlers restricted Africans and South Asians to plains to the south and east of the railway line, characterized by nonporous soil that flooded during rains, swamped, and harbored conditions conducive to mosquito breeding even in the dry season.[26] The Nairobi market (Second Indian Bazaar, shown in figure 2) at the city's center was an essential area for the South Asian community and Africans, serving as a housing and commercial hub. Lack of sanitation services, proper infrastructure, and regulation from the municipal authorities worsened the already-existing environmental issues caused by the black cotton soil, leading to many public health problems for the residents.[27] Most African male workers were migrants who earned wages and returned to their rural homes after a brief stay in Nairobi. Their European and South Asian employers paid them a bachelor's wage, which was insufficient to afford decent housing or living. Additionally, their employers, except the railway authority that built the first African housing, provided little housing accommodation for them. As a result, Africans had to make temporary homes within and on the outskirts of Nairobi. By 1921, over 12,000 Africans resided in eight overcrowded communities. They included Kangemi, Kawangware, Kibera, Kileleshwa, Pangani, Mombasa, Masikini, and Pumwani.[28]

Processing the Sources

My research for *Urban Saniscapes* initially started with examining the work of William John Ritchie Simpson in Accra and Nairobi in 1908 and 1913, when he dealt with plague outbreaks threatening to destabilize colonial rule and economies. His proposed blueprints for Accra and Nairobi, crucial to my research, hinged on his sanitation expertise, rearranging the built environments to prevent future disease outbreaks and ensure the cities' healthy growth. The Simpsonian blueprints provide evidence for ecological and environmental determinism in tropical medicine, underscoring how frequently people came into contact with vectors and pathogens based on their settlement patterns and habits, proximity to animals, and land use. However, Simpson's urban plans privileged the lives and health of Europeans over non-Europeans. A diversity of empire-wide and outside advisors, including Major Orde-Brown, Herbert Baker, Walton Jameson, Maxwell Fry, L. W. Thornton White, P. R. Anderson, and L. Silberman, followed in Simpson's footsteps, although these latter urban experts were not as discriminatory as Simpson. Maxwell Fry, for example, went so far as to expose the discriminatory nature of the Simpsonian plan in Accra that attempted to remake the city without consideration for the interests of Africans. The book draws directly and indirectly on these experts' reports, letters, proposals, and urban drawings in libraries and archives in the United Kingdom, Kenya, Ghana, and the United States.

In addition to these Western expert advisors, powerful interconnected governments and institutions linked to modern capitalism were also involved in urban policies and city-building, producing a wealth of sources this book analyzes. Robert Home and Carl Nightingale show that these governments and capitalism-associated institutions teamed up with intellectual advisors and spread cities and segregation globally.[29] During the process, they created census returns, Secretary for Native Affairs papers, gazettes, ordinances, meeting minutes, maps, drawings, city engineers and attorney general papers, medical and sanitation reports, official correspondence, and advertising brochures. The records include information and descriptions of various aspects of Accra and Nairobi, such as buildings and construction booms, open spaces, local resistance to colonial urban plans, demographics, public health and sanitation issues, infrastructure, demolition, municipal government, and "slums." When read together, they show committees, discourse, prompts, and the like, shaping colonial policies from privileging European health in the 1920s to housing and developmentalism of the 1940s embracing Africans.[30]

Taking official correspondence, for example, governors had leeway, which gave a variegated influence on urban policies and practices. The evidence defies easy analysis that the cityscape emerged from the "top" consisting of experts and officials, or the "bottom" of the everyday urban residents.[31] In the beginning story of chapter 1, a sanitation-driven layout of Victoriaborg made by Governor Hugh Clifford and the failed attempt to remove the Nairobi Bazaar as proposed by Simpson to prevent plague and malaria was a confluence of top, bottom, and in-between. Accra had a history of grassroots mobilization and legal action against colonial sanitation measures. Clifford was not interested in expanding Victoriaborg as he aimed to minimize instability in the city. The governor's decision contradicted Simpson's blueprint and his predecessors' policies of relocating Africans from their ancestral homes and repurposing the land for European residential interests. In Nairobi, South Asian communities mobilized political capital in India and London, which proved effective against settler attempts to demolish the Nairobi market. Edward Northey would also uphold the interests of the South Asian community and their business relations with African Nairobians by not relocating the Nairobi Market as Simpson proposed. This latitude of governors to decide whatever they wanted is what Kwasi Kwarteng calls "anarchic individualism" in the British Empire.[32] The urban built environment reflected Kwateng's anarchic individualism and fits it in with Raymond Dumett's "decentralized improvisation," indicative of the range of choices and tools available to governors to extemporize urban policy practices that, at times, contradicted the visions of health and urban planning experts.[33]

Reports of officials, health experts, and architect-planners contain details suggesting misleading ideas that Africans were passive recipients of European urban visions. They don't wholly reveal the inability of officials to provide housing, infrastructure, and services and distract from their offensive policies, such as collecting taxes from Africans for European health and comfort. The records also noted events of Africans ignoring, resisting, and evading social engineering, characterizing them as backward. These depictions appear in colonial sanitation records, which Stephanie Newell aptly describes as symptomatic of broader contestations for land, power, and resources involving diverse urban constituencies.[34] Yet at other times, they reveal what Africans *did* to (attempt) to cope with persistent pollution, garbage, and overcrowding in their neighborhoods. In fact, waste accumulating in African residential locations because of uneven municipal services was persistent and constituted what Rob Nixon has called "slow violence."[35]

Colonial rule's uneven application of sanitation in favor of Europeans inevitably provoked an African response and shaped the built environment in particular ways. Liora Bigon's morphogenesis idea offers insights into understanding the diverse actions of officials, experts, and urban residents that came together to (re)configure the sanitation aspects of the urban built environment, which this book calls *saniscape*. Attempts to demolish "slums," provide housing, and cleanse neighborhoods of waste, enables the understanding of the saniscape as constantly generated (re)constructed, "deconstructed, activated, deactivated, and negotiated" by various players within and outside colonial and municipal authorities.[36] While European settlers liked to think of Nairobi as a "white city" and tried to keep it as such through municipal restrictions, the commanding presence of Africans and the South Asian communities in the urban economy and politics compelled experts, including Bransby Williams and Simpson, to push for the creation of exclusive residential areas for the communities in Nairobi. Indeed, African Nairobians whitewashed their houses to prevent vectors from spreading plague-causing pathogens and petitioned the municipality to grant freehold landed property, revealing the means through which they negotiated sanitation, sought to alleviate slum-like environments, managed their social lives, and engaged the settler state in ways evocative of AbdouMaliq Simone's "multiplexity of social organizations."[37]

Conventional archival materials produced by European officials and experts documented few African voices and perspectives on sanitation. Unlike in Nairobi, the situation is better in Accra because of its extended connection with the Atlantic exchange circuits, resulting in the formation of a class of Western-educated African elites who engaged directly with colonial officials and experts. Because of these historical differences, the reader will see in chapter 1 a more direct engagement between the African elites and colonial rule. After that, Nairobi's educated elites will gradually show in the records as more directly participating in making the city. A reader looking for the exact things Africans said in direct response to the Simpsonian blueprint, for example, in Accra and Nairobi, may not see it because of the dearth of African voices in the colonial archives. However, as will be seen in the ensuing chapters, when it came to the implementation phase of colonial visions, how Africans responded to them provides evidence of their agency in making the saniscape. Regardless of how damaging archival documents portray the responses, they show that African actions spoke louder than their words.

Newspapers and oral histories are equally crucial in reconstructing African experiences and perspectives on sanitation. African newspapers covered ongoing events and meetings and editorialized the pressing sanitation concerns in African communities. Urban residents also contributed short articles and commentaries about the saniscape to newspapers to show how it felt to experience communities with inadequate sanitation infrastructure and municipal services. While expert reports in the archives document the need for sewers, drains, pipes, streets, and toilets in African residential areas, the newspapers will provide insights into what it was really like to live without these infrastructures. The papers provide complex perspectives that counterbalanced negative official descriptions of African actions.[38] Most urban residents who could not read or write relied on Western-educated Africans to read and translate the newspapers aloud. In Accra, Africans with basic literacy skills in addition to African lawyers and physicians performed this role.[39] The role of the educated elites in disseminating information through the newspapers and translating from English to local languages understood by the urban masses gave them a unique advantage in mediating information to better position them as suitable leaders to provide sanitation infrastructure and services than the colonial administration and the traditional African authorities.[40] In his autobiography, Kwame Nkrumah recalls mobilizing the masses through newspaper reading and translation.[41] Gale, in his research, found that newspapers were a valuable resource for understanding the influence of sanitation on African nationalism, as they often answered pertinent questions about the development needs of African urban residents.[42]

Similarly, newspapers gave the educated elite access to the masses in Nairobi. Although this book uses only English newspapers because of my limitation in Kenya's local languages, it is worth noting that as early as 1928 Jomo Kenyatta, the nationalist leader who led Kenya into formal independence and became the first president, resigned from his job at the municipal council to take up a position as the general secretary of the Kikuyu Central Association (KCA). One of his first assignments was to edit *Muigwithania* (the Reconciler), the first African newspaper in Kenya.[43] Harry Thuku, who was also influential in Nairobi's politics and commanded the respect of sanitation workers, recalls keeping up with newspapers and having mass meetings in Nairobi to discuss the plight of Africans under the settler regime.[44]

Finally, the African novel series provides rich insights to support specific aspects of sanitation. The fact that novelists fictionalize the saniscape based on how they experienced it toward the end of formal colonial rule and the decades following the era demonstrates the continuing importance of urban sanitation in cities. Bill Marshall, the director of Studio Africain in Accra when he published *Bukom*, indicates that his discussion of the saniscape accurately depicts the aspirations of Accra's seaside communities.[45] Equally, Thomas Akare, who worked as a journalist and became a full-time writer, used *The Slums* in Nairobi to discuss what many Nairobi Africans thought about their impoverished conditions vis-à-vis the optimism that came with nationalism and *Uhuru* (freedom and progress).[46] Although they produced works of fiction, the novelists criticized poor sanitation and development policies in the colonial and postcolonial periods.

The Saniscape in Chapters

This book embarks on a unique journey, exploring the diverse histories of Accra and Nairobi. It invites readers to delve into their distinct narratives as settler and non-settler colonial cities. Structured chronologically from 1908 to 1963 and beyond, the book shifts between local communities, colonial states, and the colonial metropole and offers a fresh perspective on the complex interplay of multiple, often competing, interests in making the saniscapes, the book's central theme.

The introduction provides a detailed explanation of the theme. Each chapter focuses on a specific period in the history of Accra and Nairobi. The narrative style of each chapter keeps the reader engaged in the unique stories of the cities, highlighting key similarities and differences. In each chapter, the discussion always begins with the Accra case, followed by Nairobi's, under each subheading. At the end of each chapter, the conclusion situates the main arguments in the relevant scholarly texts. One thread throughout the book is how Africans coped with the uneven saniscape and colonial underinvestment in their communities' sanitation infrastructure, services, and regulation. A range of options they had were openly condemning colonial racism that prioritized the sanitation of European residential areas, technocratic failure, and constructing their own sanitation infrastructures.

Using the plague outbreaks in Accra and Nairobi and W. J. R. Simpson's working visits as reference backgrounds, chapter 1 shows what Africans and South Asians did to prevent the colonial state and its medical advisors from creating buffer zones envisioned for both Accra and Nairobi by 1920. Buffer zones were swaths of land intended to insulate residential enclaves exclusively designated for Europeans, in the imagination of colonial officials, settlers, and medical experts, to prevent diseases and disease-causing vectors from Africans and South Asians spreading to them. Rather than roads, railway lines, or walls taking a relatively minor width of land to separate European housing areas, buffer zones, undergirded by the mosquito theory, required swaths of land, which threatened to displace Africans and South Asians from their homes and sources of livelihoods. Even though buffer zones were not in place as envisioned by 1920, the contours of racially defined segregated residential areas between Europeans and non-Europeans had taken shape. Once residential segregation was in place, it became easier to concentrate sanitation infrastructure and municipal services on European residential areas in both cities. As will be seen in the introduction, this unequal distribution of these public health resources produced the uneven saniscapes that Decima Moore and Oliver Lyttelton saw in Accra and Nairobi.

Covering the period from 1920 to 1940, chapters 2 and 3 overlap chronologically. However, they focus respectively on slums and demolition, making them thematically different and interrelated. Colonial discourse on slums often evoked the demolition of African neighborhoods. The two chapters mutually reinforce some critical arguments about the fluid use of "slums" from their historical origins and how that targeted African neighborhoods and allowed calls beyond official domains for "slum clearance." From their roots in Industrial Britain, various urban constituencies juxtaposed "slums" with relatively affluent residential areas and regarded "slum" dwellers not only as the cause of deplorable slum-like conditions but as threats to urban societies. Despite the overseas distance, the political and economic conditions that produced "slums" in Britain also contributed to their emergence in Accra and Nairobi. "Slums" often appeared in official records as having attributes of overcrowding, congestion, and inadequate (lack of) sanitation infrastructures and services. These most visible physical elements of the so-called slums became the basis for their demolition and urban renewal. However, the advocates for demolition, some of whom were imperial agents, colonial officials, technocrats, and African urban residents, seemed oblivious that the faith of the colonial economy and cities depended on the skilled and unskilled workers who resided in "slums." Indeed, the reappearance of slum conditions after demolition demonstrates their connection to the cities.

Chapter 2 unpacks "slums" from their origin in industrializing and urbanizing Britain. It asks who resided in the communities that colonial records and newspapers designated as "slums" and interrogates the poor sanitation attributes that made them "slums." The slum-like communities in Accra and Nairobi were components of the colonial economies. In Accra, the Ga used their skill in navigating the seas of Accra on their surf boats to move people and commodities to and from the coast. Colonial officials, commercial agents, colonial experts, and visitors arriving in Accra met the boat crew first before the rest of the city's residents onshore. The Ga accommodated migrant workers who, in turn, welcomed newcomers and made urban life and labor bearable, reproducing the labors of colonial workers. Colonial officials made little accommodation and sanitation arrangements for the African workers. In Nairobi, the Swahili house owners, for example, provided housing and other services to make the harsh conditions of Nairobi's "native locations" bearable for migrant workers who worked for the state, municipality, and private employers. The term "slum" was so fluid that British officials, technocrats, and urban residents used it to flatten various African communities. The term also distracts from colonial rule's failures to keep up with the rapid urbanization the economies had set in motion. Yet the sanitation lag resulted from colonial urban policies prioritizing European health over Africans. The "slums" of Accra and Nairobi were an invented problem at the intersection of local and global responses to commercial and industrial capitalism. While poignantly showing that "slums" were not just a temporary blight but an integral part of the cities, this chapter sets the stage for the next, which discusses the futility of colonial urban planning and public health policy that isolated and (attempted to) demolish the problem areas of "slums."

Chapter 3 questions "slum clearance" as a reasonable solution to urban squalor and epidemics. Demolition as a sanitation project did not eliminate slum-like conditions in the cities. Indeed, demolition shifted and spread the poor environmental situation that colonial officials and their technocrats set out to remove. It sometimes exacerbated the growing urban population's housing and sanitation lag. That happened because improving the slum-like problems was not the main reason despite it appearing so in official correspondence. The economic motives behind demolition were to expand opportunities for commercial capitalism and settler dominance with little benefit to Accra's and Nairobi's African residents. However, Africans' resilience was evident as they perceived the planned destruction of their neighborhoods as a way for the state and municipal authorities to exclude them from the economic opportunities of urbanization. Colonial demolition activities yielded varying results. The responses of urban residents showed they had rights through their status as Natives. Ga landowners and property owners of Pangani and Pumwani were determined to benefit from the urban economy.

Chapter 4 focuses on urban housing. Housing was a means to address the shortages following the demolition, population explosion, and backlog of accommodation needs in the interwar, wartime, and postwar Accra and Nairobi. The chapter examines the housing situation in the cities in the context of imperial and colonial reckoning of neglecting the development of the colonies. Political pressure from colonial subjects led imperial and colonial agents to realize that urban residents would no longer accept the poor sanitation, manifested by "slums" and housing shortages in their cities. Imperial and colonial agents and their technocrat advisors, who included urban planners and social workers, saw housing in neighborhood units as a means to improve the standard of life, create jobs, and alleviate the shortages. Colonial and settler agents thought that science and technology would promote research into local building materials, allowing for industrialization and mass production in the housing sector. While the colonial state in Accra continued the rehousing projects after an earthquake and later integrated the neighborhood unit, the settler state and municipality used housing and the neighborhood unit to stabilize (according to the colonial state) Africans and families in Nairobi permanently. The projects could provide neither the envisioned job opportunities and social progress nor the required housing needs of the growing urban populations.

Still, they inscribed the contours of class in the built environment. The chapter demonstrates class in the built environment by showing the distribution of private and communal toilets and baths in the cities.

In Accra, colonial urban rehousing, which integrated roads and dense vegetation to create barriers dividing the residential locations of Ga and laborers from the estates of wealthy and Western-educated Africans, envisioned the continuation of the sanitation-based racialized residential segregation in the first two decades of the twentieth century. This vision did not materialize. A dynamic Ga land tenure system, coupled with shortages and high costs of labor and building materials, proved impossible, leading to an incomplete project. In chapter 5, the settler state in Nairobi would also consider fences and barriers to control waste problems. Chapter 5 examines waste in the cities during the momentous decades of the 1950s, when urban residents, local authorities, and the state aspired to modern infrastructures and technologies to remove accumulated and stagnant waste from their communities. These waste problems stretched back to prior decades and persisted. In the 1950s, however, piled-up trash in African communities, in contrast to European residential locations, reassumed political implications in Accra, which nationalist leaders and African representatives of the Accra Town Council leveraged and discredited colonial rule for producing the city's division by waste. In Nairobi, a strike and Mau Mau brought the city's sanitation system to a collapse, with the African locations bearing the brunt. The construction of modern sanitation infrastructure to reduce waste buildup in sections of the city perpetuated an unequal saniscape and became part of the development discourse.

The epilogue summarizes the book, focusing on the role of Africans within the complex web of global, local, and regional dynamics that shaped the urban saniscape. It begins by revisiting Rendeavour's Appolonia City and Tatu City housing projects in Accra and Nairobi. These residential communities are part of a string of interventions throughout the colonial history of the cities to address urban challenges such as overcrowding and congestion, which have seriously impacted environmental sanitation. Urban residents who have the financial means and seek to escape these sanitation challenges provide a profitable market to incentivize Rendeavour to undertake such expensive housing and development projects. The epilogue recalls events in the five chapters and shows how they relate to Readeavour's urban housing and development visions.

Acknowledgments

I AM DEEPLY GRATEFUL TO THE INDIVIDUALS AND INSTITUTIONS THAT HAVE PROfoundly influenced my academic journey and played a crucial role in the publication of this book. There are many contributors to its creation, far more than I can recall, considering the lengthy process it took for the ideas to evolve. It all began at the University of Ghana, Legon, in the Department of History, where I earned my bachelor and master of philosophy degrees. On several occasions, faculty members made lighthearted jokes about the mosquito that rendered settler colonies in West Africa unfeasible. These jokes often sparked discussions about Kenya, South Africa, climate, soil, and comparative history. Those discussions planted the seed for this book in my mind. I extend my deep appreciation to everyone who made these discussions both inspirational and thought-provoking.

This book arises from my doctoral dissertation completed at Washington University in St. Louis. The research and writing process began in 2013. I am particularly grateful to my graduate school advisors, Jean Allman and Timothy Parsons, for their invaluable support. Jean's guidance predates my graduate school experience at Washington University. Although not officially my advisor at the University of Ghana, Jean's assistance during my formative years in academia was invaluable, carefully reading my papers and providing insightful suggestions for improvement.

At Washington University, I experienced firsthand what it means for an advisor to be genuinely invested in a student's success through my work with Tim. Tim went the extra mile. The extensive knowledge, wisdom, patience, and encouragement from both Jean and Tim were invaluable throughout this journey. They consistently guided me in developing a comparative history of Accra and Nairobi—two cities often viewed as distinct by Africanists due to their differing settlement patterns, land tenure systems, and power dynamics. Their collaboration as co-advisors was crucial to the project's success. Even after I completed my doctoral degree, Jean and Tim continued to provide valuable insights that shaped my intellectual journey, my success in academia, and this book.

Additionally, I would like to extend my gratitude to the individuals who have significantly influenced my intellectual development throughout this process. Like Jean, Sara Berry has been a constant presence since my time at the University of Ghana. Sara took the time to read all my writings from 2008 to the present, made an effort to provide excellent feedback, and offered invaluable academic guidance. She also taught me a great deal about social history. I also express my sincere appreciation for the steady guidance that Nancy Reynolds provided throughout my graduate studies. When I arrived at Washington University in 2012, I had little knowledge of research and writing related to cities. Nancy taught me so much through her classes and guided readings, far beyond what I can adequately describe. In memory of the late Margaret Garb, I extend my tribute for the foundational knowledge she also provided about urbanization and urbanism. Being a teaching assistant in Corinna Treitel's Health and Disease in World History class was a tremendous gift. In addition to teaching sections of the class, I frequently engaged in discussions with Corinna about the socio-economic conditions that impacted health outcomes both in the past and present, especially following the outbreaks of Ebola and cholera in Africa. These conversations were immensely valuable, and I often found myself jotting down numerous notes after our discussions. I am also sincerely thankful to Shanti Parikh and Monique Bedasse for their encouragement during my research and writing process. Despite their busy schedules, both Shanti and Monique took the time to read my work and provide crucial feedback. I am deeply indebted to the rest of the faculty and staff in the Department of History, the Department of African and African American Studies, and the Sam Fox School of Design & Visual Arts at Washington University for their immeasurable support during graduate school.

I was fortunate to receive generous scholarships and fellowships from various institutions, without which my research and writing would have been impossible. They enabled me to travel between libraries and archives in the United Kingdom, Ghana, Kenya, and the United States. They also allowed me to present my research to several intellectuals whose contributions to the book are profound. I want to express my deepest gratitude to the Divided City: An Urban Humanities Initiative at Washington University in St. Louis. This initiative, in collaboration with the Mellon Foundation, the Center for the Humanities, and the Sam Fox School, focused on the complex historical and contemporary implications of segregation. While holding the Divided City fellowship, I further explored various analytical directions and actively participated in projects such as the City Seminar, the Informal Cities Workshop, and the Alberti Program: Architecture for Young People. I also owe a great deal to the Center for the Humanities at Washington University for the fellowship I received. The center's seminar series, under the outstanding direction of Jean Allman, which included both graduate students and faculty fellows, provided an intellectual space for me to continue exploring ideas that significantly enriched my thinking. At the center, Samuel Shearer took the time and effort to workshop sections of the book and offered me insightful ideas. I express many thanks to Samuel.

I was fortunate to receive a graduate student fellowship as part of the Mellon Sawyer Seminar titled Grounding the Ecocritical: Materializing Wastelands and Living on in the Middle East. My research and writing have greatly benefited from the exceptional work of Nancy Reynolds and Anne-Marie McManus, the co-directors of the Mellon Sawyer Seminar. They organized seminars and invited outstanding scholars specializing in environmental studies and urban studies to campus, providing me access to a rich array of ideas and intellectual pathways to explore. To all the individuals I met during my time as a scholar or fellow at Washington University and in the archives and libraries, you have contributed immensely to this book, and I could not have accomplished this without you.

At Elon University, I received ongoing funding and scholarships from various departments to support the completion of my book. Notably, a two-year scholar position at the Center for the Study of Religions, Culture, and Society (CSRCS) provided me with essential resources for conducting research, gathering key materials, and holding interviews. This position included course reassignments each year, allowing me to dedicate time to writing and providing services to the university. My sincere appreciation to the center's director, Brian Pennington, whose steadfast encouragement has been invaluable. Brian also took time from his busy schedule to review portions of the book and offer constructive feedback. Additionally, many colleagues at Elon contributed in various ways, from reading the entire book to chapters and engaging in departmental and informal discussions of my ideas. I would especially like to thank David Scobey, Ryan Johnson, Baris Kesgin, Amanda Kleintop, Brian Degre, Mussa Idris, Raj Ghoshal, Michael Carignan, Michael Matthews, Charles Irons, Caylin Carbonell, Andrea Sinn, Kirstin Ringelberg, Evan Getti, Mary Jo Festle, Sumeyye Pakdil, Hui-Hua Chang, Amy Allocco, David Fletcher, and Peter Felten for their support.

Ryan Kirk, from the Department of History, Art History, and Geography at Elon University, created all the maps in the book. Despite his many responsibilities, he took the time to meticulously study the maps I retrieved from the archives and reproduce them using GPS and other modern software. He patiently supported me throughout the lengthy back-and-forth process with the press to produce acceptable versions of the maps. His exceptional generosity and grace were remarkable. As he often said, his main goal was to see the book published, and he genuinely enjoyed creating the maps.

There were others beyond Washington and Elon Universities whose contributions were significant. Patrick Umeh and Fentuo Tahiru assisted me in finding potential cover pictures. Nate Plagman, Muey Saeteurn, Leslie Hadfield, and Jonathan Roberts generously allowed me to bounce ideas off them. Zeynep Kesgin, the teenage daughter of Sumeyye and Baris, joined our lengthy intellectual discussions and created colorful bookmarks to aid my research and writing. Thanks to their support, the book was completed on time, and I am extremely grateful to them.

I have thoroughly enjoyed working with Michigan State University Press. My deepest gratitude goes to the press, especially to Caitlin Tyler-Richards, for her efforts in driving the initial publication process and for consistently offering valuable suggestions and encouragement. After establishing a great working relationship, Caitlin smoothly transitioned the process to Peter Alegi and Elizabeth Demers. Together with Judith Lakamper and Amanda Frost, Peter and Elizabeth ensured the project reached a successful conclusion. I feel fortunate to have collaborated with such a dedicated team. To the anonymous reviewers, your insightful and constructive critiques, comments, and suggestions have greatly improved the book. Thank you all very much!

I dedicate this book to my late father, Mohammed Sani Qasim. He believed that a parent's primary duty is to ensure their children achieve more than they ever did. To support my educational aspirations, he went to great lengths until his passing. This publication serves as a testament to his hopes and a tribute to his sacrifices.

Introduction

At a meeting of the Nairobi City Council, I met smartly dressed young, ambitious African city engineers and planners in the summer of 2014. I had gone there not to collect interviews but to obtain some documents for my research. Some needed documents were unavailable at the Kenya National Archives and Documentation Services (KNADS), so the archivists recommended checking with the City Council nearby. During my visit, the experts I met talked enthusiastically about a vision for urban projects to transform the city through massive infrastructural development. When it was my turn, I spoke about my research and walking tour of various parts of Nairobi. They disapproved of my presence in some places I visited. They were not happy about me going to the "slums." As a foreigner from Ghana, they gave me a little talk emphasizing the importance of avoiding "slums" like Kibera, listing the typical issues associated with them, such as crime, diseases, overcrowding, and congestion. In my experience in the city, for middle-class and well-to-do Nairobians hoping to avoid these things related to slum conditions, urban developers provide the ideal residential complex for them. This trend in Nairobi is not different from that in Accra.

Appolonia City in Accra and Tatu City in Nairobi appeal to these urban constituencies. The development and sustainability of Appolonia and Tatu cities rely on the increasing number of African urban residents who work, earn high incomes, and seek to move away from congested and overcrowded communities to residential areas with well-maintained sanitation. Appolonia City is about twenty-five miles northeast of Accra Central, and Tatu City is about twelve miles north of Nairobi's central business district. Rendeavour designed and developed Appolonia and Tatu cities as integrated urban residential areas to live, work, and play. Rendeavour is a leading urban developer in Africa. It has international expertise in media and communication, real estate and infrastructure development, finance, marketing, and law. Rendeavour's vision is to develop a well-planned residential infrastructure to support the live-work-play needs of Africans in the middle and upper classes and to ease stifling urban congestion and housing shortages. To Rendeavour, these urban sanitation problems were self-evident. However, this stated initiative of Rendeavour to help alleviate urban congestion and housing shortages targeting specific sections of urban residents is merely a continuation of a series of sanitation improvements in the cities since they became the capitals of the British non-settler and settler colonies of the Gold Coast and Kenya over a century ago. Colonial states, experts, and urban residents used the discourse of slums to depict the lag of sanitation. They imagined and used mass demolition, housing, infrastructure, and everyday municipal services and regulations to solve sanitation problems.

Victoriaborg, midway between Ussher Town and Christiansborg, was the first suburban community to emerge because of sanitation-related challenges such as congested housing development, demographic overcrowding, and a need for suitable housing in Accra. It was the first residential project of its kind in West Africa as a segregated community exclusively for European officials in 1893. The idea to build Victoriaborg for European officials came from Dr. John Farrell Easmon, the first African medical officer of health, appointed in 1884. Europeans and their wives had lived among Africans in James Town and Ussher Town, where overcrowding, sewer, drainage, and planning were critical at the time. The colonial state and its medical advisers took Easmon's idea further. They built Victoriaborg and expanded it in the first two decades of the twentieth century to accommodate the growing number of Europeans in Accra. They concentrated sanitation reforms in Victoriaborg, neglecting the African communities already lagging in drainage, sewer, and Western planning standards.[1] Governor Mathew Nathan amended the town's Police and Public Health Ordinances, enabling him to embark on a sanitation campaign to preserve Victoriaborg as an exclusive European residential area. He demolished African houses sprawling nearby.[2] Incremental development and improvement within Victoriaborg, relative to the Ussher Town and Christiansborg, made the residential community salubrious, affording Europeans amenities and environmentally clean surroundings to live, work, and play while changing the overall built form of Accra's coastline. Victoriaborg eventually comprised official buildings, bungalows with lawns and gardens, a hospital, cricket and polo fields, a golf course, and a tennis court. Meanwhile, in the African communities, demographic growth without corresponding spatial expansion and sanitation projects, like drainage and water systems, lagged, and residents continued to get ill and die from preventable tuberculosis, dysentery, and fevers.[3] In official minds, this uneven pattern of the built environments of African and European residential areas needed homogenization to transform the coastline east of Korle Lagoon (shown in figure 1) and make Accra worthy of being a British capital city. However, removing Ga from their long-established home to implement spatial homogenization was far more challenging than relocating European officials to Victoriaborg.

On the other hand, a few years later, in Nairobi, the colonial government sought to relocate Africans and South Asians from the center of the city. As in Accra, sanitation was the official justification for the relocation. As Nairobi emerged as a European settler capital, the colonial state and the settler-dominated municipality significantly influenced the land tenure. This power allowed them to relocate Africans and lower-class South Asians, including those residing in the Nairobi market or Indian Bazaar. In 1912, the governor appointed a Nairobi Sanitary Commission to investigate the sanitary conditions of Nairobi and its environs. The commission found that the city was "dangerously insanitary" because of "insufficient drainage, overcrowding, and non-segregation of races" in the market and its surrounding areas. The commission recommended a city plan that included demarcating segregated areas for Africans and South Asians who were then residing and working in the market. The commission heard testimonies claiming that Africans and South Asians in the market posed a threat of malaria and plague to nearby European areas.[4] Subsequently, the colonial state and municipality laid out Pumwani and Eastleigh for Africans and lower-class South Asians. These newly opened neighborhoods helped to decongest and improve the market and the city center. However, Eastleigh and Pumwani deteriorated over time due to inadequate sanitation. In the 1920s, Eastleigh, to the west of the Aerodrome and the southern edge of the city's sewage works, lacked roads and drains. Much later, the colonial legislature complained of a lack of drainage as the cause of pneumonia in Eastleigh. Pumwani was the first authorized African location in the Eastlands, but its drainage problems, faulty layout, and inadequate municipal services made it deteriorate over time. Before the 1940s, it appeared in official and medical reports for population overcrowding, crime, prostitution, and all the humiliating terms frequently used to describe "slums."[5]

Accra and Nairobi manifested strikingly uneven landscapes within just fifty years of being colonial capital cities. In her account of the African parts of Accra on the way to Victoriaborg in the first decade of the twentieth century, Decima Moore, the wife of future governor Gordon Guggisberg, noted the product of Easmon's proposal of relocating European officials. To Moore, the African neighborhoods of James Town and Ussher Town were unattractive because they were a mixed development of houses and huts constructed with local materials and business premises belonging to Africans and Europeans. Within a mile, Decima was impressed with what she saw as the road approached an open plain toward Victoriaborg. She passed numerous impressive buildings, including the Hospital Club, High Court, Secretariate, Treasury, and bungalows.[6] European visitors to Nairobi, such as Oliver Lyttelton, would have also witnessed a similar sharp transition passing through Eastleigh, Eastlands, and the city center on their way to the Hill in 1950. Orderly and impressively painted stone houses with wooden verandas belonging to South Asians disappeared and gave way to Eastlands, where a messy crowd of African houses mixed with shops constructed of tin, wood, and cardboard. Africans and South Asians owned the shops. As visitors crossed the breathtaking, modern-looking westernized city center into the Hill, the built environment looked familiarly European as gardens surrounded stone and multistory buildings consisting of pillars, porches, and glass and spacious homes.[7] The sanitation reform that decongested the Nairobi market and created Eastleigh and Pumwani in Eastlands disproportionately impacted where Europeans, South Asians, and Africans lived and worked.

These spatial variations in African, South Asian, and European residential and commercial areas that the visitors to Accra and Nairobi observed are what this book conceptualizes as the saniscape. The saniscape was the confluence of collision, discord, agreements, mediation, and discourse surrounding sanitation reforms that manifested in the urban built environment. It focuses on the sanitation processes that made what David Harvey refers to as the urban built environment. Harvey defines the urban built environment as encompassing all physical structures, such as sewage systems, roads, houses, schools, warehouses, offices, community centers, and others in the city.[8] The saniscape draws the reader's attention to the sanitation aspects of the city's built environment. As both the cause and consequence of the lagging development of public health infrastructure and municipal services and regulations, the saniscape untangles the sanitation impetus that drove urban renewal in Accra and Nairobi.

As seen in the preface, public health movements inspired by Chadwick, Snow, and Simon brought about drainage, refuse removal from roads, and improved water supply, all of which transformed cityscapes and positively shifted patterns of diseases and health. Victoriaborg was the legacy of Easmon's conviction that it was uncongenial for European officials to live amid African neighborhoods without drains, sewers, and the emerging standards of Western urban planning, which included regulating overcrowded populations and congested buildings. Eastleigh and Pumwani were the products of racial segregation. The settler state incorrectly imagined the nonsegregation of Africans and South Asians as the cause of poor environmental sanitation in the Nairobi market. They regarded the market lacking drains and other sanitation infrastructure as the hotbed of plague and malaria. During the early days of colonial rule, officials and their technocratic advisors aimed to set up sanitation infrastructure, services, and regulations to protect Europeans in Accra and Nairobi from infectious diseases, but pushback due to inherent racial discrimination, tensions within and beyond the cities, and the challenges of mobilizing sufficient funds, workforce, and materials to keep up with the rapid urban growth produced an uneven saniscape. The saniscape was a convergence of the policies and practices of various people within and outside the colonial state.

The concept of saniscape goes beyond just a dichotomy of the presence and absence of sanitation in each city. It allows for a spectrum of states of sanitation. Roads, drains, pipes, toilets, septic tanks, sewers, and housing were the essential elements that required robust regulation and servicing for an efficacious sanitation system in cities. The complete set of sanitation components was only sometimes present in one place simultaneously. For example, the residents of James Town and Ussher Town experienced excessive regulation for mosquito prevention despite inadequate drainage. Nairobi's municipal authority invested in Pangani's water supply and toilets to keep it afloat until mass demolition and relocation of residents. Although their neighborhoods looked different from European areas, Africans in Accra and Nairobi built their sanitary infrastructure and kept their homes in decent, hygienic order. Viewing the urban saniscape as a spectrum avoids the binary analysis of the dual city, where sanitation was available in European residential areas and absent in those of non-Europeans.[9]

Khaled Fahmy's olfactory and subaltern approach to sanitation privileges smell over sight and provides an analytical avenue to transcend the dichotomous residential view of the city.[10] Before the germ theory and the microscope, Chadwick's proposed miasmatic-based public health reforms assumed that diseases came from decaying animals and vegetables. The miasmatic idea of public health inspired engineers and city planners to envision cities with adequate drainage, well-ventilated housing, proper sewage, ample water supply, and racialized housing segregation in Africa.[11] In Fahmy's scholarship, the thoughts of sanitation reforms coincided with Haussmann's urban renovation in Paris. Fahmy argues that the changes affected the daily lives of city residents in various ways. Residents' responses unintentionally shaped smell, which the officials, planners, and engineers did not anticipate.[12] While emphasizing sight and smell equally, this book shows the saniscape as the physical manifestations of Africans attempting to cope with British colonial health reforms and city planning.

To see how the saniscape formed over time, it is worth broadly exploring the historiography and scholarship of political economy influenced by the Industrial Revolution in Europe. The partnership between the government and commercial entities was closely connected to the historical development of public health as a discipline and practice during the Industrial Revolution. The middle class in Britain successfully launched a series of campaigns to use government resources to improve urban health and enhance the overall wealth of Britain. In the process, the state became confident in medical and sanitation experts and other technocrats. Their expertise improved the health and life expectancy in Britain. The state and empire builders relied on these experts to make overseas territorial possessions stable and viable for economic prosperity.[13]

Daniel Headrick outlines the stages of European imperial penetration and occupation and provides evidence for the groundbreaking argument that Western medicine was a tool of empire.[14] In the "consolidation stage" of imperialism, Headrick demonstrates how medical innovations, which kept European officials and merchants healthy and alive in colonial territories, made it possible for technologies such as roads, railways, and steamship lines to facilitate economic exploitation of colonies for the benefit of Britain.[15] Randall Packard and Meredith Turshen have demonstrated how political and economic shifts have impacted the pattern of health and diseases among different racial groups and negatively affected Africans disproportionately.[16] Colonial rule made less housing provision for most urban Africans who lived in overcrowded and congested conditions with inadequate sanitation infrastructures. These conditions caused sanitation-related diseases like tuberculosis.[17] Gwendolyn Wright refers to the incompleteness of planning and development in African colonial cities, evident in the environment and housing of

African urban residents as "ambiguous modernisms."[18] The physical manifestation of incomplete colonial planning and development of health infrastructure and services is the saniscape. The saniscape lies at the intersection of public health and city planning.

Although this book is the first to coin and use the concept of saniscape to describe the manifestation of sanitation infrastructure, services, and regulations within the cityscape, a significant body of scholarly work has analyzed the intersection of health and city planning in some form. Philip Curtin, whose work provides an early inspiration for thinking about the saniscape, amply demonstrates the mark of sanitation on the built environment with the argument that Europeans applied their knowledge of medicine and planning in redesigning old cities and creating new ones, like Accra and Nairobi.[19] Curtin draws on Thomas Gale's extensive research that explores discriminatory and racist urban policies, which Europeans implemented to prevent sanitation-related diseases, like malaria, yellow fever, and plague, from spreading among them. The most controversial health policy was racialized residential segregation and the neglect of sanitation in African communities. This discriminatory health policy strained race relations and came to fuel anti-colonial sentiment and urban discontent.[20] As will be seen, in Accra and Nairobi, Europeans carved out their segregated enclaves with adequate sanitary facilities instead of a universal sanitation system to prevent disease outbreaks. Europeans sought to make buffer zones to insulate themselves from diseases in underserved African communities, which they came to imagine as hotbeds for contagious diseases. The relationship between this approach to city planning and race relations is the focus of Maynard Swanson's seminal article, "Sanitary Syndrome."[21] Swanson discusses sanitation syndrome as a European perception loaded with imaginations of contagious disease. The syndrome influenced the segregationist ideology of medical experts and state officials in South Africa in the late nineteenth and early twentieth centuries.[22] Racialized residential segregation and uneven sanitation reproduced a cycle of a lag in sanitation in African neighborhoods that, in turn, stocked a discourse of unhygienic African bodies and places and shaped the fear of disease outbreaks. This lag discourse invented the knowledge of Africans and their neighborhoods as slums and propelled a reconfiguration of the cityscape through mass demolition, relocation, and rehousing.[23]

The chronological endpoint of this pioneering body of scholarship gives pause mainly when analyzed in the broader context of the historiography about the improvement of European health since the Industrial Revolution. Before the microbiological basis for understanding disease and providing healthcare, deaths from infectious diseases declined across Europe. Health started to improve, and life expectancy rose following better nutrition and sanitation movements by Chadwick, Snow, and Simon, among others.[24] Within African tropical colonies, officials and medical experts used a combination of miasmatic and microbiological theories, prioritizing the health of Europeans between 1900 and 1920. Securing the health of Europeans after World War I, officials extended healthcare to African laborers because of their crucial role in the colonial economy. The historiography begs whether African health improved near the standard of Europeans when most Africans lived in neighborhoods lagging in environmental sanitation after 1920.[25] Centering the sanitation of African locations in the history of Western medicine and colonial health is essential because adequate sanitation was what provided the initial impetus for the decline in mortality and morbidity and promoted longevity in Europe. The fact that the pioneering authors terminated their various scholarly works in the 1920s does not necessarily suggest that African health improved after colonial rule started providing them healthcare.

By focusing on the sanitation conditions crucial to determining the health outcomes of the Africans of Accra and Nairobi, the saniscape builds on the scholarship and extends the perspective beyond the 1920s. Rather than healthcare, it was environmental sanitation that impacted African lives, livelihoods, and health outcomes significantly. Most African residents in Accra and Nairobi lived in congested and overcrowded conditions similar to those experienced by Europeans during the cholera years and before the sanitation revolution. Packard and Patterson discuss the disproportionately high prevalence of sanitation-related diseases among Africans living in less salubrious environmental conditions.[26] Africans suffering from a barrage of these diseases because of their living conditions did not show up in colonial hospitals and medical records mainly because they had other care options. They could use the therapeutic pluralism prevalent within the cities and throughout the colonies. An afflicted African and the support group seeking therapy shopped around various healers and chose whose service to employ for specific diseases.[27] Roberts argues that it was this African agency in healthcare that sustained the five different therapeutic traditions in Accra, one of which was Western medicine.[28] The saniscape, which crucially determined health outcomes and gave dignity to human conditions in the city, was what various urban constituencies latched onto to condemn colonial regimes and aspired to urban improvements, progress, and better living standards over the colonial period.

Urban Constituencies, Incompleteness, and the Saniscape

The historical development of the saniscape explains how the interests of different urban constituencies inscribed sanitation in the city's built environment. Reconfiguring the physical fabric of the city in accordance with sanitation dictates followed movements by the middle class to alleviate the poor living conditions that the Industrial Revolution brought about in the colonial metropole. Outside the metropole, the urban elite also embraced sanitation to improve health and the appearance of the built environment.[29] Ruth Rogaski argues that the urban elite's embrace and application of *hygienic modernity* contributed to transforming the urban built environment into "hygienic hierarchies," whereby the sanitation attributes of their neighborhoods straddled the appearance of the few British enclaves, with the most infrastructure and services, and the quarters of the everyday non-elite residents with the least hygiene.[30] In this book I call Rogaski's description the saniscape. The uneven saniscape that Rogaski describes echoes Stephanie Newell's analysis of how urban residents and officials used the concept of proximity in describing the nearness of urban districts with varying degrees of sanitation services, infrastructure, and regulations.[31] The discourse of proximity in Newell's book evoked health threats and aesthetic mismatch in the cityscape. It implied enforcing sanitation homogeneity, which could mean demolishing an entire neighborhood officially designated as a slum. As Newell notes, African elites not only deflected colonial prejudicial racial sanitation discourse on the majority of Africans but they expressed their vision of what a modern city looked like.[32] While embracing Western logics of sanitation, Accra's and Nairobi's African elites pressed their respective colonial administrations and municipal authorities for "slum clearance" and adequate sanitation services, infrastructure, and housing.

One of this book's contributions to the literature on racial residential segregation and colonial cities is the growing class consciousness over sanitation throughout the colonial period. As mentioned earlier, imperial and colonial officials and experts set out to build capital cities segregated by race and class, but they lacked the willpower and ability to mobilize enough money, workforce, and materials to keep up with the pace of urban growth. From an early date, they argued that poor sanitation threatened urban residents and that urban planning, design, and development must protect Europeans and, later, educated Africans from diseases by removing them from neighborhoods of contagion.[33] Colonial regimes concentrated sanitation reforms in areas set aside for Europeans and

African elites. As a result, sanitation and health outcomes were decidedly better in Euro-elite neighborhoods, allowing officials to deflect blame for poor sanitation and health onto underserved Africans. While African elites had shown their dislike for poor sanitation conditions, those who could afford it strove to live in residential areas with better sanitation. They increasingly found common ground by bitterly criticizing colonial racism and neglecting the urban sanitation needs of Africans. As you will see in greater detail in the ensuing chapters, Western-educated, well-paid, enterprising, and wealthy Africans mobilized for their sanitation needs earlier in Accra than in Nairobi. This mobilization for better sanitation has a more extended history in Accra because urban culture and a vibrant class of Western-educated elites date back to the mid-nineteenth century, when Nairobi did not yet exist.[34]

How uneven the saniscape became presents a detailed perspective on the scholarly interpretation of colonial power and its inability to "modernize" the urban built environment in line with technocratic and elite ambitions. Modernization originated from the European tradition of progress and change. Imperial and colonial agents, along with their technocrat advisors, including sanitation, medical, and urban planning experts, attempted to impose modernization in African colonial cities. However, the obsession with pursuing this Western order rarely yielded the envisioned outcome, not even in settler cities with the stringent form of colonial rule.[35] Gwendolyn Wright and William Bissell, for example, have argued that colonial attempts to impose modern forms and norms of urban planning and development proved incomplete, chaotic, and ambiguous for multiple reasons. When technocratic interventions attempted urban blueprints with little cultural awareness, African urban residents ignored, resisted, and modified them.[36] Colonial rule's imposition of a foreign urban order also created an African underclass.[37] Building on these perspectives on the incompleteness and ambiguity of urban colonial order, Jennifer Hart argues that the residents of Accra felt the impact of modern regulation systems used by colonial agents, technocrats, and Western-educated Africans, which informalized their everyday lives.[38] This book also builds on this body of scholarship by conceptualizing the saniscape to give attention to the sanitation part of the built environment. It examines the neglect and historical development of sanitation infrastructure, municipal services, and regulations as they manifested in colonial Accra and Nairobi.

The development impulse embedded in colonial sanitation reforms in the city clashed with the hopes of Africans to benefit from urbanization and urban capital.

In Accra, the Ga fisherfolk pushed back on colonial efforts to move them from the "slums" to safeguard their growing economic interests under colonial rule, and Ga women acquired compound houses from the colonial state to enhance their advantage in the cash economy. Similarly, property owners in Nairobi, including the women who appear in Luise White's *The Comforts of Home*, modified their houses to immobilize the settler-dominated municipality from demolishing their neighborhood in the name of sanitation.[39] They appealed for security of tenure to encourage further investments to reduce slum conditions in the African locations. Although residing in places that colonial officials designated as slums, Africans pursued innovative means for self-progress in various ways that reproduced the colonial cities and economy.[40] Colonial rule's inability to assert complete control of these African residential locations sometimes appeared in official and expert reports as straightforward poor sanitation that needed reform.[41] As Timothy Mitchell stated, this sort of intervention throughout the twentieth century was the "politics of techno-science" that claimed to use expertise to fix society and bring national and economic growth.[42] However, they did not always align with the economic and social aspirations of African urban residents whose lives, property, and livelihoods the interventions encroached on. The negotiation of these tensions by the different constituents, involving multiple people from within and outside the colonial state, entwined developmentalism and competing interests with sanitation and made the saniscape in ways that ensuing chapters explain in detail. Thus, the saniscape allows us to see the morphogenesis of Accra's and Nairobi's built environments in their own terms and as places influenced by local, regional, and global networks.[43]

Accra and Nairobi in Comparative Perspective

As a unit of analysis, sanitation allows bringing two different cities together in a single scope. Sanitation gave imperial and colonial agents, technocratic experts, and urban residents the basis to imagine and attempt to make Accra and Nairobi into "modern" capital cities. This way of transforming cities was what the secretary of state for the colonies, in consultation with the Tropical Advisory Medical and Sanitary (TAMS) committee, hoped to accomplish when he notified the House of Commons about his intent to assign William John Ritchie Simpson to design a plan for the healthy growth of Nairobi to prevent recurring plague outbreaks. He praised

Simpson as "one of the foremost authorities on bubonic and pneumonic plague" and as an "expert authority on tropical sanitation" and qualified to solve Nairobi's sanitary problems.[44] The secretary continued:

> It is hardly necessary . . . to justify the selection of Professor Simpson, who has repeatedly assisted the Imperial Governments of various Colonial dependencies . . . Professor Simpson visited West Africa in 1908 . . . in connexion with an outbreak of plague at Accra, in the Gold Coast . . . and it is no exaggeration to say that it forms the basis on which the sanitary organization of [Accra] is being built and it is to Professor Simpson's suggestions and to his experience which he acquired by his visit that much of the striking improvement in health in the European community . . . is to be attributed.[45]

The secretary used Accra to recommend Simpson as the most suitable person to resolve the acute sanitation challenges in Nairobi. This use of Accra is particularly interesting because Simpson had similar assignments in and outside Africa earlier. As will be seen in chapter 1, Simpson reorganized the health department of the Gold Coast to prioritize the health of Europeans by expanding and remaking Accra's built environment and extending the segregated European residential enclave regardless of the plan encroaching on the ancestral homes of African communities. As Thomas Gale has discussed, the attempt to implement blueprints of racialized housing segregation, like W. J. R. Simpson's, caused African resistance.[46]

While Simpson's recommendation caused a commotion in Accra when the colonial state tried to implement it, his reputation as one of the British Empire's foremost sanitation experts increased. He had gained notoriety for spreading urban segregation throughout the empire in an age of "segregation mania" when plague outbreaks threatened to destabilize the British Empire.[47] Simpson's training was in medicine at the University of Aberdeen. Later, as a teacher at that very university, Simpson taught hygiene. He became a health officer at Calcutta (India) Municipal Corporation from 1886 to 1897. Because of his distinguished achievement in preventing an imminent plague outbreak, which would have caused panic and disrupted the much-needed trade in India, Britain's most profitable imperial territory, the University of London promoted him to professor of hygiene and public health, a position that he accepted and held from 1899 to 1927. He was one of the founders of the London School of Hygiene and TAMS committee advising the Colonial Office (CO) in London on medical and sanitary policy in the tropics. When contagious diseases threatened the very existence of colonial territories, the

CO regarded Simpson's expertise as vital in stabilizing the empire and spreading segregationist ideas and practices in cities worldwide during the twentieth century. Simpson carried tremendous weight in London, where imperial planners and officers centrally directed the planning of colonial cities. And so, when the CO deputed Simpson to address the plague and sanitation in Accra and Nairobi, he carried the authority of the British Empire.[48]

Simpson arrived in Accra in 1908 and Nairobi in 1913 to advise on the healthy development of the cities in the aftermath of the plague outbreaks. His Simpsonian blueprint for Accra proposed an area for "richer natives," such as African merchants, lawyers, and physicians. Some had already built European-style houses for personal use and to rent to teachers, clerks, and other well-to-do residents. By leaving a mark on the city and demonstrating their growing numbers, elite and Western-educated Africans secured a place in the Simpsonian plan, officially adding a socioeconomic layer to Accra's racially segregated cityscape. However, the fact that wealthy and elite Africans had assimilated Western lifestyles and possessed the financial means to build (and buy) houses in Victoriaborg did nothing to convince Simpson that race-based residential segregation was unnecessary.[49] Through the CO and the TAMS, Simpson put pressure on the local colonial state to follow the urban planning recommendations of sanitation officers.[50] The endorsement of Simpson for work in Nairobi by the Secretary of State for the Colonies came after Governor Henry Conway Belfield of Kenya formally requested a sanitation expert. Simpson arrived in Nairobi in May 1913. His plan for Nairobi also instigated local controversy. Similar to his plan in Accra, he acknowledged a class-based housing segregation and demarcated a segregated residential location exclusively for wealthy South Asians in his blueprint for Nairobi's redevelopment, shown in figure 5.[51] Through the CO, TAMS, and local sanitation officers, Simpson continued influencing sanitation policies in the colonies.

An editorial in the *West Africa Times* discussing the exploitative disposition of non-settler colonies in West Africa also rouses curiosity about comparing sanitation in non-settler and settler colonies. It provides credence to the comparative framework that West African cities developed as trading ports with minimal infrastructure, whereas East and Southern African settler cities received significant investment in building and construction projects. Colonial planners of Kenya, for example, envisaged the permanent settlement and developed Nairobi's built environment with Europeans in mind. The editorial noted:

> But here, the few merchant houses we have are all so engrossed with the main business of making as much money as they can during a particular season, not one of the companies or big combines would seem to have the time or the inclination to encourage a system of helping the people to improve their surroundings by . . . observance of good sanitary conditions of living. This is one of the curses of West Africa. That all who come out to her for trade look upon their stay as of so temporary a character that no constructive or permanent schemes ever enter their plans of development to help the social advances of the people.[52]

The editorial emphasizes the unfortunate plight of the African residents of Accra. It implies that European settlers committed funds to capital-intensive sanitation infrastructure that could benefit the Africans of Nairobi. Except in Nairobi, the settler colonial state implemented better sanitation schemes exclusively for Europeans, similar to what colonial officials did in the Gold Coast building and maintaining Victoriaborg with improved sanitation exclusively for European officials. No adequate permanent schemes, including drains, sewers, and septic tanks, crucial in managing waste and preventing sanitation-related diseases, existed in the African locations to improve their social standards and promote development.

The idea that West Africa was cursed because of poor sanitation turned course during anti-colonial movements after World War II. Harold Cooper, an author, lecturer, and former British public relations officer in Lagos (Nigeria), published an article that nationalists mulled over hoisting a flag with the mosquito as "the most prominent symbol" to celebrate independence from British colonial rule.[53] Inadequate drainage and trash collection and stagnated water provided a conducive breeding environment for the mosquitoes, which caused malaria and yellow fever. The very reason that African-educated elites latched onto for criticizing non-settler colonial rule was a cause for praise. The poor sanitation bred mosquitos that made settler colonial rule difficult in West Africa. Cooper found it

> odd that an insect which has plagued the West Coast of Africa with two of its worst diseases, and against which a war of extermination is now being waged should be singled out for this tribute. But the fevers carried by the mosquito had one beneficent effect: they discouraged European settlement in West Africa and thus averted, or at any rate drastically modified, the racial conflict which today disfigures human relations in other parts of the continent.[54]

Cooper later mentioned in the article that the reason for nationalists considering honoring the mosquito was because there was "no 'settler' problem."[55] While the editorial in the *Times* saw the importance of settlers in building infrastructures to drain water and reduce mosquito prevalence in the city, nationalists, about two decades later, would revise that view and regard settlers as an obstacle to African independence from colonial rule.[56] Cooper published this article when Kenya was in the thick of a bloody freedom movement that the settler state declared as "Mau Mau."

Despite all these imperial, colonial, and newspaper references juxtaposing different aspects of sanitation in settler and non-settler colonies, no book-length project historicizes how sanitation development unfolded in these various places. In this book I compare the histories of Accra and Nairobi, the respective capital cities of the non-settler colony of the Gold Coast and the settler colony of Kenya. This book contributes to the extant scholarship that has established the differences and similarities of colonial states in Africa and provokes the central premise of colonial African historiography that settler colonies, where Europeans appropriated much of the best land and used it to dominate the colonial economy and society, were fundamentally different from territories such as the Gold Coast, where Europeans controlled much of the export and import trade but did not care to live and farm.[57] Mahmood Mamdani, for example, takes a similar approach and challenges narratives of South African exceptionalism in African studies, showing that the analysis of colonial institutions and their legacies in postcolonial states demonstrate apartheid South Africa as a generic form of African colonial state.[58] A detailed study of the two colonies' urban sanitation policies makes their distinctions even sharper while revealing profound similarities.

Land tenure was crucial in sanitation. It determined how technocrats, colonial officials, and urban residents could intervene and shape the built environment by constructing infrastructure, demolishing "slums," and providing housing. Various scholarship on the individual colonies and cities has thoroughly demonstrated the significant role of land ownership in the histories of Accra and Nairobi.[59] Through housing, better sanitation, and participation in the urban economy, African resilience and creativity reproduced the cities and shaped urban sanitation despite the little urban accommodation the colonial states made for them.

CHAPTER 1

Buffer Zones, 1908–1920

When the residents of Christiansborg in Accra faced displacement in a colonial plan to extend Victoriaborg, the exclusive European segregated enclave, before the outbreak of World War I, their options for opposing the plan ranged from openly rioting to filing lawsuits. They saw the expansion as an unjust act aimed at dispossessing them of their ancestral homeland. Hugh Clifford, who had just arrived in Accra then as the new governor, investigated resident sentiments against Victoriaborg's extension and overruled the plan. He proposed a different direction to extend Victoriaborg north of the race course, shown in figure 4, instead, where officials would likely meet less resistance. Clifford's decision contradicted W. J. R. Simpson's Accra blueprint based on the germ and mosquito theories of disease transmission. Clifford aimed to avoid local antagonism, whereas Simpson intended to protect Europeans from infectious diseases. When the colonial state was still grappling with the tension arising from the Simpsonian blueprint in Accra, Simpson was in Nairobi with a similar vision to extend the European half of the city. The Simpsonian Nairobi plan threatened the destruction and removal of the Nairobi market (Indian Bazaar), where Indians and Africans lived and conducted their livelihoods. A detailed analysis of why the Nairobi market remained despite Simpson's recommendation for removal reveals not only the official attempt to mediate local resentment but also the contributions of Africans to the property value of the market site.

Simpson's vision for European-only residential communities in Accra and Nairobi integrated buffer zones to physically distance Europeans from Africans. Buffer zones were swaths of unbuilt and built nonresidential plots separating racialized neighborhoods. Sanitation experts and colonial officials set out to curve parcels of valuable urban plots as buffer zones to insulate segregated European residential areas from tropical diseases. While segregation was vexing and generated concern and consternation in Accra and Nairobi, they paled compared to making buffer zones around them. When attempted buffer zones threatened to supplant built areas, they met resistance from African and South Asian landowners because of the threat of severe disruption to their lives and livelihoods. Unlike familiar tales about colonial authoritarianism, the so-called scientific case for racial segregation, ideally protected by buffer zones, ran afoul of the political and economic practicalities of colonial rule. By 1920, buffer zones had never gotten off the ground as initially planned to replace Christiansborg and the Nairobi market. Where buffer zones developed, it was primarily because experts and officials established them on sparsely occupied terrains, where they met less opposition.

The Mosquito Theory of Buffer Zones

Simpson's plan reinforced the contested medical belief that buffer zones would shield Europeans from mosquito-borne malaria and yellow fever. In the second half of the nineteenth century, the research of Carlos Finley and Alfonso Laveran, doctors from Cuba and France, respectively, influenced new findings that connected yellow fever and malaria to the mosquito. Their research built on the germ theory that microscopic organisms cause diseases.[1] Following these discoveries, a chain of interdependent findings appeared, culminating in a final breakthrough before the close of the nineteenth century. Patrick Manson's research linked malaria to mosquitoes, opening a new scientific field of research on the role of vectors in disease transmission. Although he incorrectly theorized that malaria-contaminated drinking water caused the disease, Mason's milestone work established his reputation as the father of tropical medicine. By 1898, Ronald Ross's research built on Manson's findings and identified the *Anopheles* out of the 1,500 mosquito species as the carrier of the plasmodium, the malaria pathogen. Additionally, Ross showed that an *Anopheles* bite and injection of plasmodium into bodies transmitted the disease to an individual.[2] In 1901, research confirmed *Aedes aegypti* as the mosquito transmitting yellow fever. The medical community took years to internalize and implement the new theories about mosquitoes as malaria and yellow fever vectors.[3] In the age of "segregation mania," combating these diseases became enmeshed with racism and nineteenth-century miasmatic theories.[4]

In Accra, colonial officials and their medical advisers justified the making of buffer zones between European and African communities based on theories of mosquito breeding places, flight ranges, and feeding habits. A scientific community influential in shaping this colonial health policy was the Royal Society Malaria Committee of Britain. The malaria committee believed that African children up to age five were the primary source of infection, contributing to the question of how far the mosquito could fly and which host it preferred to feed on. The question became a subject of research and debate. Between 1900 and 1903, malariologists floated the contested theories of mosquito prevalence in African communities and preference for African blood regardless of the physical distance between the neighborhoods in which Africans lived. While the discussions were ongoing, colonial officials and medical experts believed that if only Europeans could reside in an area far from the mosquito range, they could avoid malaria and yellow fever.[5] As part of the imperial and colonial policy to keep Victoriaborg mosquito-free and exclusively segregated to keep Europeans healthy, Governor Nathan embarked on the demolition exercise of nearby African communities he considered "slums."[6] After outbreaks of plague and yellow fever in 1908 and 1910, the Colonial Office (CO) and its metropolitan medical advisors, as well as local colonial officials and their medical advisors, made racialized residential segregation a general policy.[7] W. J. R. Simpson and the Tropical Advisory Medical and Sanitary (TAMS) committee pushed for the implementation of buffer zones as added insulation to European residential areas. By 1911 European morbidity and mortality improved, but not necessarily because of buffer zones. The calculation of mosquito flight range on which buffer zones were based was inaccurate, mosquitoes certainly bred on European premises, and some Europeans lived in their residences with African servants and their families.[8] European health improved, rather, through better environmental sanitation in their segregated areas and quinine prophylaxes (and medication).[9] Unfortunately, when Europeans relocated from African to European residential areas, the colonial administration had little incentive to undertake costly sanitation improvements in African James Town and Ussher Town, producing an uneven saniscape along Accra's coastline.[10]

Like in Accra, sanitation-related diseases were a significant factor in establishing a protected area for Europeans in Nairobi. In the minds of European settlers, officials, and medical experts, South Asians were believed to spread the plague, while Africans were thought to transmit malaria.[11] Outbreaks of plague and mosquito-borne illnesses occurred frequently, leading to municipal efforts to demolish the Nairobi market and move its South Asian and African inhabitants away from the southern region of the swamp through where the river flowed. When Simpson arrived in 1913, the city had recorded about five plague outbreaks in the Nairobi market, where congestion and inadequate sanitation services and regulations were most visible.[12] Since the market was also residential and expert opinion held that the *Anopheles* fed at night, municipal and medical discourse scapegoated residents for Nairobi's rising rate of malaria annually.[13] During World War I European settlers were afraid that the influx of migrants would cause the spread of malaria and plague incidents in the city.[14] While overcrowding and inadequate (absent) municipal services provided environmental conditions for the diseases to spread, the racist notion of South Asians and Africans as inherently dirty provided grounds for municipal effort to create buffer zones for the European residential areas on Hill and at Parklands. The idea of inherently unhygienic races was suggestive of African and South Asian habits that predisposed them and the market to perpetual poor sanitation conditions, which any official intervention was doomed to fail. But that was another one of the white settler excuses for neglecting adequate sanitation infrastructure, service, and regulation.[15] It set the stage for blaming the character of South Asians and Africans for the slums-like conditions that made Nairobi's saniscape uneven.[16]

Accra: Sanitary Segregation, Simpsonian Blueprint, African Residents

Veto Powers and Bureaucratic Infighting Regarding Buffer Zones

When W. J. R. Simpson (figure 3) arrived in Accra on February 2, 1908, his task was not to stop a raging plague in the city per se. With the help of Ga chiefs, African communicators and laborers, and local medical advisers, the colonial administration could already control the widespread transmission of the pathogen before Simpson. The chief of James Town, Kojo Ababio, for example, helped to evacuate over two hundred families in the west of Korle Gonno. At first the local colonial

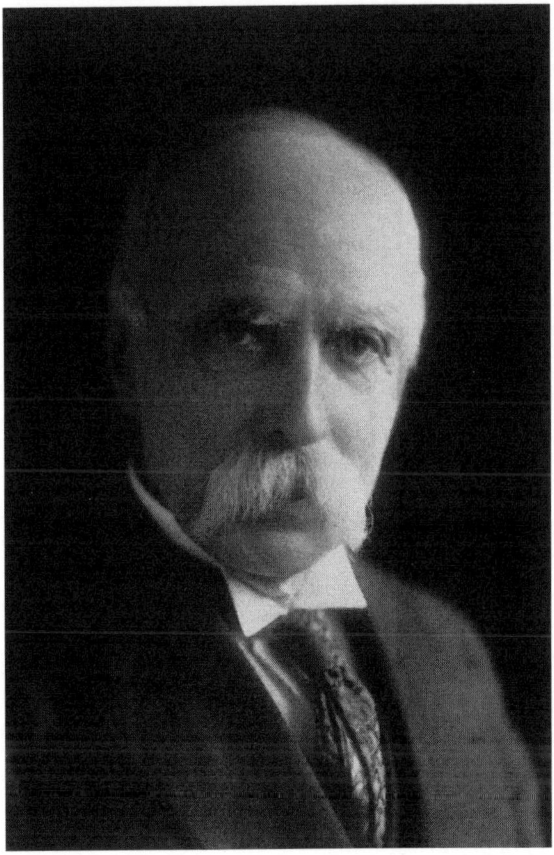

FIGURE 3. Sir William John Ritcher Simpson (1855–1931) was a physician trained at the University of Aberdeen. He was one of the founders of the London School of Hygiene and Tropical Medicine and an advisor to the Colonial Office on medical and sanitation policy. Simpson believed that racialized residential segregation was essential in keeping Europeans healthy and maintaining public health. In 1908, he arrived in Accra, accompanied by J. H. Harran, who had experience in handling plague outbreaks in Kenya. Their purpose was not to avert the ongoing plague but to advise the colonial state on preventing a future epidemic. Based on his successful work in Accra, Simpson was employed by the Colonial Office to advise on preventing recurring plague outbreaks in Kenya. By May 1913, he was in Nairobi. In practice, his segregationist proposals involved the demolition of African and South Asian housing, compulsory appropriation of their land, rehousing projects, and strict urban planning, design, and development. This blueprint for urban health caused tensions and the transformation of the cities' physical fabric. SOURCE: WELLCOME COLLECTION.

administration did not see the need for Simpson. However, since the outbreak was part of the third plague pandemic that had killed at least six million people in India and because medical experts cautioned plague recurrence wherever it struck, the CO insisted on assigning Simpson to observe the Accra situation and advise local officials and experts on how to plan a healthy urban development to prevent future breakouts.[17] Simpson's plan entailed adequately accommodating and segregating Europeans. Simpson advised Governor John P. Rodger to purchase "large portions of the land within and outside" the municipality boundary for that purpose.[18] Since local medical experts saw the sea as the southern natural boundary of Victoriaborg, Simpson's recommendation meant establishing a proper distance between European and African residential areas along the coastline of Accra.[19] Simpson attempted to persuade the officials to demolish parts of Ussher Town and James Town to create open spaces for proper drainage, sunlight, and fresh air. Nevertheless, the cost of £3,000 to buy land around James Town and the port was too high. Moreover, there was no assurance that the landlords would not sue the colonial administration if the state forcibly appropriated their land. In Asere, residents forced colonial agents back by throwing stones at them to prevent the demolition of their houses. The local police intervened and managed to calm the situation.[20] From the experience of the Ga, colonial demolition activity of African houses freed land for extending Victoriaborg and building homes to accommodate the growing number of European officials. The violent act was not a local aversion to modern sanitation and public health common in colonial records but a protection of their ancestral homes.

After returning to Britain, Simpson rationalized why European residential areas required buffer zones and attempted to implement them in Accra through the TAMS, which acted as an advisory body to the CO. Simpson's articulation of the buffer zone idea slowly took shape in the TAMS committee after his working visit to British colonial West Africa, of which Accra and Freetown were part. While in Freetown, he noticed that the Hill Station, a community exclusively meant for European officials, was protected from African homes on one side by a large undeveloped land designated for a water reservoir. However, an African residential area had spread out on the other side of the Hill approaching the European residences. Simpson thought it was ideal for all sides of Hill Station to be protected from the sprawl of African communities.[21] Immediately after his mission in Accra, Simpson announced the formation of the future TAMS committee for the CO. He made this public during a luncheon at the Exchange Station Hotel in Liverpool on December

4, 1908. A year later, the CO constituted the TAMS committee.[22] It consisted of distinguished medical and health experts, including Simpson himself, Patrick Mason, Rupert Boyce, Ronald Ross, and later Andrew Balfour. The work of TAMS proved helpful in stabilizing imperialism, and the CO later extended its coverage to all of Britain's dependencies.[23]

In the TAMS, a subcommittee consisting of Simpson and another member proposed a city plan based on a medical principle. It formulated the idea that "in all areas on the West Coast set apart for the residence of Europeans, a circle not less than a quarter of a mile across should be kept clear around the settlement, and in that circle, neither natives nor Europeans should be allowed to settle."[24] Without comment, the TAMS committee adopted the recommendation. It proposed a strict control of residential buildings within a radius of at least a quarter of a mile between European and African neighborhoods.[25] The crucial part of this physical planning of Accra was the colonial administration rigidly preventing African and European residential properties from "encroaching" each other at least within a quarter of a mile radius.[26] In practice, however, the extension of European Victoriaborg encroached on African Christiansborg, and the African houses in that neighborhood could be demolished to create buffer zones to prevent transmission of yellow fever and malaria to the expanding European settlement. While based on a double standard that allowed European encroachment on African areas, the way that local officials and medical experts applied the rule suggested a principle of medicalized city planning grounded on theories of malaria transmission that privileged Europeans at the disadvantage of the longstanding African communities. Building a Victoriaborg stretching East to West along Accra's coastline explains why Simpson urged the Gold Coast administration and health experts to demolish and decongest African James Town and Ussher Town.[27]

However, the TAMS committee and the CO relied on the senior sanitary officer (SSO) to enforce the medicalized planning in the city. With Simpson's advice, Governor J. P. Rodger and the CO added the Sanitary Branch to the Gold Coast Medical Department with the SSO as the head. The primary task of the branch was to perform public health duties. T. E. Rice, a physician, became the first SSO, heading the branch in 1910.[28] The SSO's urgency increased after a yellow fever outbreak in Sekondi, about 141 miles west of Accra, killing nine Europeans. One year before the outbreak, medical officers in West Africa organized a conference, resulting in the formulation of strategies to segregate the European population within a decade, which would require more land for segregation and buffer zones. When the yellow fever outbreak occurred, it strengthened their belief in residential segregation. The physicians held another conference two years after the outbreak to reiterate their plans. All these public health concerns empowered the TAMS committee to persuade the CO to give enormous power to the SSO, who, with his assistants of sanitation engineers, tried to carry out a contentious form of medicalized planning in Accra.[29]

Governor Hugh Clifford, who served as governor from 1912 to 1919, called out the SSO and his assistants for exercising veto powers, challenging and restraining them. The veto sparked a series of crises and exposed bureaucratic infighting and contradictions within the colony and empire.[30] Following the TAMS committee's medicalized city planning policy, the SSO could decline to sign a site plan for European homes because of its proximity to Africans. Without the SSO's endorsement, the Public Works Department could not construct urgently needed European housing even during a raging yellow fever breakout and other public health emergencies. The governor, the most powerful man "on the spot," could override the SSO only by appealing to the CO for permission. To Clifford, this SSO's veto power was an "autocracy, uncontrollable by the Governor."[31] While Clifford committed to preserving the health of European officials, he broke with his predecessors who had followed the SSO's lead, stating the SSO would

> continue to have the right, which is possessed by every officer in his position, to protest against any decision of mine, and to request reference to you; but to reverse this process, and to force me, as Governor, to be the protesting and appealing party, is, I would submit to create an impossible position alike for me and for the Senior Sanitary Officer.[32]

The exercise of veto powers by the SSO revealed the tension within the colonial state regarding the governor's ultimate power versus the role of the TAMS committee and the Sanitary Branch. Interestingly, the CO's reaction to Clifford's appeal was that it accused Major Herbert Bryan, the acting governor before Clifford's arrival, of being a bad influence on Clifford and urged the secretary of state for the colony not to allow Clifford to do as he pleased. When Major Bryan was on leave in London, the CO and TAMS committee summoned him to explain Clifford's behavior.[33] Meanwhile, the "impossible" situation the veto created gave the CO an excuse to transfer Rice, the SSO, to Sierra Leone within a year of Clifford's arrival in Accra to ease the bureaucratic tension.[34]

The Backlash from Africans, Clifford's Capitulation, and the Diversion of Victoriaborg's Extension

A curious aspect of the CO's antagonism toward Clifford involved why he decided to redirect the extension of Victoriaborg north of the race course, as recounted in this chapter's opening anecdote. It was the reaction of Africans against the buffer zones and the sanitation officer's veto authority. Clifford dispatched a lengthy appeal to the CO within three months of arriving in Accra as the new Gold Coast governor, arguing that it was crucial to reconsider medicalized planning because it was unpopular among Africans. He found that purchasing land from Africans "compulsorily" and leaving it unoccupied would likely cause strong opposition among Native landowners:

> And in the case of the people of Christiansborg . . . there is every reason to believe that the acquisition will only be effected after more or less serious breaches of the peace have occurred. Moreover, in a large number of instances, each case will almost certainly be fought out in a court of law, and in any event our cost will, if that occur, amount to a considerable sum. In view also of the material damage which this acquisition will inflict upon Christiansborg, the Government estimate of the value of the land will, in all probability, be materially enhanced by the courts.[35]

In Clifford's view, displacing residents would have been too costly. It would have provoked resistance, possibly violence, that would have required additional expense to bring under control. And it might have threatened colonial control itself. All these factors undermined the practicality of colonial rule. The tension involving where to make buffer zones with(out) much resistance revealed colonial rule's contradiction rather than the hegemony of science. The altercation between the colonial and imperial bureaucracy and the health experts was not about the efficacy of science in securing urban health. Instead, it was how colonial rule implemented the science of public health, which favored the health of minority Europeans and alienated the city's African residents on whose loyalty and goodwill the political economy depended.

One aspect of Clifford's appeal to his superiors, which also directly affected Accra's physical form, was the future spread of Christiansborg. He broke from the previous three governors, Mathew Nathan, John Rodger, and James Jamieson Thorburn, his immediate predecessor, regarding a city plan that prioritized the health of Europeans. In his campaign against malaria, Nathan had informed Ronald

Ross that the health of Europeans was of utmost importance for general urban improvement.[36] This policy explains why he amended the Towns, Police, and Public Health Ordinance to demolish African residential areas near Victoriaborg. Rodger followed in Nathan's footsteps in city planning.[37] After the plague outbreak, Rodger agreed with Simpson's proposal to radically transform Accra by buying large swaths of land within and outside the municipal boundaries to build European homes and make buffer zones. For that purpose, Rodger constituted an Accra Improvement Committee, which failed in its attempt to demolish and forcibly relocate the African residents of Accra.[38] Some Africans in these communities cooperated with official urban renewal plans after the plague and migrated west across Korle Lagoon and north of the coastline, establishing the foundations of Korle Gonno, Riponsville, and Adabaraka.[39] These new residential areas created in response to congestion and lagging sanitation in James Town and Ussher Town reshaped the city physically but not in the radical way Rodger and Simpson envisioned. Following Rodger, Thorburn also constituted a second city improvement committee that continued his predecessor's policy.[40]

It was left to Clifford to continue these policies after Thorburn retired. Clifford, however, realized that carrying out that longstanding policy and expanding buffer zones negatively impact "the future expansion of [Christiansborg] whose village will be entirely prevented if this acquisition [of land] be proceeded with."[41] He implied that his predecessors' policies of creating buffer zones forestalled the expansion of Ussher Town along the coast and contributed to its congestion. Besides congestion in Ussher Town, the policy threatened the primary economic occupation of the Ga. Fishing as a primary means of Ga livelihood was the main reason the community preferred to expand their homes along the coast rather than inland away from the sea. The CO did not take Clifford's appeal kindly, leading to severely criticizing Clifford, summoning Major Bryan, the colonial secretary regarded as a bad influence on Clifford, to the TAMS committee, and announcing that the CO would closely supervise Gold Coast officials.[42]

The CO's severe rebuke of Clifford was unsurprising because he made taxation, the most sensitive issue in the city's sanitation history, a pillar of his appeal. About two decades earlier, Africans opposed the municipal council because the colonial state wanted to use it to raise money for Accra's sanitation rather than making it a representative institution where Africans could participate in government.[43] When officials attempted to enforce the ordinance and collect taxes later, however, a widespread and fierce African uprising unleashed a "reign of terror" when the police quelled street violence.[44] The women leading the resistance believed that the ordinance and taxes were unfair.[45] On their part, Ga chiefs protested their minority position in municipal affairs and the new taxes, arguing that they paid enough indirect taxes on exports and imports to improve Accra's sanitation. As the colonial capital, Accra's population had increased following enhanced commercial and security infrastructure, contributing immensely to sanitation problems. Ga's traditional sanitation methods, which involved family and communal labor to clean individual homes and the entire city and build toilets near Accra's outskirts, struggled to keep up with colonial urbanization. Ga chiefs needed official help to clean Accra since colonial rule had claimed the city as its capital.[46] Clifford touched on the thorny issue of taxation that had shaped the colonial wisdom that enforcing adequate sanitation in the city hinged on a "high degree of tact and goodwill" by all parties.[47]

Clifford governed a colony where local newspapers were animated about taxation, the inappropriate use of African tax money for European residential comfort, and the colonial neglect of African sanitation needs. The 1914 medical report of the colony stated that as bungalows became available in Victoriaborg, Europeans moved there. Consequently, colonial officials felt little need to finance large-scale sanitation projects, such as drains, in African communities.[48] When Clifford noted that Africans were the primary taxpayers and that their money was "lavishly" used for "protecting the health of Europeans" in racialized segregated housing areas, the CO was defensive and hostile toward him.[49] To counter Clifford's argument, the CO claimed that the African residents benefited from colonial rule through the port, railway, post office, and the overall increase in land value due to Accra being the capital city. It warned Clifford not to "drag in the West African native" into it, as though residents had no agency to push back on colonial injustices.[50] To the contrary, the historical records provide evidence of Accra residents refusing to accept colonial urban sanitation reforms they deemed unjust and inappropriate.[51]

Meanwhile, the frontline role of the Sanitation Branch in displacing Africans, forcibly buying up their land, and implementing sanitation reforms over an extended period during the tenure of three successive governors was a constant source of irritation to Africans. From the time that officials and their medical advisors began to apply the mosquito theory on the ground, the local press had published severe criticism of the Sanitary Branch for scapegoating Africans. Through the so-called mosquito brigades, officially sanctioned house-to-house inspections of African communities for signs of mosquito breeding conditions and invaded Africans' domesticity. Court fines for sanitation-related offenses were one of the daily urban lived experiences of colonial rule.[52] To some residents, sanitation was "nothing but an instrument of oppression and a devise [*sic*] for affording opportunity" for colonial rule to "lord it as tyrants" over Africans.[53] Regarding the physical manifestation of sanitation in public areas within the African communities, the Sanitary Branch did not apply the same rigor to emptying the dustbins and cleaning the market as in peoples' homes.[54] The branch demolished homes to make way for streets and drains and regulated new buildings, but it undermined the integrity of sanitation by:

> constantly changing their plans; one officer recommending and constructing one kind of public work, building, or drain this year, which another condemns and pulls down the next year and so on from year to year as to involve the Colony in a waste of public money, and leave the inhabitants in a constant state of doubt and perplexity as to the integrity of the workers.[55]

In the name of sanitation, built-up areas were perpetually being (re)scripted and (re)arranged by contested and confused sanitation engineering, wasting African tax money and actually creating conditions conducive to mosquito breeding. While the physical manifestation of disagreements between medical officials and sanitary engineers on the built environment was inconvenient and annoying to the everyday city residents, it represented an indictment of colonial technopolitics.[56] It undermined public confidence in the colonial regime.

The most offensive aspect of colonial sanitation to Accra's everyday residents were the public toilets (pan latrines). The colonial state constructed blocks of buildings in perceived vantage points of the city for the public to use. Sanitary engineers designed the toilet blocks in ways meant for users to ease themselves into galvanized iron buckets. The blocks of toilets and the buckets required frequent washing and disinfection to ameliorate their offensive smells. However, this servicing was inadequate, leading to a blame game by officials, sanitation experts, and the African residents of Accra, who faulted each other for the improper use, insufficient maintenance, and lax regulation of the toilets. The toilets were largely unpopular. They lacked gender privacy, and most residents believed that their unclean conditions would expose them to diseases and render their charms ineffective against enemies. Public criticism of the toilet also faulted the lack of a waterborne sewage system.[57] Prison and Kru (from Liberia) laborers manually carried excrement from the public toilets to the tipping point. While acknowledging public complaints about the smell exacerbated by the manual labor, Clifford noted that the colonial achievement of bringing piped water to Accra was an incomplete public health measure without installing a sewage system.[58]

The primary reason for the intense urban discontent with colonial rule was not European housing segregation per se but the sanitation regime and its implications. The establishment of segregated enclaves was a long-standing practice within the Ga communities, dating back to their initial settlement in Accra centuries before the city became the colonial capital. The families and lineages that trickled into Accra lived in separate places. Over time, they gradually merged into distinct quarters. This historical context is crucial to understanding the later spatial developments in Accra. For instance, at the turn of the century, most Muslims in Accra, identified in colonial records as Hausa migrants, resided just north of Ussher Town. This pattern continued into the interwar period, with the emergence of Muslim suburban enclaves such as Adabraka, Sabon Zongo, Nima, and Kanda, among others.[59] Because of their familiarity with different communities living separately in their quarters, residents' intense resentment was not a reaction to European residential segregation by itself. It was because of the repercussions of the sanitation regulations in a racialized divided city as noted in one of the local newspapers:

> We believe the poor illiterate indigene has no objection to the segregation of the Whites; neither does the average educated aborigine worry, but for the fact that he has the suspicion that he is to bear the brunt of taxation, get nothing in return but the abominable conditions of life we have been endeavouring to depict. . . . Every yard of gutter tells a tale. One has only to look at the dustbins &c., [*sic*] to convince oneself that they have no interest in their [sanitary engineers] work. We invite the Department to watch the big drains during the heavy rain to satisfy themselves of our grievances.[60]

Once racial housing segregation was in place, it became easy to channel funds toward improving exclusive European residential areas while neglecting those of Africans. Segregation was undoubtedly racist, and it caused dissatisfaction. But it at least benefited Africans in one respect. If removing Europeans had done anything for the African communities in the short term, it at least helped to ease congestion and disease transmission. As the *Gold Coast Nation* indicated, decongestion helped prevent Africans from contracting pathogens that Europeans acquired, mutated, and spread.[61] However, European segregation helped to reinforce racialized discrimination, leading to inadequate sanitation infrastructure in African communities, as officials neglected the construction and servicing of drains and dustbins in James Town when British officials moved out of the community.

While Western-educated Africans used the newspapers to confer about the city's inadequate sanitation, they could mobilize residents against the colonial state and its medical advisors. They were part of the urban Africans who felt the adverse impact of the lag in sanitation. The newspapers engaged and condemned the very scientific explanation undergirding segregation itself, thereby undercutting any possible rationale for buffer zones. They challenged the science as "the Mosquito Eropaganda."[62] European merchants and missionaries who stayed within the African communities and European officials who moved to Victoriaborg with their servants and mistresses did not help the medical cause for buffer zones.[63] European traders still residing in the African communities lived in "palatial" houses surrounded by clean environments while their African employees lived in congested housing conditions.[64] This urban physical pattern was not as clear-cut to fit into the dual city concept of explaining colonial cities elsewhere.[65] Europeans lived in African residential areas and vice versa. Residential segregation, ideally protected by buffer zones, was unwelcome because it required expropriating even larger parcels of land that residents used for multiple purposes, including residential and farming. It was not uncommon for Africans to call out sanitation experts and protest compulsory land acquisition for buffer zones. The press followed and informed about ongoing land acquisition negotiations between officials and African land custodians. The African-run *Nation*, for example, promised to expose any "trace or semblance of exploitation" of collusion not in the interest of the ordinary urban resident to mobilize protests.[66]

However, coming from the perspective of Africans, the newspapers' tone showed a social distance from the mass of Africans who had no Western education. The classism in the newspapers revealed itself when Western-educated Africans pushed back against official criticisms that painted Africans with a broad brush as "unsanitary" and "completely beyond any sanitary control."[67] The *Nation* noted that officials regarded the "native no matter his attainment or antecedent" as "impregnated with microbes to an extent which makes it deadly for his white neighbor to breathe in the same atmosphere."[68] The newspaper revealed the implication of buffer zones on Accra's saniscape:

> Think for one fleeting moment of the havoc this false teaching has wrought in the Gold Coast! As a working hypothesis, it has proved a deadly fiasco . . . it has

> discouraged European builders to make use of sites in vicinities where respectable natives live.[69]

Discouraging Europeans from living near "respectable" Africans who had developed a taste for Western culture had an adverse impact. Since the official policy was to protect European health, their bungalows near wealthy and Western-educated African residential areas would have compelled the colonial state to construct drains, regularly empty dustbins, and regulate buildings in the neighborhoods of these high-class Africans.

In light of the intense controversy over buffer zones to insulate Europeans from Africans and the sanitation officer's veto, Clifford revised the original plan for extending Victoriaborg east along the coastline (see figure 4). Unilaterally selecting different sites north of the race course for the extension of Victoriaborg in contravention of the SSO and the TAMS committee, Clifford violated protocol by not seeking permission from the CO. This singular action on his part was crucial. It redirected the extension of Victoriaborg toward the northern edge of the municipal boundary. Clifford's decision was foundational in developing a wealthy residential corridor northeast over Accra's twentieth-century history.[70] It saved the colonial state from the backlash from Christiansborg's residents.[71] Clifford selected sparsely populated sites to create open spaces between European residential areas and those occupied by Africans to reduce the risk of inflicting "material damage" upon Christiansborg residents. Following the veto of the SSO and displacing established African settlements would have had "serious breaches of peace" between affected Africans and the colonial state.[72] The veto was not only a liability to colonial peace but also challenged colonial rule's practicality. It empowered the SSO to

> issue to the Governor and to the Heads of other Departments what amounts to instructions, which must be obeyed pending an appeal to you. He himself meanwhile is not subject to instructions of any kind, save purely executive matters. He, as in duty bound, has only to consider the abstract question of what is desirable, viewed solely from theoretical point of view of a sanitary expert. Considerations of practicality, of administrative convenience, and of financial possibilities do not enter into his calculations. . . . Such advice will always be valuable; but its adoption on all occasions without modifications as necessity may compel the executive government to make—owing to other matters which are not within the purview of the Senior Sanitary Officer—is impossible, unless the work of the Colony is to be notably impeded and frequently brought to a standstill. Yet, at the present

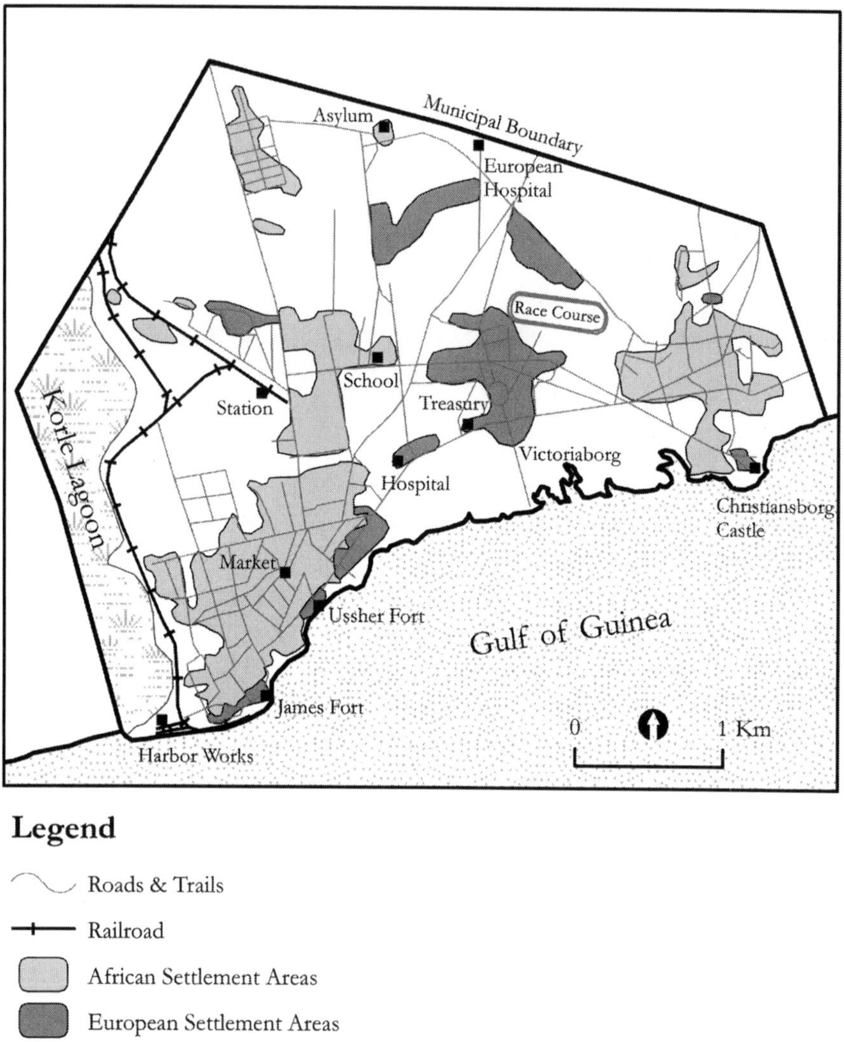

FIGURE 4. Governor Hugh Clifford's redesign showing the diversion of European Victoriaborg's extension north of the Race Course. African opposition to the earlier colonial plans, which threatened to displace them from their ancestral homes, was crucial in shaping Governor Clifford's decision. The earlier extension plans had threatened African Christiansborg to the east. MAP CREATED BY WASEEM-AHMED BIN-KASIM

> time, the advice of the Senior Sanitary Officer is binding on the Governor until and unless he appeals to you.[73]

Clifford's question to the CO and its TAMS committee was how he was supposed to rule as governor if he had to obey the SSO, whose primary duty was narrow in scope to ensure the health of Europeans. As governor, he was responsible for the whole colony, including the heads of departments and the different communities. To have everyone see him subordinated to and helpless before the excesses of the SSO undermined his authority. Thus, the veto was impractical to colonial rule.

Nairobi: Sanitary Segregation, the Simpsonian Blueprint, and the Market

Collision between the Settler System and South Asians and Challenges to the Destruction of the Nairobi Market

Although Nairobi manifested a physical division, its African, European, and Indian residents lived in relatively loosely defined, racially segregated areas by 1908. From its beginnings, social class had become more visible than race in the physical layout of Nairobi's built environment. The division among Europeans was particularly apparent, with senior railway authorities controlling the desirable land south of the Nairobi swamp, as shown in figure 2. Within the railway-controlled south, the senior officers lived on "the Hill" separately from subordinate South Asian and European staff who, to facilitate operations, lived near the railway infrastructure.[74] Simultaneously, the civil officials controlled the land north of the swamp. An uneven saniscape in the areas controlled by the two European authorities was visible moving across the swamp from the north toward the south within the first decade of the city's history:

> The offices and headquarters erected by the Railway authorities were princely compared with the buildings erected by government across the swamp. Lack of funds and shortage of staff for the task in hand forced Ainsworth to put up corrugated iron building of a shabby and unfinished appearance. The first of the Railway houses on the Hill to be completed, an "elaborate affair."[75]

As seen in the preface, Colonel John Ainsworth was the provincial administrator who transferred the province's capital from Machakos to Nairobi to control urbanization. Where Ainsworth and staff lived and worked sharply contrasted with the railway organization's property. The distinction between the areas, however, reflected wealth rather than race. The city itself needed universal planned development, including networks of drains and sewers. When the capital of Kenya was relocated to Nairobi in 1905, the city's physical layout gradually transformed because another authority besides the railway oversaw the city's growth. The shift in the seat of colonial power to Nairobi enabled the civil officials to lord over the railway authorities, taking land the railway authority previously controlled. As a show of their power, the civil officials moved their offices south of the swamp.[76]

Also, in the south of the swamp was the Nairobi market, located in a prime area. The market was the most prosperous economic place in the city. The market appeared in the colonial records as the Indian Bazaar because a few wealthy transnational South Asians owned the property. However, most South Asians who lived and did business in the market were poor. Still, Africans also resided and did business there.[77] Serving residential and business functions for poor South Asians and Africans, the market stretched over nine acres from its eastern boundary on Government Road to the west toward the railway line. A central street ran through the bazaar, east to west. Narrow passages divided blocks of shops, some built of concrete blocks and iron, resting on stone plinths about two to three feet high.[78] The market's strategic location and dense population lent the city an "eastern" character, starkly contrasting the European settlers' vision of Nairobi as a "white city." That was a constant source of irritation for the settlers. The market's proximity to the European business and residential areas also generated intense unease among colonial officials and settlers because of recurring plague outbreaks. Complaints that the market was the most unsanitary section of Nairobi and, thus, the primary cause of diseases led the Colonial Office to assign W. J. R. Simpson to investigate and recommend modern sanitation for the city.[79]

Local colonial and imperial sanitation experts who believed the Nairobi market to be a hotbed of the plague feared the disease would spread to their European residential areas from the market. For that reason, the Simpsonian blueprint for Nairobi envisioned the cityscape made of "separate quarters for Europeans, Asiatics, and Africans," divided by a "neutral belt of open unoccupied country of at least 300 yards in width between the European residences and those of Asiatic and Africans."[80] Simpson's vision incorporated Bransby Williams's earlier city plan, but it was similar to Accra's reorganization of the sanitation department to enforce race-based residential areas separated by buffer zones to prevent the encroachment of the residential areas on one another. Africans and South Asians would have

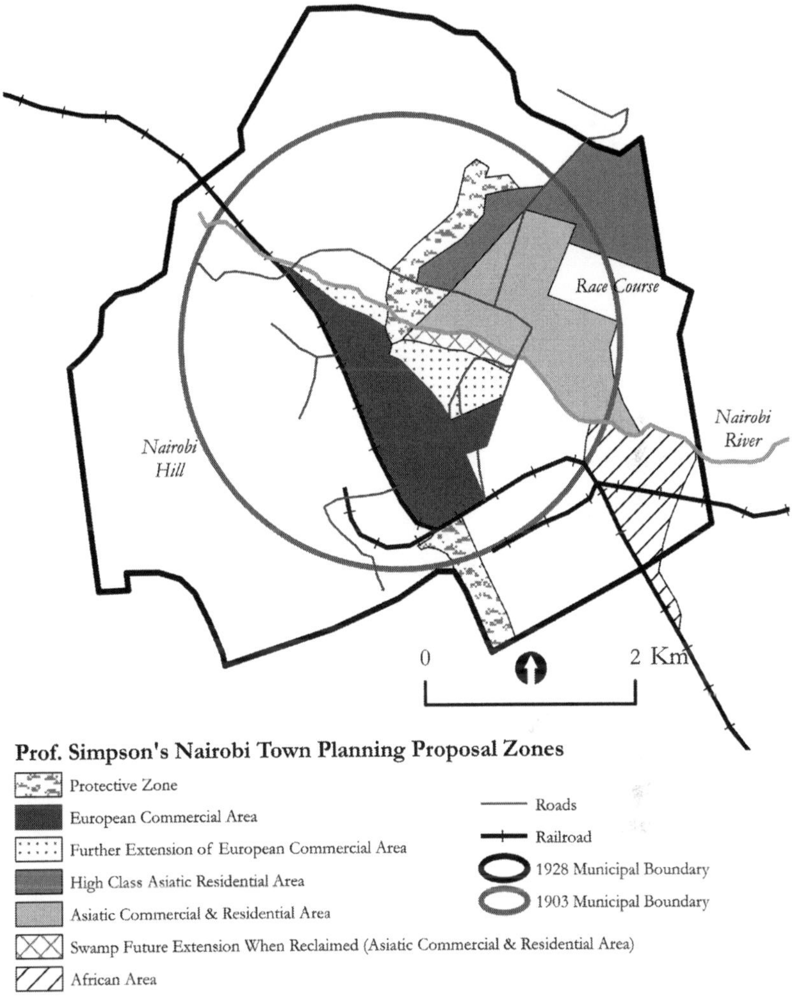

FIGURE 5. William John Ritchie Simpson's Nairobi blueprint protected European residential areas to the west and northwest with a nonresidential commercial area and natural boundaries such as the Nairobi River and swamp. It provided residential locations intended to separate wealthy South Asians from the poor members of the community. The plan also provided an African location. MAP CREATED BY WASEEM-AHMED BIN-KASIM

separate residential areas outside the south of the swamp. While European settlers insisted Nairobi was a European city, and Africans were rural people with no place in the urban environment, Simpson insisted Africans required a residential location because of their meaningful impact on the social and economic life of Nairobi.[81] In Simpson's blueprint, there was no green belt, but the Nairobi River divided the African and South Asian areas. Still, there were two of them that separated the European residential areas on the Hill and Parklands to the north, prioritizing European health. To further bolster their protection, the two green protective zones were linked to an imagined nonresidential European commercial area, which extended from the northwest to the southeast (see figure 5).

While Simpson proposed destroying and removing the market and its residents and repurposing the land for European commercial use, he also considered allowing wealthy South Asians to establish their stores there so long as the market remained nonresidential. In his words, "the standard and mode of life of Asiatics, except the highest class, do not consort with those of Europeans."[82] Simpson's redesign of the market site arouses curiosity because, at the time, he was evaluating the debate about the feasibility of converting a prime urban site into an unbuilt green buffer zone in Accra. His repurposing of the market incorporated Accra's perspective that an unbuilt buffer of prime land lost too much money and cost too much to maintain, employing labor to clear weeds, keep it clean, and prevent it from becoming a mosquito breeding ground.[83] It would have been a waste to leave the most commercially lucrative center in the municipality unbuilt. He therefore envisioned it as a nonresidential European commercial area. His vision seemed plausible because part of the land stretched east to west, covering a European commercial area. The land was connected to the Nairobi swamp and river, two separate green lands, and the Municipal Forest to provide a protective buffer zone for the European residential areas on the Hill and Parklands shown in figure 5. Repurposing the market to create a nonresidential European commercial area would help strengthen the buffer area provided by the swamp and river, an essential physical boundary to the European residential district. His plan addressed growing concerns about the rising rate of malaria in the city. Experts believed that malaria transmission mainly occurred at night, which justified the creation of a nonresidential commercial zone for Europeans. In Simpson's mind, this plan could reduce the risk of malaria infections since the Europeans would spend shorter hours in their stores in the commercial zone during the day.[84] The residential areas of African and South Asian communities were to the east and south of the buffer zone. Thus, similarly to Accra, the Simpsonian blueprint for Nairobi aimed principally to protect European health and lives.

The most controversial element of the Simpsonian proposal was removing the Nairobi market and repurposing the site for a nonresidential European commercial zone. One of Simpson's primary problems with the market was that it doubled as a residential and business location for the South Asians and Africans. Similar to Accra, Simpson's proposed solution to sanitation for Nairobi was segregating South Asian and African residents from one another. His statement regarding the "demolition, gutting out, and clearance" of the market as a means of residential segregation was radical and quite frustrating to wealthy South Asians who owned land and held substantial investments in and around the market.[85] Based on his perceptions of cultural differences and racism, Simpson made derogatory comments about the African and South Asian communities, implying that they were inherently unclean and could not be improved. However, municipal neglect of regulation, infrastructure, and service, coupled with the market size being too small for the demographic density, contributed to the market's deplorable environmental sanitation rather than any inherently unclean habits of the residents. Seven years earlier, before Simpson arrived in Nairobi in 1913, Bransby Williams, a British sanitary engineer, had recommended that if demolishing was impossible, it was essential to decongest the market, construct sewers and drains, and provide piped water. The municipal council, dominated by settlers, was reluctant to undertake the proposed expensive sanitation project. By 1913, the condition of the area had worsened. This was evident from the report of the sanitation commission appointed by the governor, which consisted of European officials, settlers, and health experts. The commission reinforced Bransby Williams's sanitation recommendations. Simpson's extreme view of the market and harsh proposal lay in his idea that sanitation improvement, other than demolition and removal, would be futile. To him, the place would revert to unsanitariness even with municipal intervention.[86]

Ultimately, the market remained in place after Simpson's recommendations. A lack of political will, the resistance of South Asian property owners, and the distraction from World War I posed an obstacle. In May 1914, the colony's chief secretary forwarded the Simpsonian proposal to a six-member subcommittee of local officials, some of whom were part of the commission that recommended remodeling the market as a pathway to better sanitation. After the subcommittee reviewed the Simpsonian blueprint, it reaffirmed an earlier view to incorporate the desires of wealthy South Asians and to consider the high cost of a complete demolition. In its report, the subcommittee wrote that:

> Conversion, to be effective, means expropriation. All the arguments against expropriation of the Bazaar apply with equal force against the conversion of this area into European quarter a scheme which besides being unfair to the Asiatics is unnecessary.[87]

The subcommittee preferred to keep the market in place against Simpson's proposal. However, its approach to improving sanitation was to create open spaces and install drains and sewers while removing the Africans and overwhelmingly poor South Asians to residential locations across the swamp. The subcommittee intended to make the market a wealthy district regardless of race. It envisioned the market as a commercial area of rich, land-owning South Asians and European businesses.

For his part, Alibhai Mulla Jeevanjee, as one of the wealthiest South Asians with significant investment in landed property in and around the market, posed another challenge to the Simpsonian blueprint. Jeevanjee was a Bohra merchant who founded the *African Standard* within three years of Nairobi's existence. He received a contract from the railway authority to provide labor and equipment during the construction of the railway line. He brought nearly 32,000 South Asian laborers, artisans, and clerks to work for the railway authority, and over 6,500 of them stayed in Kenya. Some of those who remained in Nairobi after the railway line was completed stayed in the market on Jeevanjee's land. Jeevanjee had received vast swaths of land in and around the market in return for helping Ainsworth, who headed the underfunded civil administration and a thinly spread supporting staff, to construct the colonial offices and quarters during the relocation of the provincial administration from Ukamba to Nairobi. As a significant property owner in the heart of Nairobi, his interests collided with those of settlers, which he attempted to offset by advocating for more South Asian representation in the municipal body. With that increase in representation, he aimed to alleviate the drainage and other sanitation problems in the market through an influence of budgetary allocation for public health.[88]

Jeevanjee negotiated a delay in implementing Simpson's plan with Governor Henry Conway Belfield, although the governor denied committing to that.[89] Additionally, Jeevanjee created a map that redesigned the market to be more inclusive and less racially segregated than Simpson's original plan (see figure 6). He proposed repurposing the market to cater to Nairobi's middle class. However,

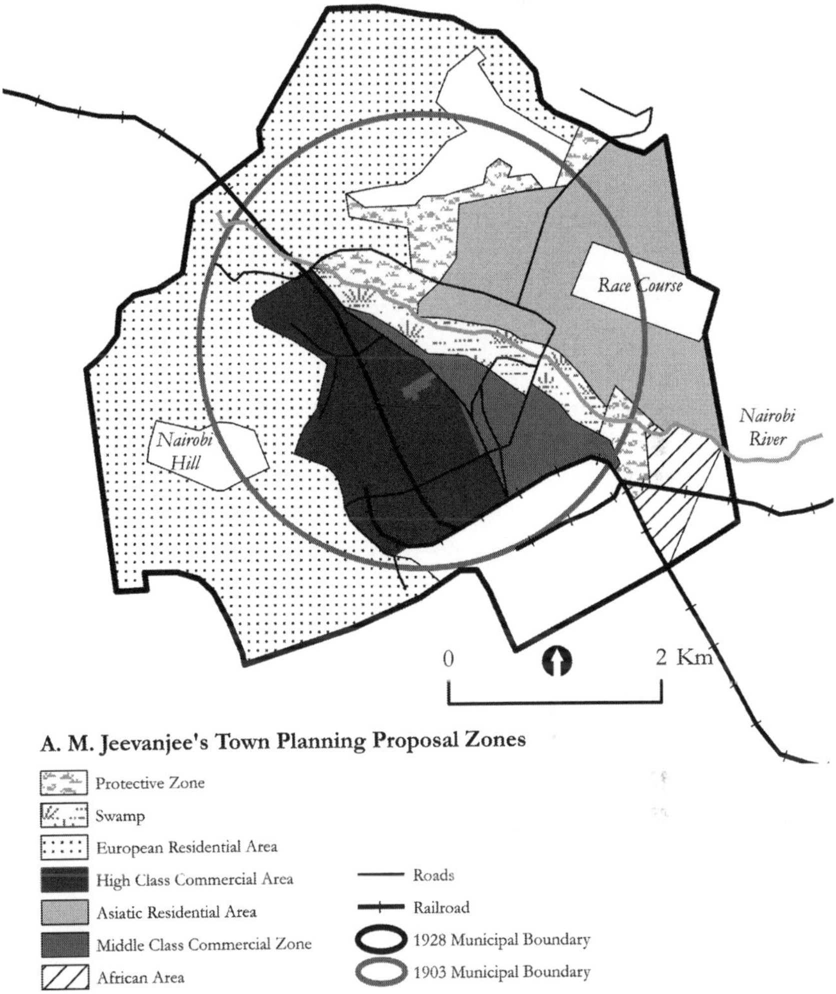

FIGURE 6. Jeevanjee's counter blueprint for Nairobi primarily focuses on commercial areas based on socioeconomic class. However, it envisions racialized residential areas separately for Africans, Europeans, and South Asians. MAP CREATED BY WASEEM-AHMED BIN-KASIM

Simpson rejected the map. During the war, the influx of South Asian migrants to Nairobi increased, leading to calls from Europeans for the market's demolition. They claimed that the poor environmental sanitation of the market would worsen and increase the likelihood of a plague outbreak. The governor reinforced Simpson's idea of establishing a sanitation administration to address the market's demographic growth, sprawl, and Nairobi's overall sanitation. Jeevanjee became concerned that the officials would destroy the market while following Simpson's sanitation reform idea.[90]

In his effort against the market's destruction, Jeevanjee was quick to correctly argue that the appalling market conditions resulted from municipal neglect. His argument challenged Simpson's rationale that South Asian and African residents were inherently dirty. Jeevanjee was not far from the truth. Jeevanjee's position seemed to fit in with the settler-dominated municipality's longstanding plan to expropriate the land where the market was located. As mentioned, Bransby Williams had mapped out a drainage system that would have facilitated wastewater flowing away from the market. And the local sanitary commission reinforced Bransby Williams's plan just before Simpson's arrival. Simpson himself validated Bransby Williams's market-improvement proposal. The municipality shelved those recommendations and said it had no money to implement them. It neglected drains and sewers, regular waste removal, building regulation, and population growth for years. The logical outcome of the neglect was making the market a hotbed for contagious diseases, thereby inventing a pretext to confiscate the site legitimately and dispossess the South Asian property owners.[91] Jeevanjee gave the municipal land officer a tour of the market to prove his point about municipal neglect. The South Asian property owners fulfilled their legal requirements of paying rates and building their property by their leases and sanitary regulations. Municipal authorities approved their shops on the site. So, Jeevanjee expected no less from the municipality than to fulfill its obligation of providing sanitation infrastructure, services, and regulation.[92]

In the meantime, South Asian property owners in the market agreed with the settler state to collaboratively check the market's congestion and sprawl. Under the agreement, officials and municipality asked the South Asian community to report the immigration of poor Africans and South Asians into Nairobi and the market. On the other hand, they were to encourage skilled South Asians to move into the city and colony. The agreement also included a request to property owners to refrain from subdividing their land.[93] While the tension over the market seemed to have eased, Jeevanjee's grievance against the settler system escalated. In June 1917, the state informed Jeevanjee, through the acting chief secretary, of new legislation reinforcing the Hill as an exclusive European residential location. Officials told Jeevanjee to stop his plans to build on Hill plot No. 363 if he intended the house for his personal or "Asiatics" residence.[94] This instruction was the expression of European fear that the South Asian community would spread west into European residential areas. A Jeevanjee house on the Hill would open the floodgates for other wealthy non-Europeans to acquire and develop property there and move in. The fact that Jeevanjee's plot got official attention to the extent of prompting the discussion of legislation suggests that issues on sanitation, segregation, and buffer zones were, in part, questions over property. The legislation raises questions about who could own, live, sell, lease, and buy land and landed property in different parts of the city. The central issue was not who owned the yet-to-be-built house but which race would live in it. In fighting back, Jeevanjee declared that the governor had approved his building plans in a meeting two years earlier. The governor, however, denied that such a meeting ever took place, was not aware of Jeevanjee's residential plot on the Hill in the first place, and could not even imagine sanctioning the construction.[95]

Jeevanjee's challenge to the state's plan to racially homogenize the market had enormous implications compared to how it appeared on the surface. It questioned the very idea of the city as a European settler capital, touching off a flurry of deputations, instructions, petitions, and clarifications crisscrossing Kenya, South Asia, and Britain, seeking answers to two main questions: Was Kenya a "white man's country"? And whose interests would dominate in Nairobi? Settlers had declared Kenya a white man's country, where the interests of European settlers superseded those of the South Asian community. In July 1919, secretary of state for the colonies, Alfred Milner, expressed his support for the Simpsonian blueprint, prioritizing European needs in the House of Lords. But the rationale he offered was social rather than sanitation related. He argued that segregation in Nairobi would create comfort, convenience, and peace, as it did in British India. Like the Ga of Accra, South Asians were also familiar with segregation in India before coming to Nairobi. To Milner, segregation in and of itself was not the primary issue. Like Accra, the problem in Nairobi was the sanitation meanings of the Simpsonian blueprint. It entailed forcibly removing the South Asian community for the health of Europeans. It meant destroying the market and converting the site into a nonresidential commercial zone, which would doubly serve the interest of Europeans as a buffer and market. Why must Europeans have all the best places in Nairobi?

The Nairobi Indian Association and Jeevanjee enlisted the support of pressure groups in India and the Government of India. The Government of India, which consisted mainly of British civil servants, had considerable influence in 1919 due to India's contributions to World War I and the rising strength of Gandhi and the Indian National Congress. The growing popularity of the nationalists in India made the European officials of the Government of India extremely sensitive to discrimination against South Asians throughout the empire. It criticized Milner for contradicting an earlier position of the CO that officials would not consign "British Indians" to inferior status. The government further referred Milner to his previous stance about British authorities treating the races in the empire equally.[96]

Revising Simpson's blueprint and redesigning the market could not quickly resolve the messy controversy entangling the settler state, the South Asian community, the Government of India, and CO. Managing the conflict required a reexamination of the idea of Nairobi as a European city, an idea that privileged settlers over landed property in the salubrious part of the city. The colonial state substantially revised the Simpsonian plan during the governorship of Sir Edward Northey. The market remained in situ rather than demolishing and relocating it, separating European and Indian commercial districts by only a street, not a whole buffer zone as Simpson envisioned. The market would witness a renewal and decongestion activity piecemeal in the interwar period. Yet there was still the sticking point of wealthy people, like Jeevanjee, in the South Asian community acquiring landed property and building their houses on the Hill and in other environmentally suitable parts of the city reserved for Europeans. As the Government of India noted,

> They have only asked that they should be allowed to acquire suitable residential sites, which hitherto have generally been denied them. The only exception are the few Indians who have been brought up to live in European style.[97]

The Government of India promoted equity in residential plots between wealthy South Asians and Europeans. As part of this effort, they called for a Royal Commission to investigate discrimination in Kenya.

The events surrounding the collision of European settlers and South Asians partly explain why the British government issued the Devonshire White Paper of 1923. Also known as the Devonshire Declaration, named after its author, Victor Christian William Cavendish, who was the ninth duke of Devonshire and the secretary of states for the Colonies, the paper stated that wherever the interests of Africans clashed with those of Europeans or South Asians, African interests should take priority. Across the continent in Accra, the declaration validated, in theory, Governor Clifford's earlier push to bring the interests of Africans to the fore over the extension of Victoriaborg and the creation of buffer zones.

It is essential to contextualize the declaration as a paradigm shift in the imperial system resulting from tension arising from local sanitary segregation in the colonies. Clifford's disregard for the veto powers of sanitation officers to keep peace in Accra was part of these tensions.[98] Back in Nairobi, by declaring the "paramountcy" of African interests, the Devonshire White Paper weakened the position of South Asians vis-à-vis Europeans and did little for Nairobi's Africans. Since the declaration prohibited racialized residential segregation by legislation, the Kenya colonial state, without law, openly prevented Africans and South Asians from Parkland and the Hill neighborhoods. They regarded the two places exclusively for European residents.[99] The White Paper attempted to silence Jeevanjee and his South Asian supporters hiding behind African interests.

The Missing Presence of Africans and the Market's Resilience

Although Africans were critical to the market's profitability and ultimately contributed to the lack of official will to demolish and relocate it, the debate about the market in the city overlooked their role. While a few South Asians owned the land and many dominated the market's population, Africans lived and worked in and around the market. When the sanitation commission proposed the residential segregation of Nairobi's "natives" and Indians in the market, it noted that "numbers [of Africans] reside in the Bazaar and in River Road" to emphasize that the African residents were significant. African women doing sex work rented accommodation in the market. Some Africans sublet verandahs to retail their wares, and others rented spaces for a stay while working in the city.[100] Despite being paid bachelor low wages by their South Asian employers with little allowance for housing and regardless of the challenging living conditions, such as a lack of toilets and municipal services, Africans served their South Asian employers as shopkeepers. They were also cultural brokers between South Asian owners and the market's prominent clients, who were Nairobi Africans. Although fluctuating, the population of Africans residing in Nairobi exceeded 15,000. That was more than the combined population of Europeans and South Asians, about 1,600 and 6000, respectively.[101] By 1921, most Africans were predominantly male migrant wage earners living in eight communities in and around Nairobi, including Kangemi, Kawangare, Kibera, Kileleshwa, Pangani, Mombasa, and Masikini.[102] The market was conveniently located for most Africans, who formed the bulk of its customers and (re)produced its core functions. However, the widespread belief among European settlers that most Africans were rural in character aimed to promote the notion of Nairobi as a white city. It explains why they failed to factor in the city's teeming African community in the South Asian and European competition for dominance.

The sanitation commission and the South Asian community acknowledged this crucial "native" role in the market. The commission's discussion to relocate it integrated the idea of choosing a site that would continue to appeal to and draw Africans. In this way, the commission aimed to assure the market's shop owners that the relocation would not jeopardize the trade with their African customer base. Also, although not mentioning Africans as the market's shopkeepers and clients specifically, Jeevanjee observed that the reason for the municipality's determination to dispossess South Asians and repurpose the market site for a European commercial area was because of its prime location, its advantage of attracting numerous Africans, which enabled the South Asian shop owners to keep a reliable business and accrue substantial profit.[103]

Multiple testimonies, from those of colonial officials to experts at the commission, noted that Africans were the market's primary customer base. The testimonies explain why the commission seriously considered that a site for a new market must be near the route Africans plied in and out of the city.[104] However, the cost of compensating the South Asian property and shop owners was too high for the settler system to bear. It was located in a suitable and profitable part of Nairobi. Eventually, the settler state was unable to expropriate the market. Regarding the inability of the settler-dominated municipality's failure to compensate the South Asian shop and property owners, Governor Belfield stated:

> Apart from the question of expense, which must prove an insuperable obstacle for some time to come, is not now considered essential, because, when an alternative situation in the new Asiatic trading area becomes available, it is anticipated that there will be a partial emigration from the present buildings, which will give an opportunity to compel the renovation and improvement of the better-class premises, whose owners may for some time to come elect to remain where they are.[105]

Governor Belfield rejected Simpson's recommendation to demolish and relocate the South Asian community south of the swamp and Nairobi River. However, the governor's decision was silent on the market's African clients and cultural brokers, who were essential to its profitability and resilience. They were crucial to the value of the market, which made the compensation of the South Asian shop and property owners too expensive for the settler system to implement demolition and relocation. For that matter, Africans seemed officially silenced in their role, preventing the complete removal of the market as Simpson envisioned. They contributed to stopping the racialized homogenization of the market area and converting it into an exclusively nonresidential European commercial center.

Conclusion: Buffer Zones and the Practicality of Colonial Rule

To prevent Europeans from getting sick with transmissible diseases like malaria, yellow fever, and the plague, the CO and its TAMS committee, along with the colonial states, used the germ and mosquito theories to justify creating racialized residential segregation. The use of infectious diseases as an excuse for residential segregation, which was already in vogue in the Cape Colony during that period, is what Maynard Swanson refers to as the "Sanitary Syndrome."[106] Referring to the global reach of the so-called syndrome exhibited by European colonizers as "segregation mania," Nightingale shows that European government officials, medical experts like Simpson, and businesses were the agents for the wide spread.[107] Based on Jama Mohamed's and Godwin Murunga's research, rather than attributing the widespread outbreaks of contagious diseases to the supposedly inherent nature of Africans and South Asians as imagined by Europeans, the global movement of these agents and the internal transformation within the colonial territories, such as urbanization and population movement, that came in their wake to facilitate economic exploitation caused the epidemiological problems for which Africans suffered disproportionately.[108] Yet British officials and medical experts latched on to the prevalence of the diseases in the cities to pathologize and segregate themselves from subjected Africans and South Asians. The experiences of the subjected people in Accra and Nairobi were similar to those of French colonial *indigène* in Kalala Ngalamulume's scholarship.[109]

Residential segregation was a deeply resented aspect of British colonial rule in African cities. In stark contrast to Nairobi, Accra had a more extended history of urbanization where vociferous Western-educated Africans challenged "scientific" segregation, calling it out in their editorials, comments, and articles as European propaganda. In their critiques, these elites inadvertently betrayed their class interests. They gave up their desire for a social distance from the rest of Accra's urban population due to their education in missionary and colonial schools. However, they revealed the impact of segregation on the cityscape. Theories of transmission of diseases like malaria and yellow fever discouraged the development of European housing near wealthy Africans. Since imperial and colonial policies prioritized Europeans' health, the absence of their housing near African residences meant the underinvestment in sanitation in those neighborhoods. Indeed, as Victoriaborg improved in amenities and Europeans moved there, the colonial state and municipality paid little attention to the sanitation of African communities. Over time, the resulting stark contrast in the city's saniscape manifested along racial lines. In Nairobi, the struggle over the uneven racialized saniscape was more apparent between the wealthy South Asians and the settler state. Not only did Jeevanjee, one of the wealthiest South Asians, mobilize his political capital to challenge the underinvestment in sanitation in the Nairobi market, but he also proposed a new map that prioritized the development of the city along class lines, challenging Simpson's blueprint. He even started developing a residential property on the Hill reserved exclusively for Europeans. Zarina Patel demonstrates this role of Jeevanjee, her grandfather, as a challenge to colonialism.[110]

No matter how intense the controversy surrounding racialized residential segregation, it paled in comparison to the creation of buffer zones in Accra and Nairobi. People had practiced residential segregation across time and space, and the Africans and South Asians in Accra and Nairobi were familiar with it.[111] Segregation separated European areas from those of Africans and South Asians by the width of a street, wall, or railway line. However, buffer zones to insulate the segregated enclaves in developed urban areas were more problematic. The zones required more significant swaths of land than needed for a railway line, wall, or street. Before colonial attempts to repurpose parts of Accra and Nairobi for buffer zones, African residents had lived in segregated quarters, and some South Asians, who preferred to live in exclusive residential areas for cultural reasons, were familiar with segregation in India. However, at the turn of the twentieth century, the sanitation implications for segregation undergirding buffer zones differed. They were inherently racist and discriminatory against non-Europeans. Colonial rule used the germ and mosquito theories to justify buffer zones. In Accra, officials and medical experts pathologized African bodies and residential areas and imagined them as threats to Europeans and the political economy. Their counterparts in Nairobi and Kenya's settlers, who controlled the municipality and lived in and around the city, regarded South Asian and African communities similarly. Colonial rule in both cities looked to buffer zones to insulate European communities in their residential enclaves.

European segregated areas, ideally protected by buffer zones, ran afoul of colonial rule's political and economic practicalities. In Accra, European officials and experts disagreed about the feasibility of, and even the need for, racially segregated residential and commercial areas far from Africans, and merchants and missionaries were openly opposed to them. Displacing Africans to make buffer zones was too costly and provoked resistance, possibly violence, which would have required additional expense to bring under control. It might even have threatened colonial control itself, as evident in Governor Clifford's protest. Clifford's protest, which resulted in the rerouting of the extension of Victoriaborg, laid the foundation of a prosperous residential corridor north of the race course. Crucially, African mobilization against prior colonial plans to displace Africans from their ancestral homes and repurpose the land for buffer zones and European residential enclaves gave momentum to Clifford's protest. In Nairobi, pressure from well-to-do South Asian merchants weighed against the complete demolition of the Nairobi market because of the lack of sanitation. But that was not enough to prevent the market's destruction and relocation. The municipality and colonial state were unwilling to pay the high cost of compensating South Asian land and shop owners for the destruction and relocation of the market. Interestingly, the market's value hinged on the numerous Africans who provided the most clients and served as cultural brokers and shopkeepers. Ultimately, the settler system allowed the market to remain in the same place, contrary to Simpson's vision for Nairobi. Because of these challenges, buffer zones did not appear in the areas as envisioned, revealing the incompleteness of colonial urban planning, designing, and development. The process of making buffer zones and the inability to achieve them as envisioned reinforces Bissel's argument that colonial plans to (re)make cities reveal "incoherence, incapacity, and incompleteness."[112]

The incomplete development of sanitation infrastructure, services, and regulation in Accra and Nairobi manifested in the cities' uneven saniscapes. Sanitation in European locations was decidedly better than those of Africans and South Asians. These unsatisfactory sanitation conditions in African residential areas deteriorated further during the interwar period. The next chapter connects the emergence of "slums" in Accra and Nairobi to the persistent sanitation challenges of urban development and the political economy of colonial rule.

CHAPTER 2

Slums, 1920–1940

Official depictions of the so-called slums as disorderly and out-of-place in modern cities often gave the misleading impression of the African communities as accidental byproducts. However, "slums" were built-in components of colonial urbanism and the colonial urban order. The African residents who lived in these communities were crucial part of the daily urban economies. The "slums" were mutually determined with the rest of the city while physically and socially contrasted from it, at least by some colonial officials and technocrats. Although for their gain, the African residents of Accra tapped into longstanding expertise and welcomed migrant workers. Officials, municipal authorities, technocrats, and commercial agents used the labor of these migrant workers to build, maintain, and run the colonial cities and economies. Similarly, the African communities of Nairobi rented and provided various services to most African migrants working for the settler state, municipal council, and private employers. The resulting congestion, overcrowding, and inadequate sanitation in the communities were the most visible attributes that colonial official correspondence and expert reports described as slums. The idea of this chapter, that "slums" were invented problems in Accra and Nairobi, delinks colonial perceptions of the places as the result of failings of the people residing in them and instead ties them to the confluence of local and global industrial and commercial capitalists order that gave little attention to the environmental sanitation of urban residents. This chapter considers "slum" districts of the urban saniscape as parts of the city rather than isolated outposts.

Colonial descriptions of African communities mirrored the slum discourse in nineteenth-century industrializing and urbanizing Britain. The term "slum" invoked material and intangible characteristics in British industrial cities, including moral depravity, criminality, squalor, and diseases. The definition of the term, first as criminal, became public in James Hardy Vaux's writing in 1812. The term became British slang for taverns and eating houses, places for loose talk and suspicious activities, and evolved, incorporating defective dwellings and neighborhoods. During the cholera years, it took on layers of meanings suggesting fear of contagion, death, and poverty.[1] Although these conditions existed in pre-industrial Britain, they became sharply associated with modern cities because of industrialization and urbanization.[2] Newspapers and novels further popularized the term until it assumed semi-slang synonymity for "rookeries," "feverdens," "little hells," "devil's acres," and "dark purlieus."[3] As its meaning spread, journalists and novelists dropped the quotation marks. By the 1880s, they were using "slumming" as a verb.[4]

Patrick Geddes, known for pioneering urban planning and sociology initiatives, observed an inherent relationality about "slums" and modern cities. He lamented their development as part and parcel of nineteenth-century city building. Cities showcased progress, modernity, and wealth, yet so much deprivation was inscribed into their physical and social fabric.[5] The cities were the physical manifestations of capitalist and proletariat relations. In London, the capitalists and powerful employers used menial and casual workers who received low wages for their labor to maximize their profits. These employers then reinvested their earnings into commercial and industrial apparatuses, which contributed to transforming the city. However, the workers with little money to improve their living standards watched as their communities deteriorated. A further influx of people seeking employment in London and residing in the communities only worsened the situation, adding overcrowding and deterioration to the neighborhoods. Thus, the poor areas amid London's industrial and commercial affluent districts forged it as a metropolis divided along class lines.[6]

"Slum" communities stood out and engaged official and public attention because of their physical characteristics, the social status of those who resided in them, and the imagination of people outside the locations. Wealthy London residents, some of whom may never have seen essential features of a "slum," created the image that defined the communities as aberrations when juxtaposed with respectable and affluent residential areas nearby. They invented them as a problem based on their imaginations of what was tolerable. In particular, disease and revolt toppling their socioeconomic status drove the fears of the wealthy residents about "slums." Additionally, the spatial contrast between "slums" and affluent areas was so glaring and disturbing that it attracted sustained journalistic coverage and impelled missionary and humanitarian outcry for intervention. Like Geddes, journalists and humanitarians bemoaned the contrast of deprivation amid economic progress in London. However, the cities' insatiable demand for labor and the resulting exploitation of workers circumvented chances of achieving a somewhat spatial homogenization to bring the physical features of "slums" somewhat on par with the affluent areas. In the political circle, what constituted a "slum" remained vague, and the legislature and judiciary failed to define its main characteristics, allowing for the fluidity and arbitrary use of the term. However, in public and expert domains characterized by contested, transactional, and situational use of the term, "slums" were congested neighborhoods where houses were medically unfit for habitation and the residents were a threat to society.[7]

By the turn of the twentieth century, the public linked the continued existence of "slums" with worsening social, moral, and medical fears and called for their demolition. The public outcry stemmed from a confused belief that widespread slum conditions were the "consequence of failings in the inhabitants." In the popular view, the residents constituted a particular "order of society that was undisciplined, thriftless, dangerous, and intemperate."[8] This pervasive view of the communities was what health and planning technocrats promised officials and municipalities to transform. British colonizers exported these longstanding convictions about "slums" to Accra and Nairobi, where they invented them as aberrations, although the cities lacked industries characteristic of those in Industrial Revolution Britain. However, the urban growth of Accra and Nairobi cannot be decoupled from Britain's attempt to promote industrial development and job opportunities for its growing urban population in the colonial metropole. In the empire's wealth flow network, Accra's and Nairobi's worsening congested living conditions and sanitation challenges were also the overseas products of Britain's industrial and urban revolutions. They acted as conduits for consuming industrial finished products and facilitating raw material extraction. Regardless of the distance between the colonial cities and Britain, the economic machinery that socially and spatially divided urban residents in British cities also facilitated a similar reality in Accra and Nairobi. However, the lack of heavy industries and entrenched racism added unique layers to the "slums" in Accra and Nairobi. Official records of the communities, comprising shoddy housing, irregular layouts, overcrowding, and inadequate (nonexistent) drainage, sewage, and water supply, revealed racism, cultural biases, lack of political will, and insufficient funds for urban parity.

The rest of the chapter charts the course of urban growth and overcrowding in interwar Accra and Nairobi. Looking first to Accra, it discusses demographic growth in James Town, Ussher Town, and Zongo. The housing shortage and deterioration of sanitation conditions provided the context for slum discourse in British colonial correspondence and African newspapers. Turning to the African communities of Pangani, Pumwani, and Kibera in Nairobi, this chapter examines similar processes of demographic growth, congestion, lagging sanitation development, and "slum" discourse. The discourse often portrayed the African communities as disorderly, diseased, and out-of-place in modern capital cities. The fluidity of the term made it applicable to various settings, but it flattened unique socioeconomic and cultural realities about the "slums" in Accra and Nairobi that (re)produced the colonial capitals. Also, the language frequently juxtaposed the African communities with segregated European areas. However, the communities, relative to exclusive European segregated areas and the rest of the colonial cities, show that the so-called slums were built into colonial urbanism. The "slums" provided and reproduced the laborers that built and maintained the colonial city to generate wealth for the absorption of the metropolitan cities and economies.

Urbanization and Congestion in Accra: James Town, Ussher Town, and Zongo

Migrant Workers and Accra's Built Environment

As the capital of Gold Coast, Accra needed a steady supply of skilled and unskilled African workers to build and maintain the necessary infrastructure to keep the city and colony functioning. Most of the Ga were content with their longstanding sources of livelihoods. While welcoming migrants for centuries, they considered colonial menial work demeaning and refused recruitment. However, they leased houses and land to urban migrant workers.[9] Housing the migrant workers, especially in James Town, provided another income stream for the Ga communities.[10] The colonial state was the most prominent recruiter of workers through its public works departments. Railways also served as a significant employer. The municipal authority, firms, and individual urban residents also attracted workers. Among the African urban workers, laborers rarely saw their housing and sanitation needs filled by their employers despite their crucial roles in building and maintaining the city and economy.[11] Colonial reliance on unskilled workers disproportionally fell on the Northern Territories of the Gold Coast because the area had late exposure to Western education and missionary apprenticeship in skilled work. The laborers, some forced by their traditional chiefs, were responsible for constructing and maintaining roads, drains, bungalows, public buildings, and recreation grounds.[12] Accra's skilled African workers came from the western, central, and eastern provinces as well as Ashanti and outside the colony. Official records put them in a rather broad category as having the "natural aptitude" for acquiring a "high standard of proficiency in the use of machinery" because they were from places with an early advantage of technical facilities and apprenticeship from colonial and Christian missionary education. The concentration of migrant workers in the cities, in turn, attracted ancillary populations whose entrepreneurial work in cooking and selling food, petty trading, and transactional sex sustained urban workers.[13]

The rapid development of Accra's physical infrastructure through Governor Gordon Guggisberg's Ten-Year Development Plan significantly increased the number of migrant workers in the city in the 1920s. Guggisberg unveiled the plan in 1919 amid a public call for infrastructure. For example, cocoa farmers in Accra's interior appealed to expand rail and road networks to enhance the transportation of their surplus cocoa accumulated because of wartime production and demand increases.[14] Farmers' pleas for infrastructure in the Gold Coast fit in with calls in the colonial metropole to build "land fit for heroes" of the Allied victory in World War I. Gold Coast cocoa farmers aspired for improved transportation infrastructure to take advantage of the longstanding Atlantic trade network and increase their wealth through increased cocoa production and export.[15] Luckily, the Gold Coast government had generated sufficient revenue during the war by exporting cocoa and manganese to Britain. Cocoa exports through the Accra port augmented British capital and set in motion an economic revolution, evident in the frequent repurposing of much-needed houses into warehouses for storing cocoa beans.[16] Increased construction activity meant that officials added to the importations of building materials from Britain, such as cement, roofing sheets, and steel, contributing to expanding the metropolitan economy, employment, and urbanization.[17]

Since Accra was the export and import trade bottleneck, it received the most significant budget allocation in Guggisberg's development plan, providing work opportunities and attracting migrants. The physical transformation brought about by migrant workers was hard to miss in the 1920s. W. J. R. Simpson, the plague expert discussed in chapter 1, observed sixteen years later during his second working visit to advise on another plague outbreak in Kumasi, north of Accra, that "the Accra of 1908, with some exceptions, [was] almost unrecognizable in 1924."[18] The improvement committee set up by Governor Rodger demolished African houses on Otoo (High) Street, filled in ponds and quarries, and made open spaces.[19] Accra's wealthy Africans received new housing in Adabraka. Victoriaborg also obtained golf and race courses and recreational spaces, among other amenities. For James Town and Ussher Town, the colonial administration cut through them with newly constructed roads. New business premises close to the seaside communities and new African communities in Korle Gonno, Korle Bu, Mamprobi, and Sabon Zongo spread out across the city.[20] The period also saw further construction and extension of paved roads and monumental infrastructure, including Selwyn Market, Korle Lagoon Bridge, Korle Bu Hospital, and Achimota Secondary School.[21] These physical changes were possible with migrant workers in Accra. Regarding the export revenue and the construction projects, one medical report from the Great Depression recalled that the "colony in its prosperous days moved too fast in its expenditure on social services." The report noted an observation of a Gold Coast medical doctor who indulged in self-gratification for colonial accomplishment in the Gold Coast compared to Kenya during a visit to East Africa.[22]

Congestion, Overcrowding, and Health Outcome

Health experts pointed to the growth in population as the reason for Accra's overcrowded and congested conditions. The opportunities in urban work opened alternative income streams for Africans and drew the city into the global capital network, although wages were low. When the Great Depression occurred, and job opportunities shrank, an official admitted colonial rule's inability to prevent the influx of African laborers into the city. Some laborers traveled long distances from the Northern Territories to Accra. Others came from mines because they preferred to live and work in Accra. And when they could not find jobs, they could stay if they chose to.[23] By 1921, Accra's population of 38,049 sprawled beyond the boundaries of the seaside communities. Ten years later, it was about 61,558.[24] To officials, however, Accra's overcrowding would ameliorate if migrants only returned to "their villages and live on the produce of their farms."[25] The demographic impact of migrant workers was significant, and an official revealed colonial inability to control urbanization and overcrowding. When Accra Town Council reduced municipal services during the Depression, population growth connected to urban wage work compounded the poor environmental sanitation in the city.[26] Medically, the loss of wages and overcrowding contributed to high incidents of tuberculosis in the Ga and migrant communities.[27]

Although African entrepreneurs took advantage of the acute housing shortage and invested in real estate, more was needed to accommodate migrant workers. A large single room was an asset because house owners could make more money by providing bed space for the increasing number of lodgers and the large "floating" population.[28] Colonial discourse of the inferiority of local houses and municipal regulations favoring permanent buildings expanded the demand for cement and other materials from industries in Britain.[29] Accra Town Council recorded that the permits issued between 1927 and 1944 showed entrepreneurs' and developers' interest in lodges to lease for migrant workers' short-term stay. The licenses for lodges increased from 100 to nearly 250. However, there were fluctuations in the requests for permits to alter existing buildings and to build makeshift accommodations. The Depression and personal economic hardships slowed the pace of new construction despite an influx of laborers looking for work. As a result, the new buildings that came during the building boom of the interwar years did less to help alleviate overcrowding in James Town, Ussher Town, and Accra's suburbs.[30]

W. J. R. Simpson, during his second visit to Accra, and the Gold Coast press, underscored the relationality of the overcrowded African areas and the rest of the city. Simpson noted that it was no use to demolish congested places and make roads to open them up at enormous expense, only to allow other crowded places to emerge nearby. The newly congested communities springing up showed that the colonial state and the municipality had trouble housing workers from the Northern Territories and French colonies engaged in demolishing houses and constructing roads.[31] The colonial state made little provision for its urban migrant workers. Like Simpson (and Patrick Geddes), the local press disapproved of the congestion amid the transformations that characterized Accra's saniscape. Despite the prosperity from wartime trade, the African communities remained underserviced, whereas the state spent £130,000 on "palatial bungalows for officials."[32] The construction and maintenance of roads and bungalows in these affluent official residential areas were employment avenues, drawing African migrant workers who sought accommodation in James Town, Ussher Town, and Zongo, incrementally causing overcrowding and overstretching what little sanitation was available in those communities.[33] The physical surroundings of the neighborhoods where laborers lived contrasted with the residential and official areas where they worked. From the laborers' perspectives, in their daily work experience, they moved across an uneven saniscape comprised of overcrowded and congested underserved communities to privileged, well-maintained, and regulated European official residential areas.

As seen, the Ga seaside communities of James Town and Ussher Town on the coastline of the Atlantic Ocean had a hallmark of fishing and salt-making for centuries before Accra became the capital of the Gold Coast. They were tight-knit communities that lived in close quarters contingent on historical factors, including for security reasons. The construction of Victoriaborg and its zoning as a European residential area also prevented Ussher Town from spreading along the coast. The inability to spread out along the coast maintained and exacerbated the congested conditions in Ussher Town. Because of the resulting congestion, Ussher Town often appeared in colonial records as a "slum," with all its inglorious associations of disease, subversion, and blemish. In the mind of officials, Ussher Town threatened urban health and disfigured a city that was supposed to be a British colonial capital.[34] Officials invented Asere, a quarter in Ussher Town, as the "most urgent problem" among the city's "slums."[35] The colonial system often viewed these African neighborhoods as occupying land suitable for constructing storehouses and business buildings. Thus, Ussher Town, for example, wasted a valuable site that could have boosted the political economy.[36] Bounded by Akrashie Street to the north, High Street and Market Street to the south, Quartey-Kojo Street and Bukom Square to the east, and Bannerman Road to the west, Asere came under the scrutiny of the local African press, which helped to spread the official depiction of it as a slum.[37]

Asere's proximity to famous places like Bukom Square and High Street, Accra's main thoroughfare, made it visible to many African motorists and pedestrians. Those who saw Asere and could write their experiences for publication in the newspapers criticized the poor infrastructure and the inadequate (absent) municipal regulation and services based on a contrast to the nearest district, "the great emporium of Accra trade" along High Street. To them, Asere and Bukom Square were a mismatched, out-of-place area in a colonial capital city. They saw Asere as a problem because of its proximity and relationality to the wealthy district. Sanitation in the two areas was uneven.[38] As will be seen in the next chapter, this discourse of relationality opened up the possibility of spatial homogenization through demolishing and remodeling Asere and its environs to match the upscale district nearby.

Regardless of the affluence of the district near Asere, the choice of the Ga to preserve their ancestral home was an informed decision. What officials saw as a straightforward slum was quite more in the view of the Ga residents. Asere, and indeed the rest of Ussher Town and James Town, was home and a source of livelihood. Living near the ocean was economically advantageous to the fisherfolk whose livelihoods were connected intimately with the sea. Residents could travel easily to and from the beach, where they safely docked their fishing canoes. Even officials acknowledged that the coastline was "the only beach in Accra where sea-going canoes [could] be beached with any degree of safety."[39] They wanted to be near relatively calmer waves to facilitate their occupation.[40] Also, living along the coastline ensured they remained in communion with their ancestors buried in the ground below. Yet, at the risk of aggravated congestion and concomitant health outcomes, the communities provided housing accommodation for migrants drawn to employment opportunities in the growing colonial and urban economy.

As evident in colonial records, officials failed to acknowledge the Ga contributions to (re)producing the colonial economy and city by providing places for migrant workers to stay. Because it was not official policy to house its employees, Africans working for the colonial state found accommodation in the seaside neighborhoods, especially James Town.[41] Like the fisherfolk who used the urban economy for another income stream, Ga landlords who took advantage of increased housing demand invested in large rooms to accommodate as many migrant workers as possible.[42] As demand exceeded supply and rents increased relative to low wages, landlords rented bed space to accommodate more people.[43] Groups of employees pooled their money together to rent houses with "very poor conditions for which they usually pay an unduly high rent."[44] By pooling money to make urban living somewhat bearable, renters could save money from the meager wages to live.

As the built-up areas extended in response to the housing needs created by the population influx, it became challenging for the Ga to follow traditional practices of building toilets in the nearby environs outside the settled areas. They could only travel a limited distance across the sprawling city to ease themselves. And the public toilets within the city were uncongenial. Logically, they constructed private enclosures as toilets, compounding the congested nature of their built-up area of the city.[45] Coupled with overcrowding, which overstretched the little amenities available in the communities, the congested built area did give the Ga communities a slum-like appearance.[46] But the overcrowded population and congested development in the communities were partly the demands of the colonial urban economy. In the official hurry to scapegoat Africans, they occasionally pointed the finger at African extended family systems and traditions as the cause of overcrowding and congestion. In 1935, the Medical Department reported that the resulting "slum" conditions from overcrowding were attributable to "the habit of an employed person providing for his relations who [were] out of work." At times, officials unfairly labeled Ga as lazy for refusing employment as colonial laborers, creating a labor gap that colonial rule filled with migrant laborers and in so doing caused overcrowding.[47]

Living along the coastline became even more crucial as the urban economy depended on shipping. It gave some members of the Ga communities a compelling reason not to relocate. The port in Accra was not deep enough to harbor ships, so they anchored some distance from the coast, opening a new income stream for fisherfolk. Their skill set as canoe men and their ability to mobilize crews were crucial to shipping. They signed contracts with M. Customs and other lighterage (shipping) companies operating in Accra to ferry people and their loads, exports, and imports to and from the ships. People arriving in Accra by ship, including governors and colonial officials, met the Ga boat crew first before Accra's residents. However, exactly when ships arrived and departed was uncertain, which explains why the contract between the companies and the fisherfolk was brief—less than a year.[48] Although seasonal, the fisherfolk and their canoes became indispensable to the expanding colonial bureaucracy and commerce. The community recognized the importance of their role and looked forward to shipping arrivals and departures.[49] It made economic sense to live near lighterage companies. Describing the proximity of the built environment of lighterage companies and Ga homes, the deputy director of health services noted a "curious mixture of old and new" where large and modern commercial premises were close to "fetish houses and a collection of hovels inhabited by illiterate primitive people."[50] The biased British mind, filled with a false sense of cultural and racial superiority, did not appreciate Ga ritual and customary urbanity, which did not conform to Western zoning of urban residential, commercial, and religious functions.

Most colonial migrant laborers, primarily male, lived in different sections of Accra. Zongo, which was north of Ussher Town and predated the establishment of Accra as the capital city, was one of the sections. The community was a melting pot of different ethnicities, including Hausa, Yoruba, and Ga. Additional migrant communities, like the Sisala from the northwestern part of the colony and Zabarima from the French territories, who arrived in Accra to take up colonial labor, resided in the Zongo. In the context of the Depression, sanitation experts and colonial officials debated not how much the migrant enclaves were overcrowded but rather how bad the sanitation had become. Officials thought that congestion in the city would be reduced if migrants returned to their villages to live on the produce of their farms. In other words, Accra's official approach to overcrowding and sanitation was passive in contrast to Nairobi's, as will be discussed in this chapter, which routinely ordered the police to raid African locations to search, arrest, and deport the unemployed. According to their version, if the unemployment and hardship accompanying the Depression could force migrant laborers to return to their home origin and farm the land for foodstuff, congestion would self-correct in Accra.[51] This seeming apathy in controlling migrants reveals a colonial weakness in forging capital cities and African working classes as envisioned. By World War II, fifty-four new communities, including Adabraka, Sabon Zongo, and Nima, had sprouted farther north.[52] Colonial records of these communities as "kindred tribes" indicated the accommodation and support systems that established Zongo residents put in place to help newcomers adapt to urban life rather than being from the same ethnicities. Together with the lack of municipal services and regulations, this social system contributed to overcrowding, congestion, and poor environmental sanitation in the migrant communities.[53]

While overcrowding posed health problems in the African communities in Accra, the continued influx of migrant workers was essential to the colonial economy as it filled the critical labor gap left by the Ga community. The Zongo residents' initiative to welcome and support newcomers to the urban setting not only reproduced their numbers for the labor but also provided shelter and helped to (re)generate the energy of the laborers. The colonial state did not provide houses for most laborers, making this local initiative significant.[54] For example, congestion and overcrowding in Zongo correlated with the construction of new roads in Accra.[55] Yet migrants' presence in their numbers overstretched the limited amenities Accra offered its African residents. Officials recognized this crucial role of the immigrant community and discussed ways to intervene in their housing. Colonial officials regarded them as impoverished and transient, needing help:

> From the point of view of public health, it is necessary to properly house these "strangers." As they are aliens and nomadic, they cannot be expected to build their own permanent houses: nor can the local chiefs or private enterprises.[56]

Colonial officials saw housing as critical to health. Because the communities built their houses with temporary materials such as mud and thatch, in contrast to permanent concrete, officials offered to help appropriately house them. Their housing condition made them susceptible to diseases like tuberculosis.[57] At a general meeting of the Accra Town Council in January 1935, three out of four members voted for a proposal to the colonial state to adjust building regulations to favor Zongo inhabitants to build their houses with temporary mud and thatch materials since cement and other permanent materials were too expensive for the laborers.[58]

The connection between the health of Accra's African residents and their physical living conditions caught the attention of the local press. Newspapers, like the *Independent* and *Times*, juxtaposed the deteriorated and congested African communities and European spacious and stately residential areas and noted that the disproportionate impact of Accra's uneven saniscape on Africans was proof that the colonial system did not care about the disintegration of "native society and the undermining" of their health.[59] They observed the congestion more nuancedly and challenged colonial officials' conventional excuse that the lazy habits of Africans and extended family systems caused poor sanitation.[60] To them, the African neighborhoods were a "standing disgrace to the government and municipality."[61] The colonial state did admit it was "difficult to improve the conditions under which . . . labor [was] housed."[62]

Because of the suspicion among African residents, which colonial officials and experts had cultivated in them in the first decades of the twentieth century (as described in chapter 1), colonial rule found it incredibly challenging to go into the seaside neighborhoods and appraise the sanitation conditions unaided by educated Africans. The African press played a crucial role in laying the groundwork for officials to get into the communities and collect data as a start for any meaningful intervention. The press also helped to bridge the communication gap between officials and the communities.[63] However, in the 1930s, it became apparent that the colonial state needed more funds and the will to help improve sanitation and somewhat level Accra's saniscape. It used the Red Cross and a team of student volunteers at Achimota Secondary School to survey African communities. But that official "slum" initiative faced African criticisms. To the *Times*, the extent of the problem exceeded "the scope of voluntary service."[64] The severity of the congestion and squalor necessitated official and expert intervention rather than relying on voluntary services from the Red Cross and students. It cemented the view that the colonial state was unwilling to commit funds to the health of the African communities in the city.

Urbanization and Congestion in Nairobi: Pangani, Kibera, and Pumwani

African Workers, Settler Control, and Development

Similarly, as the capital of Kenya, Nairobi also needed regular skilled and unskilled African workers to build and maintain its infrastructure. Most of Nairobi's African wage workers came from Native reserves or Native land units, ethnically demarcated physical spaces tied to social groups outside the city. The idea of the reserve as precisely African spaces legitimized settlers' concept of the "white highlands." The reserve system restricted subsistence farming and pastoralism, forcing Africans into wage labor.[65] Over time, Christian missionaries and apprenticeship facilities gave some Africans the primary education and technical skills to help run the colonial bureaucracy and economy.[66] Nairobi's Africans included menial laborers, apprentices, shop assistants, soldiers, police, warders, and domestic servants.[67] By 1926, officials approximated the African population in the city as 18,000 against 2,665 Europeans and 9,199 South Asians.[68] These Africans, staying in the urban neighborhoods, officially known as "native locations," became incredibly diverse along ethnic, religious, and class lines. The Kikuyu were the largest group of Africans in Nairobi, most of whom had not received a Western education and worked as low-paying laborers. The Swahili and Luo residents occupied skilled positions that paid better. Nairobi's non-Kikuyu emerged predominantly as the African middle class dominating the African Advisory Council.[69]

After World War I, Nairobi also witnessed an increase in migrant activity despite Kenya being less fortunate than the Gold Coast in the wartime export trade and revenue to develop urban infrastructure. Kenya exports, restricted to copra, hides, and wattle bark, were remote to the Atlantic trade network. These exports were not as highly demanded as cocoa, and there was a higher chance of German battleships sinking commercial ships plying the long distance between Britain and Kenya.[70] The trade restriction notwithstanding, Governor Edward Northey, Guggisberg's counterpart, was determined to "see things move out of the stagnation into which they had fallen," spurring a robust construction activity in Nairobi.[71] To increase revenue, Northey's administration approved the expansion of the municipal boundary and tightened control over land and property to maximize rent and rates. He obtained additional revenue from loans and concessions from the railway organization.[72] Activities attracting laborers to Nairobi were evident in the reports of the municipal engineer and medical officer of health. They observed fluctuation in the requests for permits for new buildings and the alterations to existing ones. The permits rose from

93 in 1919 to 266 in 1925, then dropping to 184 in 1926. There were some buildings for which African and non-African entrepreneurs and developers never started and completed during the periods despite obtaining permits. Regardless of the fluctuations and finished buildings, the request for permits indicated (anticipated) growth in urban demography, demand for housing, and urban economy.[73]

The interwar transformation of Nairobi's cityscape was visible. Significant improvements occurred in the construction of roads, connecting the city center with property in the suburbs. In 1926, Herbert Baker and Walton Jameson, an architect and a town engineer from Kimberley (South Africa), reinforced the plan to connect the different parts of the city. Other construction projects concentrated on improving the central business district. The Nairobi market and its environs gradually witnessed a redevelopment by private Indian property owners, colonial administration, and local government.[74] By 1933, the building of Nairobi's Capitol Theatre, Albert House, extensions to the New Stanley and Norfolk Hotels, the Desai Memorial, the new Municipal Market, the Bhora Mosque, and the Rhamtulla Walji Trust Building improved the city's appearance.[75]

Despite colonial and municipal reliance on African workers for urban development, Nairobi made minimal provisions for Africans who provided the labor for these developments. The living conditions and surroundings of Nairobi's African residents in Pangani, Pumwani, railways, and municipal housing also lacked essential public services, similar to those in Accra. The communities needed regular waste-collection systems, clean toilets, and drain maintenance.[76] After juxtaposing the spatial dynamics of race in Nairobi as Europeans residing in the best land, South Asians in the second, and Africans in the poorest, R. Mugo Gatheru described the toilets in the African locations:

> Public lavatories were very very dirty. Some of them did not have running water. Instead, they had hard tins like dustbins in which people "eased" themselves. There was an inescapable offensive smell when these bins were full of faeces, and especially when the municipal workers who removed them were late (as they always were). One public lavatory was used by over a thousand people. Those public lavatories which had running water were constructed in a particular manner. There was a large narrow trench inside them which was about one foot deep and the water ran in it as if in a small canal. The water flushed automatically but the capacity of one lavatory was not sufficient for the number of people who wanted to use it. Consequently the water system was always defective and the faeces,

therefore, could not be flushed away. Having no alternative, people would then continue "easing" themselves until the trench was full up.[77]

The sizeable African population that the settler system forced to live in the locations overstretched an already poor toilet facility. The flow and manual removal of human excrement often broke down. The resulting stagnant waste posed a public health danger to the African communities and their South Asian and European employers. Chapter 5 details how stagnant waste and settler imaginations of possible germ warfare encouraged the construction of septic tanks and sewers.

The municipality conducted raids in the locations out of fears of perceived crimes and imminent epidemics from African communities. Unlike Accra, where officials wished the migrant workers would return to their various hometowns and farm the land, the settler-dominated municipality in Nairobi took a different approach by occasionally deploying the police to round up "illegal" Africans and forcibly deport them back to their respective reserves.[78] A way of identifying illegals was through the kipande, a labor registration system that enabled the settler system to attempt to curtail the movements of Africans. It enabled the settler system to harass and dehumanize Africans. The kipande was a small metal case worn around the neck. It contained a document listing the bearer's home district, location, registration number, father's name, ethnicity, approximate age, employment record, wages, rations, and fingerprints. Fingerprints were a crucial feature of the kipande because of their importance in facilitating identification. Africans who left the Native reserve were required to wear the kipande around their necks. The municipality used this system to enforce the policy that Africans legitimately employed in Nairobi regularly returned to the reserves after completing their contracts. Officials also intended to use the kipande system to ensure that few women came and lived in Nairobi. However, the state justified the system as a control measure for political unrest, epidemic disease, and the weakening of the color bar. During the Depression, this strenuous and unwelcome urban control kipande project proved futile. The movements of Africans into and out of Nairobi were challenging to check. African migrant workers begrudged officials and the municipality for the kipande and restricting their choice to reside in Nairobi.[79]

African Locations in Nairobi

Pangani was a thirty-acre plot of land located north of the intersection of Eastern and Park Roads. It was a destination for the Swahili since Nairobi's foundation.

Early residents asserted that the state officially allocated the land to them. They were employees of European travelers and settlers who worked as safari porters, gun-bearers, and safari domestic servants. However, the municipality maintained no record of the claim to the land. Having been in Pangani for a long time, the residents had no apparent ties to a village or "native reserve" where officials could repatriate them to reclaim the land. They were officially a "detribalized" community. To the dismay of the state and municipality, their resilience transformed Pangani into a de facto African neighborhood. The community showed their courage and determination to create a space for themselves in a city settlers envisioned as exclusively white.[80]

As early settlers and property owners, the Swahili Muslim original residents of Pangani made their living from Nairobi's growth, providing lodges and subletting plots to accommodate the increasing numbers of African migrants. On the other hand, the growing urban population provided an income stream for Pangani pioneers, some of whom engaged in transactional sex and alcohol sales.[81] The women pioneers of Pangani made significant contributions to the colonial economy since the inception of Nairobi. However, due to the colonial notion that urban labor was a man's job, official records undervalued the women's presence and contribution to the city. In 1931, an official census that differentiated between pioneers and migrants revealed that half of the 320 African residents were women. Among these women were Kikuyu, Maasai, and Kamba, who ran their businesses, including bars and lodges, that catered to migrant laborers.[82] Women provided comforts of home, reproducing men's energies so crucial to the colonial economy.[83] It was obvious that the community was diversifying, and migrants seemed to be "detribalizing" and replacing the pioneer populace. Pangani's mixed and detribalizing African community posed somewhat of an administrative challenge for colonial native policy, which was supposed to differentiate, categorize, and tie Africans to specific places outside Nairobi to conveniently deport them to when the need arises.[84] That challenged the settler notion of Nairobi as European.

Kibera shared characteristics similar to Pangani in many ways. Located south of Ngong Road, Kibera comprised a vast parcel of about five thousand acres. It was initially inhabited by discharged Sudanese veterans of the King's African Rifles. The land was a reward officials gave to the veterans for their past service and as a recruiting ground to enlist their sons.[85] Contrary to official expectation, however, residents fell out of their control, and the place became noted for alcohol sale, trading stolen property, and prostitution. By 1931, the inability of the police to control the residents made them anxious about "the dangerous situation," mainly because of its proximity to Nairobi's European residential areas.[86] To justify the eviction of residents, officials provided figures to show that migrants were dominating the original Kiberans:

> But figures given to us indicate that out of 571 houses only 251 belongs to Sudanese ex-askaris or their dependents. The remainder are said to belong to a heterogeneous miscellany of persons who have penetrated the settlement from time to time. More than half of these householders are said to be women, of whom the majority are of questionable character.[87]

According to the official view that more than half of the population was "illegitimate," Sudanese served to undercut residents' argument that the land was a reward for their service to the Crown. However, municipal attempts to evict residents failed. Kiberans tapped into their network in Britain to block municipal dispossession plans.[88]

Unlike Pangani and Kibera, Pumwani, located east of the central business district, was the officially designated residential community for Africans. The colonial state and municipal council initially intended to use it to reduce congestion in the Nairobi market and segregate the Africans from the South Asians. In 1922, the settler state established the location many years after experts like Bransby Williams and W. J. R. Simpson successively advised it to establish an exclusively African residential area. Except for domestic servants in and around Nairobi, the municipality required all Africans, including those in Kileleshwa, Mombasa, Masikini, and Pangani, to relocate to Pumwani.[89] According to the law, European and South Asian employers were responsible for building suitable housing for Africans in Pumwani, except for domestic servants exempted by the governor. They could live on their employer's property in European and South Asian residential areas. When the municipality opened Pumwani for development and settlement, it provided water service and waterborne sewage, a brick dispensary, an office to commemorate African servicemen, a native affairs office, and a beer shop, among other amenities. Missionary organizations, such as the Roman Catholic Church and the Church Missionary Society, constructed and managed churches and schools in Pumwani.[90]

Despite opening Pumwani as an exclusive African area, the municipality was reluctant to grant residents the security of tenure to encourage them to invest substantially in real estate and improve the surroundings. Not granting Africans tenure and accepting them as permanent Nairobians disincentivized the residents from investing in the community, leading to deteriorated environmental conditions. As Pumwani's population increased, causing a housing shortage, it required matching infrastructure, services, and regulations to maintain sanitation. However, the combined impact of inadequate sanitation and lack of tenure compounded congestion and poor environmental conditions. Lack of tenure gave the municipality enormous leverage. It could evict residents and auction off the property at the slightest provocation. The reasons for eviction ranged from late payment of ground rent to something as petty as finding Africans in possession of liquor on the property. On the part of the African residents, tenure insecurity was discouraging enough to build their houses using cheap, temporary materials despite having the means for concrete and masonry buildings. At least they lost little investment in the likely event of an eviction. Within twenty years of Pumwani's existence under the circumstances, it metamorphosed and officially mutated into a "slum."[91]

The physical appearance of the African locations of Pangani, Kibera, and Pumwani expressed not only a deficit in sanitation but also the inability of employers to house their African employees and preserve Nairobi as a "white city." While African railway employees and wealthy Europeans with domestic servants fared relatively better, shacks used as backyard houses for African domestic servants contrasted with the rest of their affluent property. They detracted from the otherwise spacious and splendid European residential property.[92] African entrepreneurs in Pangani, Kibera, and Pumwani, including many women, demonstrated remarkable resilience by housing most African workers in and around Nairobi despite the sanitation challenges outside the railways and accommodations for European domestic servants.[93] One reason accounting for settlers designating African locations as "slums" was that the residents built their mud houses from temporary materials. Settlers designated the homes as hallmarks of "slums." However, mud houses were the main distinguishing factor when comparing African locations to the residential areas of the South Asian communities whose houses were composed of masonry buildings. Sanitation infrastructure, services, and regulation set both African and South Asian neighborhoods apart from the segregated European enclaves. As in African locations, a similar pattern of "putrescent garbage and slope, accumulations of rubbish and offal, stagnant potholes, choked drains—and so forth" was common in the South Asian communities. Despite this commonality of poor sanitation, settlers and officials attributed the disreputable "slum" label to the African location. The depictions made the locations easy targets for demolition and removal. Locations made of mud houses could be destroyed without accruing considerable financial and legal liability.[94] The concept of a slum emerged due to politically convenient factors.

Nairobi's municipal engineer's observation about the hygienic habits of Africans challenged the idea that the sanitation lag in the locations resulted from their inherently dirty living conditions. The engineer questioned colonial oversimplifications associated with African locations. The conditions were not because of the material and quality of African buildings. The houses themselves were "clean tidy and free from insects" known to transmit pathogens.[95] However, the absence of maintenance and regulatory culture created slum-like conditions, including congestion and deterioration. The colonial and settler systems were culpable because they refused Africans land tenure to encourage them to invest in their houses and surroundings. Municipal regulation and service were inadequate. Additionally,

> surfaces of all roads and lanes and of all open drains, the strict enforcement of sanitary regulations concerning the disposal of waste water and refuse; and the maintenance of efficient services for scavenging, conservancy, and watering—these are the essential requirements for healthy and sanitary housing.[96]

Outside and around individual houses, the filth in open areas, roads, drains, toilets, and waste containers revealed the dereliction of municipal services and regulations. Contrary to European portrayal of their bodies and houses as pathological, Africans kept their homes hygienic. The idea of African locations as "slums" was an invented problem to which the municipal authority was culpable.[97]

Overcrowding and unemployment impacted the quality of housing and the African communities. Pangani, Kibera, and Pumwani were the main housing options for single African men who earned low wages and could not own homes. So, workers pooled their money to rent rooms designed originally for a single person or far fewer people.[98] Around 1935, the Kenya Land Commission, which had a colony-wide mandate to address the land question in Kenya, disclosed that the residents wanted something "done to reduce the cost of houses to natives."[99] Employers without housing for their African employees could also have increased wages to afford rent and sanitation services. At the end of 1937, the *East African Times*, for example, reported four thousand Africans sharing two hundred single-occupancy rooms. Some residents were unemployed and job searching. A municipal survey in Pangani registered thirty unemployed male Africans out of 205 in 1938. And in Pumwani, there were twenty-five out of 240. However, this was about the lowest possible number of unemployed Africans because most had returned to their respective "reserves" at the end of the year after completing their contracts as was officially required.[100]

As the most prominent employer of Africans, the settler state was the worst culprit for overcrowded housing conditions. It provided little housing arrangements for most of its employees. Because of the housing scarcity, it kept a priority list, privileging African interpreters and "office boys" over menial laborers.[101] The municipality's public housing in Kariokor on Quarry Road was unpopular among Africans because the conditions there were uncongenial. The building consisted of blocks of dormitories with sitting rooms, cubicles, and kitchens for male workers. The dormitories were too expensive and offered little value for individual rent. The rents of four and seven shillings for rooms with one and three beds were prohibitive even for firms and individual employers that used the facility to house their employees. Those who remained in dormitories supported one another, saved money, and made the rent manageable by pooling their money for single-occupancy rooms. The more occupiers, the less the monetary burden on renters for housing. In 1937, six Africans shared a single room in Kariokor. While the overcrowding in the room was evidence of inadequate municipal regulation, it increased the pace of the deterioration of dormitory amenities. Due to these realities in Kariokor, the employers and Africans avoided the dormitories and preferred Pangani, Pumwani, and Kibera, where the municipal council restricted African entrepreneurs who catered to crucial housing needs.[102]

Yet the physical attributes of Nairobi's African communities were not the sole reason official records depicted them as "slums" and threats. At times, the description of the communities was gendered and took on the shape of "black peril" phobias. But this was because the settler system made them so. The labor system in Nairobi needed men more than women. In some instances, the number of Kikuyu men could be five times more than that of women. The large number of unmarried men present fueled constant fear of sexual threats posed by male Africans against European women and children. Also, the description of African neighborhoods as poor in turn precipitated concerns about a class struggle that was likely to lead to a revolution whereby poor Africans would rise against wealthy European settlers and upset the colonial order. In 1937, members of the Nairobi Rotary Club and Associated Chamber of Commerce, high-profile colonial officials, including the governor, and the press wondered together about the similarity between the deteriorated conditions of poor British in the colonial metropole and African Nairobians and the possibility of a revolution in Nairobi. Signs of a class struggle pushed a section of the European community to appeal to settlers in paternalistic and invasive terms to tackle slum conditions, unemployment, and diseases in a "revolutionary" spirit.[103] The local characteristics, which influenced official and settler understanding of Nairobi's "slums," revealed the insecurities of the wealthy and ruling minority seeking to maintain their exploitative political and economic dominance over the settler colonial society.

Conclusion: Urban Migrant Workers, Host Communities and the Capital Cities

High population density, tight-knit development, and inadequate (lack of) sanitation infrastructure and services in the Ga seaside communities, Zongo, and the so-called native locations in Nairobi appeared in colonial official correspondence and expert reports as neighborhoods characterized by some of the most visible attributes of slums in industrializing and urbanizing Britain. Yet what constituted a "slum" was fluid at various times and places, even in its British origins, describing communities with deteriorating physical structures, poor sanitation that gave conducive conditions for the multiplication and transmission of pathogens, poor people, and socially-defined unacceptable behavior. The wobbly characterizations of "slum" were problematic. The unstable attributes of "slum" made it easy for officials and urban residents to apply it to the African communities of Accra and Nairobi despite the peculiar absence of industries similar to those in Britain and the racism attached to neighborhoods. From their British origins to their application in African cities, officials and urban residents perceived them differently based on race, class, culture, and ideology, making it a relative concept with uncertain boundaries. Alan Gilbert notes that communities became designated officially as "slums" because of neglect and old housing quality which did not transform along Western lines compared to modernizing neighborhoods nearby.[104] Not only did African residential districts in Accra and Nairobi look different from European areas because of poor municipal services, but their built environments manifested traditional architecture and building materials. Their relatively poor sanitation conditions, including overcrowding, congestion, and deteriorated (lack of) infrastructure and municipal services, cannot be decoupled from the physical appearance of the wealthy Accra and Nairobi districts. The contrast in the saniscapes was similar to the observations of Geddes and journalists in Britain in the nineteenth and twentieth centuries. Whether in Britain or the colonial capitals, "slums" were products of modern cities, which were driven by industrialization, commerce, and capitalism. This relationality of slum-like conditions with affluence associated with capitalist accumulation and commerce underpins Mike Davis's argument about the "slums'" global emergence and spread in the second half of the twentieth century.[105] However, as this book has shown thus far, the spread of slum-like condition was underway before that period.

Negative portrayals of African locations as slums in the cities distract from the aspirations and positive contributions of the people who experienced the cities and the colonial political economy. As John Parker and Naaborko Sackeyfio-Lenoch have demonstrated in their various books, while Ga had founded Accra, controlled land tenure, and exerted enormous influence in the historical development of the city through lineage, family, chieftaincy, and colonial courts, they welcomed migrant populations.[106] They were critical in building and maintaining Accra's infrastructure and commercial activities. When the colonial state could not provide housing for their laborers, the Ga did. They had rented housing to accommodate European officials and merchants before the colonial state built Victoriaborg. They even stepped in and utilized their long-standing fishing expertise to facilitate the onshore and offshore movement of imports and exports, thus overcoming a significant environmental obstacle to shipping and commercial capitalism. Migrant wage laborers also housed, socialized newcomers and made working in Accra bearable for them by providing housing. In many ways, the plight of migrant communities in Accra parallels those of some Kikuyu, Swahili, and Luo in Nairobi. Timothy Parsons directs our attention to these people living in Nairobi's "slums."[107] While many African Nairobians were desperately poor, living in locations that lacked adequate sanitation, they aspired for opportunities in education, social advancement, and personal enrichment by working as domestic servants, laborers, railway workers, retailers, and entrepreneurs.[108] John Lonsdale and Luise White, in their respective works, inspire an essential discussion about the relationship between the city and the country, property ownership, and urban wage labor through the lives of African Nairobians providing for their families in rural areas, acquiring and maintaining urban property, and making urban life tolerable for migrant laborers. Their struggles and contributions drove the colonial city and its economy. However, these efforts and their impact appeared far less in colonial records than the official depictions of deplorable slum-like conditions in which they resided.[109]

This chapter applies White's political economy approach to the "native locations" in Nairobi to analyze the "slums" of both Accra and Nairobi. White demonstrates that the work of prostitutes was a labor process that reproduced male energies for wage work.[110] In the same way, through housing and making urban life somewhat tolerable for workers for whom the colonial states and municipal authorities provided little accommodation but depended on their energies and skill to build and maintain the infrastructures of health and trade, the so-called slums (re)produced colonial Accra and Nairobi. The chapter conceptualizes "slums" as built-in components of the cities even as colonial records associated them with disorder. On this point the chapter reinforces Hart's argument that officials and technocrats invented disorder based on systems and structures that privileged European commercial interests and visions of a modern city.[111] Yet commercial capitalists and officials relied on cheap labor from the overcrowded and congested communities to run the colonial economy and build and maintain the cities. Thus, there was an order in what seemed like disorder in the cities. As Simpson observed in Accra, the improvement in Accra's sanitation reproduced unsanitary conditions nearby. Like the Ga chiefs who requested the colonial state to invest in the sanitation of Accra's African communities because of its role in slum conditions in the previous chapter, officials and African-run newspapers noted the poor housing and environmental conditions under which colonial workers and urban residents lived. Nairobi's labor system depended on men (and women) whose poor living conditions compelled European officials and settlers to equate them to Britain's poor during the Industrial Revolution and to call for action to tackle diseases and unemployment in the "slum." The "slum" communities continued to provide critical services to Nairobi's residents beyond the colonial period.[112]

The African-run newspapers on the Gold Coast compared African and European residential areas, revealing the discontent of the Western-educated elites with colonial underinvestment in the sanitation and health of the Africans. Coincidentally, condemnation of this uneven saniscape grew louder in the interwar years, when the growth of Accra nurtured profound political changes and anti-colonial nationalism.[113] As Parker has noted, the historiography of Gold Coast politics and nationalism recognizes this fundamental shift during this period.[114] It was ironic that *The Tools of Empire*, which eased European colonial occupation in the Gold Coast and laid the foundation for colonial rule, also spread discontent among Accra's residents and fueled anti-colonial sentiments.[115] Interestingly, in 1937, European settlers and officials discussed the likelihood of a revolution in Kenya because Africans resented slum conditions in Nairobi and the associated threat of diseases. The discussion foreshadowed a series of urban struggles that culminated in the "dirty war in Kenya over a decade later."[116] Anderson traces the urban causes of the dirty Mau Mau war to the impoverished "slum" side of Nairobi's saniscape.[117] As the next chapter will show, British slum discourse provided colonial officials with language to justify the (attempted) demolition of African "slum" communities. Africans found the demolition exercises to be invasive, disruptive, and self-serving. Rather than alleviating slum conditions as per colonial imaginations, demolition instead shifted and exacerbated them.

CHAPTER 3

Demolition, 1920–1940

International Housing and Town Planning Congresses in Europe, which contacted the Colonial Office (CO), reinforced William Simpson's recommendations for demolishing slum-like locations. The congress's European conveners portrayed "slums" as global urban problems requiring destruction, replanning, zoning, and rebuilding. Correspondence between London and the colonies also endorsed "slum clearance" to remake colonial cities.[1] The global and imperial urban renewal initiatives resonated with colonial officials, local authorities, and Western-educated African elites who approximated conditions in the African communities to "slums" in nineteenth- and twentieth-century Britain. Demolition appealed to them because of the history of recurring outbreaks of contagious diseases, such as plague and yellow fever, attributed to slum conditions. When steady population growth worsened sanitation in African locations, officials, local authorities, and elite residents embraced the idea of demolition as a global remedy. They advocated for the destruction of crowded and squalid neighborhoods.[2]

Mass demolition, initially seen as a logical solution to the distressing conditions of "slums" in cities, ironically became a tool that perpetuated the very conditions it aimed to eradicate. Endorsed by medical and sanitation experts, demolition, often recorded in colonial archives as "slum clearance," was a compelling solution to eliminate urban squalor and contagious diseases. However, it ended up shifting and spreading these very conditions, raising the question of whether officials and municipal councils truly intended to eliminate "slums" through the destruction of houses and neighborhoods. As will be seen in this chapter, it became evident that slum clearance had other motives. Officials used poor sanitation to stoke fears of the communities as hotbeds for epidemics and blight in modern, western-like cities. African residents of both cities opposed demolition despite the different power dynamics, land tenure, and histories of settlement of Accra and Nairobi. While the fisherfolk retained control of their neighborhoods despite aggressive colonial demolition efforts, Pangani residents made various unsuccessful attempts to preserve the community. For the Africans in these neighborhoods, demolition was not a straightforward sanitation project but a tool for marginalizing them from urban economic opportunities. This chapter compares Accra's Asere and its environs with Nairobi's Pangani in the interwar period and beyond. The challenges African residents posed to settler and non-settler states highlight the complexities and difficulties in realizing colonial visions of "modern" colonial capital cities.

Demolition as a Sanitation Measure?

Accra: Asere, the Seaside Communities, and the Expansion of Port Infrastructure

Referring to a plague outbreak outside Accra, in Kumasi, a city about 126 miles north, the Medical Department complained about James Town's and Ussher Town's sanitation, noting the threat of plague still existed in the "congested slums."[3] Western-educated African elites expressed this opinion about overcrowding, especially in Ussher Town. They urged the colonial state to take action, pointing out that significant efforts were being made worldwide to eliminate "slums" and other areas plagued by disease. Like colonial officials, they also made a note of Accra's sanitation that it had "some dangerously bad areas which ought not to be permitted to exist longer than it [*sic*] is reasonably possible: as long as they continue to be, public health danger."[4] These calls reinforced the earlier town improvement committee proposals following the plague outbreak and the botched Simpsonian blueprint for purchase of vast swaths of land for buffer zones. With the cooperation of the quarter's traditional authority, colonial officials demarcated plots in Kaneshie, three miles northwest, to relocate residents and allow for a tabula rasa to remake

Ussher Town.[5] The improvement would have included street construction and widening, open spaces, and infrastructure required for the colonial entrepôt port capital to function profitably for the colonial economy. Officials envisioned the plan as a continuation of the sanitation-driven remodeling and expansion of Accra's built environment. It spread out Accra's dense demographics from the seaside communities, forming the suburban Riponsville (Kwali Worko), Adabraka, and Korle Gonno and transforming the physical layout of the coastline.[6]

Just as some African residents favored decongestion, others were determined to continue forging their lives and livelihoods on their ancestral Ga homelands along the coastline.[7] Those determined to stay posed a problem to colonial and imperial port city remaking.[8] The residents who opposed the relocation from their coastal neighborhood viewed the move beyond sanitation reasons. Through the Asere (in Ussher Town) Conservative Association, they expressed their determination to conserve and safeguard their most ancient rights, privileges, and customs embedded in land tenure and the longstanding homes and fishing occupation, salt making, and trading on the lands along the sea.[9] The land and their homes were legacies, revered as "family gods, the bones of buried ancestors and powerful magnets to a mind so saturated . . . with religion of the animistic kind."[10] While this newspaper depiction of the rationale had demeaning undertones, it underlined the determination of Ga lineages, families, and individuals to remain in the communities because of their spiritual and cultural connections to the land. They had developed a strong attachment to their land for centuries before colonial rule. From this perspective, their relocation deprived them of a significant source of livelihood and their ancient rights, privileges, and customs. As expressed by the Asere Conservative Association, the intransigence of Ga landowners was profound. It drew out official attempts to relocate those resolute. Ultimately, they rendered colonial repurposing and renewal plans for the center of Accra incomplete.

In 1927, four months before the Accra Town Council members' meeting to consider the government's proposal to demolish Asere and relocate the residents, the Asere Conservative Association directly appealed any plans on the part of officials to change their status quo. Addressing Governor Alexander Ransford Slater, the association referred to its constitution and insisted it would "co-operate with and assist the Government *when the occasion warrants it.*" However, it continued with a note of education on "the nature and circumstances of [their] Native Institutions, Customs, and Conventions":

> We feel sure that you will always preserve and safeguard to us our ancient rights privileges customs of our Constitutions such as have been instituted by our forefathers since the foundation of the Ga nation and we earnestly pray that your Excellency will neither tolerate nor encourage any innovation or subversion of such our constitution for the constitution of every country is the foundation of the law. And it is our ancient birthright.[11]

As already mentioned, that ancient birthright, to which the association referred, embraced religious and cultural attachment to their ancestral lands on which they built their homes and to the sea from whence they obtained their source of livelihood. However, with the support of the Western-educated African elites, officials were relentless in their efforts to acquire and repurpose the site. Governor Slater directed the council to proceed with the mass demolition and relocation plans.

In the 1930s, the council decided that Chorkor, within the neighborhood of Korle Gonno, was a suitable site to move the fishing and salt making industries. This set the stage for friction between the colonial state and Asere. The environment in and around Korle Gonno, where officials envisioned the location of the local fishing and salt-making industry, had become a subject of intense debate.[12] It needed adequate sanitation, infrastructure, or services to match the population density. Without scaling up infrastructure and municipal services, poor environmental sanitation would be exacerbated because of the concentration of additional population and the Ga industries. There was a double standard in zoning the industry near Korle Gonno. The smells and wastes from the industries and its aesthetic appearance, in the minds of the colonial officials, were not suitable for the center of their capital city, representing British modernity. However, they were acceptable near the African communities of Korle Gonno.[13] Environmental racism could not be more explicit.[14] The sanitation in Korle Gonno had become hazardous twenty years after the colonial state established it following a plague outbreak. The neighborhood's poor sanitation was easily noticeable compared to the well-maintained European quarter nearby. The *Times of West Africa* reported:

> The town of Korle Gonno, especially the south-western and western sections of Korle Bu hospital which are inhabited by the native populations are in a deplorable state owing to insanitary conditions. Weeds, mud and pool abound in the vicinity. No proper roads are constructed, and there is no layout, which gives a distinct contrast between the well laid out and tarmetted roads leading to Korle Bu hospital and adjacent roads around the European and residential quarters.[15]

Across the lagoon toward the west, the uneven saniscape was striking. The lack of a satisfactory town plan caused the haphazard development of buildings and poor roads and drains in the African communities. This caused waste and surface water to collect, resulting in muddy grounds, weed growth, and mosquito infestation. An influx of migrant workers during World War II in Korle Gonno would worsen these poor conditions. While some migrants rented open spaces "to accommodate shacks of all kinds," others slept at open verandahs.[16] One experienced a sharp contrast from the community toward Korle Bu (Gold Coast) Hospital, the largest medical facility in British West Africa, where officials constructed a tarmac road leading to the hospital. The European residential area near the hospital manifested a well-planned community also with tarmac roads.

To prevent slum-like surroundings from emerging in Korle Gonno, the colonial state needed to do more than allocate undeveloped land, layout building plots, create open spaces, or demarcate roads. As will be seen in Nairobi, after establishing a new residential community, regular municipal service and regulations were crucial in keeping public spaces clean and preventing people from building in unauthorized spaces. Suitable roads with drains prevented muddy grounds and enabled waste and surface water to flow away from residential areas, thereby preventing mosquito breeding conditions. These regulations and services were inadequate in Korle Gonno, which explains why sanitation in the place came under media scrutiny when officials proposed moving the fishing and salt-making industry to the location. The move would have created a corridor of squalor along the coastline west of the lagoon, starkly contrasting the hospital and its nearby affluent community. While using poor sanitation in Asere and its surrounding area as a justification for demolition, the colonial state, often pressured by the Accra Town Council, was cautious. Following past experiences, including that of Governor Clifford, mass demolition and relocation were sure to receive anti-colonial sentiments and possibly violence. It was a fine line officials walked, to be ruling restless urban residents and risk destabilized commercial activities in the name of urban renewal. Additionally, mass demolition would have involved spending money not only to deploy the police and army to quell widespread rioting, but also pull down buildings, haul debris, and relocate people.[17]

An opportunity for demolition came when an earthquake struck Accra in June 22, 1939. The earthquake lasted about one minute and shook Accra and its surrounding areas in the evening. After the major tremble, officials reported 149 African casualties, sixteen of them dead. Many houses collapsed. Minor tremors and heavy rainfall continued for days after the quake. The hardest-hit communities were James Town, Ussher Town, and Christiansborg.[18] Continued aftershocks caused more buildings to collapse. For safety reasons, official crews went about demolishing damaged houses. Governor Arnold Hodson's remark about the official post-earthquake plans revealed that the colonial state had longstanding plans to demolish the African communities:

> My policy is, therefore, directed towards securing at the same time not only the reparation of the earthquake damage and the rehousing involved therein but also the clearance and re-planning of those congested areas which would have had to be dealt with by "slum clearance" schemes in the near future. . . . It may be mentioned that in preparation for the introduction of slum clearance schemes in Accra, a matter which has long been in the mind of Government, several layouts had already been set out on the outskirts of the town.[19]

Clearly the earthquake caused significant damage, which allowed the government to initiate a planned demolition and relocation exercise. Before the disaster, plans were in place for new residential areas on the outskirts of Accra. For over fifteen years, officials had tried unsuccessfully to demolish and relocate the African communities. After the earthquake, officials believed that the "disaster had one happy effect in that . . . the unhealthy congestion" in the center of Accra had disappeared.[20] The colonial state wanted to demolish the Ga neighborhoods to expand the port city's economic facilities.

Ironically, in the site plans for rehousing Africans displaced by the earthquake, the colonial state failed to include sanitation infrastructure and services, further raising questions about the seriousness of colonial rule in improving Africans' health and living standards. Officials had criticized Ga neighborhoods for congestion and poor sanitation for decades before the earthquake. And yet, Governor Hodson's blueprints that anticipated the demolition of Asere and its environs had no toilet facilities. Colonial obsession with "slum clearance" did not necessarily mean they were interested in providing sanitation for Accra's African residents.[21] Malcolm MacDonald, the Labor member of Parliament and secretary of states for the Colonies, queried the governor:

> The figures of cost mentioned in your dispatch, viz. 120,000 for the temporary scheme and 500,000 for the permanent scheme, are apparently exclusive of some expenditure which is likely to be entailed, such as the cost of providing roads and

> drains, and connections with water and electricity supplies; and I would wish fully inclusive estimates of cost, however approximate, to be furnished as soon as they can be given, together with an indication as to how much of the outlay proposed is expected to be recovered. If cognate schemes for any areas beyond Accra are envisaged, I would wish similar figures to be given for each area.[22]

Understandably, due to the urgent need to house homeless Africans sheltering in railway vans, school buildings, and other makeshift structures during heavy rains following the quake, officials probably rushed new post-earthquake designs without costing sanitation infrastructure and services therein.[23] However, given the urgent sanitation need in central Accra, which has been commonplace in colonial records since the declaration of Accra as the capital city, it was crucial to prioritize sanitation if officials were genuinely interested in the public health of African communities and preventing "slums." The colonial state was more interested in moving Ga residents from Accra's center than providing them with roads, drains, and piped water. The lag in sanitation planning for African residential communities caught up with the government during and after World War II and prompted a large-scale rehousing scheme.

Nairobi: Pangani and the Show of Settler Dominance

After 1920, medical officials declared Kenya a plague-endemic city. They held that the Africans living in Pangani and Pumwani, where most of Nairobi's workforce resided, suffered high rates of mortality and morbidity. A report of recurring plague incidents detailed the causes as "insanitary premises," which consisted of dilapidated mud and wattle houses overcrowded with Africans. To European settlers, the default solution to prevent the pathogen from spreading was to cleanse the neighborhoods through demolition.[24] Ewart Grogan, a settler who pushed demolition as a solution, was a wealthy European settler in Kenya who had earned a fortune from timber concessions. He owned much land and was vocal about the city's economic, political, and social issues. He played a vital role in the settler campaign for Kenya's autonomy from the CO. Grogan and European settlers of his ilk held significant power in the municipal authority. Settler feelings of threat to their health based on a judgment of poor sanitation in the African locations could bring about mass demolition of those houses.[25] Increased demolition activity in and around Nairobi, including in Kilileshwa, Masikini, Mombasa, and Kaburini, led to the migration of many African Nairobians to Pangani, which would later become the focus of official and municipal sanitation and demolition discourse during the interwar period.

In December 1922, the Nairobi District Commissioner submitted a report recommending the destruction of Pangani and detailed the compensation for the residents. This report intensified discussions about Nairobi's sanitation and the health threats that Pagani posed. However, demolition was only sometimes a unanimous decision. The report received endorsement and opposition from officials, the municipal council, Pangani residents, and nongovernmental organizations. The question of demolition, as a potent cleansing measure, divided Nairobi's European communities. The city's municipal engineer expressed doubt about demolition, stating that medical experts and settlers "repeatedly urged as the only solution of the sanitary problem," and "yet it [was] never done, or rarely, because for general application such a measure [was] out of the question." Further, the engineer argued that "in any case, it [was] not the solution to the problem, but only the creation of another problem, namely rehousing the dispossessed in such manner" to avoid "similar conditions" in different neighborhoods.[26] The engineer saw how the demolition of Pangani, without providing adequate housing for the displaced residents, only served to shift the unsanitary and overcrowded conditions to other locations within the city. When the demolition victims moved to newly constructed or laid-out neighborhoods, it was crucial to have proper sanitation infrastructure and services in place to prevent the emergence of slum-like conditions. Unfortunately colonial officials, municipal authorities, and private employers provided little to no housing and sanitation for their African workers. Unsurprisingly, as the populations that Pangani absorbed relocated to Pumwani, it, too, developed slum-like conditions.[27]

The mixed reaction to Pangani's destruction made it difficult for the municipality to take swift action. Dragging out the debate of demolishing Pangani worsened the sanitation and provided an added justification for the destruction of the neighborhood. There was no need to invest in infrastructure and services other than water and toilets to keep it livable until demolition and relocation arrangements were ready. Demolition took over a decade to finally accomplish.[28] Until then, residents lived in a precarious situation. Sometimes it seemed inevitable that officials and municipal authorities would demolish; at other times there was silence. The absence of a clear policy decision led to insufficient investment in sanitation infrastructure, services, and regulation, resulting in "slow violence" in the community.[29] The argument for demolition stated:

> The location at Pangani appears to us to be deleterious both to the health and morals of the natives. It is badly overcrowded and has a notable preponderance of undesirables. The sanitary conditions are not such as ought to be permitted in Nairobi and are a menace to the town. No substantial amelioration could be affected without a condemnation of a large proportion of the houses.[30]

The demolition was motivated by sanitation, overcrowding, and peculiar Nairobi issues. An overwhelming presence of Africans in Pangani threatened the settler idea of Nairobi as a "white city." Demolition aimed to preserve settler dominance by consolidating African residential segregation in Pumwani and making Africans easy to regulate.

Besides consolidating segregation and controlling Africans, the destruction had other benefits for the municipal authority. It considered the Pangani site a suitable residential location for the South Asian community. If only the South Asian community could be segregated and consolidated in that part of the city, it would help toward compartmentalization of the city along race lines. There was also an economic benefit. As relatively cheaper and more popular housing options were available in Pangani, the municipality had difficulty controlling rent and filling vacancies in its Kariokor housing facility, Nairobi's first public housing on Quarry Road. The Kariokor property, primarily a building of brick dormitories, was unpopular.[31] They instigated extreme hatred elsewhere in the British empire to the extent of contributing to riots in the 1930s and laying the foundation for a shift in imperial housing policy.[32] Filling municipal housing by demolishing African locations was a familiar Municipal tactic, previously deploying the gambit in Kaburini and Kileleshwa. It prohibited licenses for affected house owners who sought to rebuild lodges legitimately in Pumwani through vetting and selecting reputable African lodge owners with a respectable track record to reduce the number of eligible candidates further. In seeking a self-serving end, municipal African policy invented housing shortages and the accompanying high rent and overcrowding.[33]

Despite Pangani residents improving their properties to mitigate claims that their community was a health threat, the municipality eventually demolished the neighborhood. Residents, many of whom were women who provided the comfort of home and reproduced the energies of Nairobi's male workforce, kept their homes and surroundings hygienic.[34] They regulated close-quarter physical developments to enable light and air flows and prevent "fleas and such like vermin . . . the usual symptoms of ignorance and neglect common to insanitary slums."[35] There was "plenty of space between the huts and the very nature of the huts themselves, particularly of the roofs, generally ensure[d] no small measure of ventilations."[36] Six years after the municipality marked Pangani for demolition, residents attempted to immobilize the action by doubling down on community regulations on haphazard development.[37] Where closely built houses existed, house owners with the financial means were "proud men who [had] kept them [houses and surroundings] beautifully clean with white-washed interiors." They had the financial incentive to keep their homes clean, as these homes served as the preferred lodging option for most unattached African migrant workers. Accommodation for these unattached male laborers was particularly profitable because single rooms could take in many men in Nairobi for short stays. But the Pangani property owners could only go so far. The municipality was determined to flatten neighborhood, which it had neglected. Regular municipal services were absent to prevent an appalling eyesore. Near the clean and spacious buildings there were overflowing toilets and drains filled with excreta and urine. When demolition was underway, C. V. W. Anderson, president of the Nairobi Rotary Club, lamented the ongoing destruction of Pangani without providing replacements for the displaced residents.[38] Despite residents' efforts to make their houses hygienic, the municipality had cleared the neighborhood by the outbreak of World War II.[39]

Incomplete Mass Demolition and Local Responses in Accra

In July 1939, two days after the government revealed its intention to reconstruct the earthquake-ravaged neighborhoods along Western sanitation lines with infrastructure such as roads, open spaces, and drainage systems, the *Independent* published an article assuring the public that the land on which individual houses stood would continue to belong to owners. The article addressed residents' concerns that they would lose their land and community.[40] African landowners had little trust in the British regime regarding land. Officials had attempted to place land under colonial control through the Lands Bill of 1897, and mass dispossessing was at the heart of racialized residential segregation and the making of buffer zones.

The press had also fueled these worries with editorials and articles supporting improving the physical environment and sanitation in the African communities to fit Accra's status as a colonial capital city. Accra had witnessed significant growth due to the expansion of trade, government offices, houses, stores, and warehouses that took up much land.[41] Officials could use extra land to expand port facilities and infrastructure for commercial and security purposes.[42] During the earthquake (and throughout the colonial period), the media on the Gold Coast played a significant role in shaping the opinions and actions of ordinary Africans. When the disaster struck Accra, the governor and colonial administration regularly met with the press to communicate official relief plans. Journalists, lawyers, and clerks who were literate and fluent in English and the local Ga language mediated between the fishing community and government, attending meetings and translating proceedings.[43] Ga neighborhoods and lands continued in an entanglement of a renewed official effort to rebuild Accra along Western lines to benefit the colonial economy. The official justification for the colonial urban vision was sanitation.

Sanitation reforms focused on Asere and its environs. The community was a nagging headache to "technocratic colonialism" not necessarily because of its opposition to sanitation but due to the self-serving colonial goals that did not align with its interests.[44] Before the earthquake, Asere was the permanent home of Ga families and lineages, with over 2,822 residents living on seven acres of land divided into 126 plots. In the official view, the community was on a prime site suitable for constructing stores and business buildings near the Harbor Works, Customs Office, and sea. The Accra Town Council, dominated by European colonial appointees rather than elected representatives from Accra's African communities, frequently urged the state to demolish Asere citing congested physical development and poor sanitation.[45] Just four months before the Accra earthquake, the African councilor Jones Nelson urged the Accra Town Council to remind the government to demolish Asere:

> A more definite policy with regard to slum clearance in Accra be laid down by government and that . . . since the outbreak of plague in 1907 nothing has been done in the matter of slum clearance in Accra. He was aware the scheme would involve heavy expenditure, but if some vote was made yearly by government for slum clearance an appreciable amount of work would be done in a few years.[46]

The councilor was partially correct that the cost of demolition, which included compensation and rehousing, restrained the government. Interestingly, the councilor alluded to a sustainable way of improving Accra without mass demolition and relocation of communities, which was a savings fund dedicated to constructing sanitation infrastructure, providing cleansing services, and maintaining an effective regulatory body to prevent unauthorized construction on waterways in particular.

Sanitation reforms required a committed state and local government genuinely interested in the health of urban Africans. But the colonial state was fixated on "slum clearance."[47] However, officials remarked the actual challenge that, "one of the obstacles to dealing with the [demolition] problem" was "the difficulty of inducing the fishermen, who [were] the principal inhabitants of the slum area" to relocate.[48]

Ga opposition to colonial post-earthquake rebuilding blueprint was a complex issue involving multiple factors. A preliminary survey a year before the disaster had shown that "the conflicting considerations . . . of this problem in [Accra were] numerous," and for that reason, a "prolonged and close investigation [was required] before definite schemes [could] finally be formulated."[49] One consideration was the piece in the *Independent* in July 1939, which reiterated that the attachment to land meant more than an economic means of livelihood. Each resident had a "strong attachment . . . to his square foot of land" because it was intricately connected with "the family gods [and] the bones of buried ancestors."[50] It suggested that lineages, families, and individuals held on to their land to prevent severing their connection with their gods and ancestors if relocation and the repurposing of the neighborhood were to occur. However, some residents relocated to Kaneshi from Asere, contributing to the reshaping of the city.[51] Another reality was that the earthquake's aftermath magnified the generational divide over land and urban reform. Officials had to contemplate the remark of the acting deputy director of health service, W. M. Howells, about the surrender of the older fishing members of the community when he said, "In every large centre [principally Accra] in the Gold Coast the local Authorities" were "keenly alive to the urgent necessity for the removal of their congested slum areas."[52] The older generation, traditional official holders, like the chiefs, seemed more understanding of the government redevelopment scheme. They hoped to benefit from land transactions and the rebuilding of Accra by acquiring property and wealth to compensate for the diminishing authority of traditional power, which was their primary source of riches until colonialism.[53]

Through the paramount Ga chief (Ga *manche*), Nii Tackie Obii, the older generation and chiefs (*manchemei*) broadcasted, reiterating and expressing support for the official justification for mass demolition. They underlined its importance as the logical solution to ending congestion and disease epidemics in the community. From the chief's broadcast, it was clear that there were behind-the-scenes meetings and negotiations involving the government, the council, and his other chiefs and traditional officeholders:

> Those of my listeners who are associated with the inhabitants in some of these congested areas will readily agree with me that the proposed rebuilding of these areas is not only a measure towards bringing the inhabitants to present day living but an utmost desideratum.[54]

To modernize Accra and provide better amenities, the state needed to demolish and rebuild the congested neighborhood to match it with the appearance of the nearby upscale neighborhood, the modern High Street business district. To accommodate the changes, the proposed new layout of Asere would include thirty-three plots and broader streets. Most Asere residents would lose their plots under the new plan. The colonial state, European traders, some African merchants, and Syrian and Lebanese businesses would directly benefit from streets, shops, warehouses, open spaces, and other envisioned material developments.[55]

Like the Ga chiefs, a series of articles and editorials in the press also supported the modern rebuilding of Accra. The *Independent* envisioned a "new Accra" built from the "ashes of old Accra."[56] Reinforcing Manche Nii Tackie Obii's statement that demolition was of "utmost desideratum" in bringing residents to present-day living, the *Independent* pleaded with residents to consent "in the interest of progress and the will to build an Accra to be proud of."[57] Also, the editorial stated that "we [had] so progressed that it ought to be easy for us to bring ourselves to a frame of mind which [would] see wisdom in planning."[58] Despite this overwhelming support for the colonial state, the press suspected colonial-driven modernization. When the *Independent* published an editorial about negotiations on land sale involving residents and African chiefs, the "government stepped in, stopped the deal and proposed their own scheme of acquisition." Demolition and post-earthquake urban reform appeared as an excuse to implement longstanding plans, such as the Simpsonian blueprint.[59] The newspaper stated that colonial officials were "jealous of the stools [chiefs on behalf of their respective constituencies] as owners of the lands," noting that officials intended to introduce a "scheme of acquisition to deny those stools the satisfaction" of owning and developing land in central Accra.[60] The proximity of Asere and the neighboring Ga residential areas to the center of Accra and High Street rendered the land very valuable, and the government went to great lengths to prevent the chiefs from acquiring the property. Yet other ways the communities showed their suspicion of the colonial state were evident. After the government allocated houses to the affected people outside Accra, the heads of families suspected they might lose their property. As a result, they rented out or left their new accommodation to their kin and moved into makeshift camps near their earthquake-devastated community. Staying nearby allowed them to remain closer to their property and keep a watchful eye on it.[61]

Mass grassroots mobilizations impressed on officials that there was widespread resistance to rebuilding Accra as envisioned evident in the sharp division between the younger and older generations of Accra's fisherfolks. Ata Ampafio, the head representative of the fishing community, called a meeting of fisherfolk on July 12, 1939, to discuss the government's proposal to relocate the fishing industry. The meeting aimed to reach a consensus on accepting the government's recommendations, but the deliberations ended in a deadlock.[62] Otoo, the most proficient representative of the young fisherfolk, respectfully expressed that they disapproved of the location recommended by officials for establishing the fishing industry. According to Otoo, the sea at Chorkor was very rough, making it challenging to carry out fishing activities.[63] The fishing community's lives and jobs were at risk due to the unpredictable sea and changing tides near the proposed site. They were correct. A memorandum sent to the secretary of state revealed that "Asere, which [was] inhabited by mainly the fisher folk," was situated "in close proximity to the only beach in Accra where sea-going canoes [could] be beached with any degree of safety."[64] Ata Ampafio, friendly to the colonial state through the district commissioner, disbanded the meeting and announced the chiefs would settle the matter among themselves. Later, the Ga chief instructed the unyielding youth faction of the fisherfolk to "bear everything coolly as it would be to [their] interest and safety" to move from Asere.[65] But fishing around the proposed site was dangerous, according to officials' memo and the experience of the younger generation in the fishing community.

At a well-attended meeting that included community members, the press, and government representatives, a persuasion of the community became a threat. During the meeting, an official representative, suggested that relocating to a proposed site in Chorkor would be in the community's best interest. The new site would provide ample space for fisherfolk to dry and mend their nets and women to build ovens to cure fish without state and council interference. As an incentive, the official promised rent and tax breaks for those who would move. Chairing the meeting, Nanka Bruce, an African physician and journalist, also stated that the congestion in Accra cramped residents and inhibited the smooth operation of the fishing industry. He explained that the "object of the [relocation] scheme was not to take the fishermen away from the rest of the Ga" but "to give them a place to work in."[66] When the attendees at the Ga meeting responded in a discouraging manner, Nanka Bruce's tone turned threatening:

> Times had changed and buildings were being erected in all the open spaces and the fishermen would soon have no space to mend their nets, etc. The town of Accra . . . was being laid out afresh and the fishermen would have to move whether they liked it or not and if they could all be together in one place, it would be all better.[67]

The threat betrayed the classist imagining of Westernized, modern-looking buildings replacing the Ga urbanism in Accra. It solidified the widespread belief that landowners would lose their land under the post-disaster reconstruction plan.

Meanwhile, homeowners impacted by the earthquake asked when the colonial state would release the money promised to repair and rebuild their homes. In their desperate attempt to possess the land, the colonial officials pledged to offer them loans payable on flexible terms, hoping to obtain the goodwill of residents. The money was not forthcoming as land negotiations between officials and the communities dragged on. The delays stirred animated discussion as people waited too long.[68] In the Accra Town Council, the unofficial African councilors reminded their European official counterparts that "when the demolition of buildings commenced after the earthquake, the people believed that government would give loans to enable them to rebuild."[69] The *Independent* collaborated with the claim of the African councilors:

> Soon after the earthquake the Ga Manche accompanied by prominent representatives of the people had an interview with the governor in connection with this very subject of the demolition of houses, and as far as we can recollect. His Excellency made promises to rebuild Accra and help the people repair their houses by means of loans to be repaid on easy terms within thirty or more years. This promise and assurance given by the head of the administration were warmly welcome and became the passionate talk or conversation everywhere.[70]

This editorial in the *Independent* raised expectations of Governor Hodson's so-called promise to the people to rebuild their homes. The promise became the subject of widespread discussion. When they pressed for it through their elected representatives in the council, the European president of the council, appointed by the colonial state, stated blatantly that the governor had reconsidered the decision to advance loans for rebuilding.[71]

While the elected councilors desired improved sanitation and beautification of Accra, they opposed the demolition of homes without providing alternative housing for their constituency members left homeless. Officials had cited that quake-affected homes were too dangerous for habitation and authorized the demolition of over one thousand buildings. They sent demolition gangs to knock down houses "indiscriminately" even before any satisfactory plans to rebuild Accra and rehouse displaced people. Even homes with minor damages were needlessly demolished by the gangs, contrary to official statement that they would only tear down unfit houses. This turn of events happened because of officials' frustration following the lengthy meetings and the unsatisfactory progress in acquiring the land.[72] When the demolition of buildings in Accra peaked in January 1940, the unofficial members of the Accra Town Council demanded an immediate halt to the activity.[73] The editors at the *Independent* published this extraordinarily perceptive viewpoint:

> The feverish activity going on in the demolition of those buildings that have been allowed to stand for so long is quite another matter. Slum areas and unsightly buildings have for a long time marred to a certain extent the prestige of Accra as the metropolis of the Gold Coast. Evidently, government appears to be making good use of the opportunity afforded by the earthquake to make a clean sweep of all the architectural, sanitary and unhygienic eyesores which these slums areas represent.[74]

They evoked the inglorious "slum" that officials used to describe the African neighborhoods. It noted that feverish demolition activity targeted them because of poor sanitation. The demolition activity wanted to eliminate the community and transform the center Accra by rebuilding it in a Western style city, fitting a British colonial capital. Officials weaponized "slums" in an attempt to achieve their aim.

The press, too, requested an immediate halt to the ongoing demolition activity. For example, in the case of the Asere community, the press had previously pressured officials to demolish it. However, the press changed its stance after the earthquake, as officials had failed to provide alternative housing arrangements despite carrying out mass demolitions. This was especially concerning because the city had experienced housing shortages and a surge of migrants due to World War II, both from within and outside the colony:

> No one will quarrel with government for doing now what it should have tackled long ago. Most of the buildings coming under the category described are hardly fit

> for human habitation. In point of sanitation and hygiene they are a clear disgrace to a progressive community. We ourselves have never let the opportunity pass without taking government to task for their delinquency in its continued existence. . . . But the catch in the whole thing is that having delayed taking action for so long, an undue haste is being introduced which must be a source of hardship and suffering to many people. Had government undertaken the work of clearance a few years ago there would not have been the necessity for the feverish building operations going on merely to provide shelters as a preliminary step: Government would have been in the position to tackle the task of clearance and of providing proper accommodation in new layouts with far less haste and greater thoroughness and efficiency.[75]

The press, as the colonial state's modernization ally, switched sides because officials were insensitive to the housing shortage following demolitions. Officials aborted the demolition activity because of public outcry. As homeowners rebuilt, CO reminded Hodson of his intention to "turn the disaster of the earthquake to a good by the rebuilding of the town in a manner worthy of the capital of one of the larger British Colonies," reinforcing colonial objective to not rehouse Africans in upgraded neighborhoods, but to transform Accra into Western style city to facilitate the colonial economic and political ends.[76]

From this post-disaster earthquake experience of attempting to use the catastrophe as an opportunity for "slum clearance" and remaking Accra, the colonial government described the city planning in Accra as a "monumental problem."[77] Land tenure was the primary challenge. Not only did officials underestimate the degree of opposition to mass demolition and rehousing but they also took city planning for granted, relying on a handful of colonial officials and technocrats in the Central Board of Health to make blueprints.[78] After facing opposition in 1939 and 1940, the governor requested a town planning expert from the CO, which assigned Major E. Maxwell Fry as the government's town planning adviser.[79] Fry observed that the worst slums in Accra were at Ussher Town, where Asere was, and James Town—the areas hardest hit by the earthquake. Fry complained about the stench from the fishing industry operated by the fisherfolk of Asere. Five years after the earthquake, officials still continued trying to persuade residents to relocate to Chorkor in Korle Gonno. The frantic demolition did not achieve the envisioned plan.[80] Due to the legal complications and pushback, which Clifford had warned about, and the failure of official planning schemes, the lands commissioner acknowledged the embarrassment to the colonial state. In confessing this humiliation, the commissioner revealed the weakness of a colonial state previously thought to be very powerful.[81] One of Fry's observations about Accra's built environment was the prior sanitation implications for city planning:

> Town planning in Accra rests on a basis of built-up area and open space that has been the work of successive Medical Officers in time past. The partition of the town by building free zones was done for hygienic reasons and on behalf of the European community.[82]

Fry's reading of Accra echoed the impact of Simpson, the TAMS committee, and the sanitation officer's veto after the plague outbreak, no matter how incomplete their plans materialized. He reinforced earlier views of Accra's Western-educated elites of health inequity through medicalized city planning because of the privilege technocrats and officials gave Europeans in planning, designing, and developing Accra.

Cleansing Pangani, Legalized Violence, and African Nairobians

The process of Pangani's destruction was prolonged, revealing how settlers hindered African urbanization, which nevertheless was vital to the city's economy. The outcry against the demolition exercise echoed beyond Kenya's geographical boundaries and significantly restrained the plan to demolish the location without legal compensation.[83] In 1922, two months after the Nairobi district commissioner submitted his report on the destruction of Pangani, an article in the *East African Standard* quoted the *Bombay Chronicle*, an India-based newspaper, that the "white man in Nairobi [had] by legalized violence effectively smothered the right of the native peaceable residence in Nairobi."[84] The settler mantra of poor sanitation and contagious diseases justified the demolition exercise, a familiar tactic against Nairobi's South Asian community. The proposed demolition of Pangani was very similar to their experience less than a decade earlier when W. J. R. Simpson legitimized settler desire to destroy the Nairobi market, which housed poor South Asians and Africans and provided an indispensable source of livelihood. As mentioned in chapter 1, the South Asian community's struggle against the proposed demolition reached India and CO. It was not a coincidence that the *Standard* featured the quote when the council turned on Pangani just after destroying other African locations in and outside the city. In their eagerness to destroy Pangani and consolidate the segregation of

Africans, Nairobi's settler-dominated municipal authority ignored the sanitation implications of mass demolition suggested by the city's engineer. Although Pangani was technically a squatter location, the Nairobi municipal authority could only demolish it slowly, revealing the weakness of the settler colonial state.

During the 1930s, several activities took place to prepare for the demolition. In 1932, the municipal authority approved the destruction of five houses to make way for the building of Fairview Road. In 1935, the Kenya Land Commission, working for the colonial administration on a colony-wide assignment, surveyed Pangani to determine the cost and impact of demolition. They interviewed households individually and recommended the gradual destruction of Pangani over an extended period to allow time for the municipal authority to compensate and rehouse the affected residents.[85] Filled with optimism about the commission's work and its position in favor of the Pangani's destruction, one councilor "assured[d] . . . members that something was really being done and that the matter [demolition] was not being left in abeyance."[86] The same year, the municipal council appointed the Pangani Assessment Board, which chose Juma bin Mbawa as the community representative.[87] The commission and board conducted separate tours of Pangani at different times and interviewed households. Based on their findings, they recommended that the municipal council compensate affected residents, demolish homes slowly on a case-by-case basis, and provide new housing. This approach differed from the council's expectation of a quick demolition.[88]

Unlike the Ga fisherfolk in Accra, who successfully prevented a complete removal from their homes, having been the longstanding landowners, the residents of Pangani could not stop the council's removal. They could only claim tenure security by insisting that Colonel John Ainsworth gave them the land as a "gift."[89] Juma bin Mbawa refused to sign the board's recommendations and chose not to submit a minority report as a form of protest against the demolition. The board struggled to explain the absence of Juma's signature and report. Eventually, it most likely concocted the excuse that it was because of Juma's Islamic faith.[90] Pangani house owners, motivated by their business venture and the community the neighborhood afforded unattached men, "intensely dislike[d]" Pumwani where the municipality intended to relocate them.[91] To Pangani house owners who feared losing their tenants after being relocated, Pumwani was more suitable for family living and not ideal lodging for a community of unattached male migrants.[92] Further, the municipal council had discouraged house owners by declaring it would set down rules to have "reputable" Africans who had established "respectable" lodges to build houses and continue their business in Pumwani, implying that not all Africans who were interested in continuing the industry would be allowed.[93] Despite opposition, the council proceeded with demolition and relocation despite the resilience of the house owners.

Pangani house owners could have prevented their neighborhood's erasure if they had tenure security. Knowing the importance of tenure in protecting their homes and investments, Pumwani residents mobilized and petitioned the council to reconsider their status as tenants-at-will and grant them tenure security. As tenants-at-will, Africans were liable to be evicted and their property confiscated and sold by the council upon violation of municipal laws.[94] The council could evict African house owners for minor offenses or the crimes of their tenants, and their property was frequently confiscated or destroyed without any compensation or legal consequences.[95] The council could also expel Africans to prevent them from staying long enough to make claims of legal rights to land. This policy strengthened settler control and reinforced the belief that Nairobi was a "white" city. The sanitation implication of tenants-at-will was extensive. It discouraged African entrepreneurs from investing in lodges to accommodate the growing African workforce needing housing. Without tenure security and accommodation, the Africans made makeshift shelters and stayed in overcrowded conditions in and around Nairobi's boundaries. Because of the insecurity without tenure, Pumwani African residents petitioned the council in 1935 and explained:

> In the case of this area, there is at present no security of tenure, and we feel, as a matter of our own practical experience, that there can be no real incentive to effort or to economic well-being or to thrift in towns unless we can feel—each of us who wishes and endeavours to be thrifty and to own our own house in our Town—that we are secure in our title to the house (and land) which we own.[96]

Eight enterprising Africans signed the petition, wanting to reside in Nairobi permanently and expand their real estate portfolio. However, the lack of security was discouraging. When the deputy mayor, the district commissioner, and council members considered the petition at the Native Affairs Committee meeting, they stated that "the present facilities available for the erection of houses and residence in Pumwani [were] all that [could] be considered" and that the council would not "alter existing conditions under which stand permits [were] granted."[97] They denied resourceful Africans the opportunity to prosper in business, rejected the petition, and effectively upheld the conditions that gave rise to slum conditions in

Pumwani. Africans investing substantially in developing the land the council could seize without compensation or legal implications was not wise.

The municipal council believed that the demolition of Pangani would be a simple task. However, disagreements arose between the state and the council regarding compensation for homeowners. The Kenya Land Commission, appointed by the colonial state, argued that residents were entitled to compensation because the state and the council allowed Pangani to develop and expand as an African residential area. The commission believed that the colonial state had a paternalistic duty to "direct and control" Africans who were under European "tutelage." Since the colonial regime failed in its paternal responsibility to Africans, they owed them some form of payment. Therefore, the commission recommended an average of £15 for each house owner. This amount was a revision of £5 that the Nairobi district commissioner proposed thirteen years earlier.[98] Conversely, the council claimed that Africans who built houses without proper permission had no rights. It authorized the demolition without compensation.[99] When the council consented to provide compensation, it appointed the Pangani Assessment Board, which was sympathetic to settler interests. Not surprisingly, the board proposed £11.12 as compensation.[100] The commission's proposed compensation of less than £15 was not enough to cover the cost of rebuilding in Pumwani, where the council was seeking to consolidate the residential segregation of Africans. One Pangani house owner, who had lived there for twenty-five years, paid a monthly £5 fee to the council in addition to the hut tax. According to this house owner, the cost of building a house in compliance with the municipal regulation was £60.[101] The compensation payments offered to homeowners for constructing a house were insufficient. As a result, the government and land commission suggested offering loans to make up the difference in the price of the building. However, the council opposed the proposal of providing loans to Africans.[102] If the state gave African homeowners the financial ability to rebuild their homes and lodges, the council would have difficulty maintaining control through real estate enterprise and preserving Nairobi as a settler city.

Africans affected by the council-driven demolition filed lawsuits for damages. The council had rushed to tear down Pangani houses to make way for South Asian developers while its representatives and the Attorney General's Office were still drafting clauses to legalize evictions and demolition and punish violations of urban building regulations.[103] The attorney general declared the demolition action carried out by the municipality illegal and ordered the council to compensate the affected residents, opening the floodgates for further lawsuits from affected Pangani residents. In 1939, some residents sued seven years after the council demolished their homes.[104] The council's legal troubles with Africans increased afterward. New legal cases one after another surfaced as residents who suffered similar fates felt emboldened and stepped forward for compensation. The claimants believed they also deserved payment since they lost identical houses at the exact location because of the council's demolition exercise.[105] In light of these complications and ongoing legal action against the council, the compensation amount was increased to £50 following a new valuation.[106] Although the council succeeded in demolishing Pangani, the legal actions, together with compensation payments to Africans and the pace of destruction, were demoralizing to the settler-dominated local authority, which liked to think of Nairobi as its city.

Mayor C. Udall acknowledged the council's inability to maintain Nairobi as a European city, as envisioned by settlers. In response to two successive articles in the *Standard* in July 1943, which condemned the "slum" conditions, Udall noted that the "number of Africans and Asians who desire[d] to reside in Nairobi [was] much too great for the supply of their accommodation to be undertaken by the Municipal Council."[107] Interpreted differently, it was a mistake to demolish Pangani simply because the council could not accept the reality of being overshadowed by its African business competitors. While the statement revealed the council's incapability to provide housing for migrant laborers, it suggested that the idea of regulating the African presence in a confined, segregated neighborhood and maintaining Nairobi as a "white city" was a difficult task to accomplish. At the same time, Mayor Udall shifted part of the blame for the "slums" to the colonial state:

> In saying this it must be pointed out that there is no restriction to the immigration of artisan labor from outside the colony and no restriction of movement of natives from their own reserves into this town and having in view the present excessive overcrowding it cannot be justly contended that it is the duty of the Municipal Council to provide housing for all and sundry.[108]

Mayor Udall expected the state to impose more rigid control on the movement of Africans into Nairobi, which it could not do. The state's inability to prevent unrestricted African population growth demonstrates settler colonial weakness in fully controlling African mobility into and within Nairobi.

During World War II, the number of migrants coming to Pumwani, the authorized African location in the capital, significantly increased. This led to a further housing shortage, resulting in exacerbated congestion and unsanitary living conditions. Overcrowding worsened the already inadequate accommodation and sanitary facilities. When all the rooms were occupied, migrants and residents attached makeshift structures to existing housing and built them in the open spaces of Pumwani and on the outskirts of Nairobi, where infrastructure and services were absent.[109] The reduction of houses due to the destruction of Pangani caused severe shortages and overcrowding in Pumwani. In 1941, a census conducted in Pumwani revealed that the houses designed to accommodate 171 Africans "illicitly" sheltered 481 people. Severe housing shortage and increased urban population growth made Pumwani, the authorized destination for African migrant workers, worsen sanitation.[110] The destruction of Pangani happened barely three years ago, and now the council was considering demolishing Pumwani as well. G. C. W. Ogilvie, the officer responsible for designing and building African houses for the council, believed that the growth of commercial and industrial activities had caused large groups of African migrants, which led to social, hygienic, and economic problems. He believed housing was the root of sanitation challenges.[111] Overcrowding stretched the underserviced Pumwani and its inadequate sanitary infrastructure. Rather than alleviating poor sanitation, the council's decision to demolish Pangani shifted and exacerbated it. Seeing this problem, officials discouraged the council from demolishing Pumwani. The lesson was that demolishing houses in Pumwani, although the neighborhood had metamorphosed into a "slum," was unwise without alternative housing. The settler state needed to implement a long-term housing initiative to prevent the resurgence of slum-like conditions before mass demolition.[112]

Conclusion: Demolition, Spread of Slum Conditions, and African Resilience

Official reason for "slum clearance" was urban renewal and development aimed at eliminating blight, cleaning up cities, and preventing contagious diseases. Rather than less dramatic measures like warnings, summons, fines, surveillance, and inspections, mass demolition would showcase colonial power and promote healthy urban growth and order. The demolition of slums could prove that Accra and Nairobi were seats of British colonial and settler power. However, while "slum clearance" was not always successful or complete, it worsened congestion and squalor. Having been the product of the decongestion of James Town in the aftermath of the plague outbreak, Korle Gonno manifesting poor sanitation conditions in the interwar period was evidence that demolition and relocation to a new area without infrastructure, services, and regulation served to spread slum-like conditions. That relocation did not eliminate the slum conditions in James Town and its environs. When the Nairobi municipal authority demolished Pangani, most of the African population moved to Pumwani, where severe housing shortages and limited sanitation services and infrastructure worsened slum-like conditions. Overcrowded houses, makeshift accommodations in open spaces, and overstretched sanitation facilities became the physical manifestation of Pumwani. African locations on the outskirts of Nairobi, also characterized by makeshift structures, lacked sanitary services.

This chapter reinforces Jennifer Hart's point about how the state and municipal authorities "effectively informalized" African urban culture using sanitation regulation and order. It adds that colonial neglect of constructed sanitation infrastructures and the built environment contributed equally to the "(in)formalizing" process and the making of the African parts of the saniscape. The set of material and immaterial essentials that made sanitation efficacious in the city was not always available in new African residential locations that officials and technocrats laid out for the victims of demolished neighborhoods, recreating the very slum-like attributes often condemned. Delays in implementing the essential sanitation infrastructures, services, and regulations to keep the new neighborhoods salubrious raise questions about whether "technocratic colonialism" was serious about alleviating poor sanitation in African communities. Hart's idea of informalizing African urbanism provides the framework for analyzing demolition as a mechanism by which colonial officials, technocratic experts, and Western-educated Africans advanced the interests of the colonial economy and visions of a modern city, thereby promoting urban inequality.[113] Thus the processes of informalizing African urban cultures embraced the sanitation manifestations and implications of the built environment.

Accra's seaside African communities occupied prime lands near harbor facilities in the network of British-controlled port cities. Home notes that these port cities together were crucial in consolidating the trade network in the British empire.[114] In the official view, the Ga communities obstructed the expansion of port infrastructure, including transportation, warehouses, and other commercial infrastructures strengthen this network of ports. The view aligned with technocratic and official interests in open spaces for health, aesthetic, and security reasons. However, officials trying to demolish and relocate the communities became a drawn-out process. Demolishing was symptomatic of colonial attempts to consolidate power over the

Ga, who had long held the coastline as their political and sacral urban center.[115] To see the perspectives of Africans who received Western education about sanitation and demolition, Timothy Burke provides valuable questions and answers in a different colonial setting. The acquisition of a deep desire for something previously unavailable in Burk's book could be restated as the aspirations of educated Africans for a Westernized Accra that it lacked.[116] Colonial sanitation discourse, disparaging African settlement patterns, and everyday lives also shaped the opinion of this class of Africans. Due to their exposure to Western cities traveling in Britain, education, and Christianity, they believed in colonial visions to transform Accra from Ga urbanism to Western cities. They could not, however, bear widespread homelessness resulting from uncontrolled colonial demolition. The elites spoke out against the colonial officials and the European-dominated Accra Town Council. They urged them to stop the indiscriminate destruction of African homes, ultimately contributing to the incomplete flattening of the neighborhoods.

Settlers holding up sanitation reforms in the black soil areas of Nairobi has been a prominent trend in the city's history since its foundation. Because of the unhealthy environment in the areas, officials and medical experts even debated moving the city. Godwin Murunga discusses these delays and persuasively demonstrates that the settler regime deflected their inability to make the environment salubrious and neglect of it, blaming the African and South Asian residents as being inherently unhygienic.[117] Pangani's history and demolition also went through similar processes. The demolition activity stalled because the council and officials avoided compensating house owners and providing alternative housing for the many African-wage workers in the community. Left to the settler-dominated Nairobi municipal council alone, Pangani residents would receive little to no compensation after swiftly demolishing the neighborhood. The residents displayed resilience by staking their claim to the land and improving the hygiene of their houses, some resorting to legal action after the council demolished their homes. Complete removal of the neighborhood took a long time, and the compensation increased significantly, against the interests of the council that imagined Nairobi as its own.

Addressing housing and sanitation challenges also hinged on controlling the influx of African migrants into the city. Timothy Parsons's examination of Nairobi's African locations shows the ineffectiveness of settler attempts to control Africans' mobility and maintain a tight spatial compartmentalization.[118] Parsons's argument fits into the broader historiography of colonial rule that there was no absolute control system even in Africa's most stringent settler state.[119] Gwendolyn Wright succinctly notes that no matter how marginal people and their places of abode were, they resisted or ignored the most absolute form of control. This resistance resulted in the "incompleteness" of colonial urban visions.[120]

In Accra and Nairobi, African urban residents recognized and expressed the implications of mass demolition and relocation to their lives and livelihoods. As the young members of the fishing community observed, fishing on the seas around Korle Gonno was perilous because of the strong ocean currents. Official correspondence affirmed the viewpoint of the fisher group. Not only were the lives of the fisherfolk at stake, but continuing the fishing tradition bequeathed to them by their forefathers could take a severe hit. Their ability to speak to colonial power thwarted colonial urban vision. Ultimately, they asserted ownership of land adjoining the sea, and officials could not force them to move across the lagoon. The residents of Pangani were not so fortunate because the municipality did not accept their claims to the land and eventually demolished their homes. In the official view, the residents could not prove land tenure. It was not a coincidence that Pumwani residents, observing the demolishing in Pangani, appealed their status as tenants-at-will. Lacking the security of land tenure, Pumwani residents investing in quality property for personal use and migrant workers to lodge was not a wise decision. The municipal council could evict Africans at will and seize or demolish their property for any infringements. The Pumwani petitioners requested the council change regulations and secure their house and land ownership. This appeal was not just about securing their status in Nairobi but also addressing the root causes of the poor environmental conditions in Pumwani. Without secure property rights, there was no motivation for Africans to invest in improving sanitation in Pumwani.

After demolishing, colonial and settler rule providing adequate housing was the next hurdle. The next chapter continues the demolishing story by exploring housing to alleviate the shortages during and after World War II. Like officials, African communities in the cities identified housing shortages as a serious sanitation problem. These shortages, exacerbated by demolitions, worsened the backlog of decades-long need for African housing. This situation placed housing within a more significant shift in imperial policy in the late 1930s, which the Labour governments implemented by 1945. Labour government reluctantly acknowledged the need for healthy spaces for a permanent African urban population. This change was part of the second colonial occupation, the beginning of the development era, the prominence of post-war experts, and the rise of the Western welfare state. The next chapter analyzes the extent to which these shifts originated from colonial subjects and Africans. Providing housing during this period and the events surrounding the gesture reflected the mistaken belief of the Labour Colonial Office that reform and increased prosperity, brought about by state-driven centralized planning, could save the British Empire and diminish popular support for African nationalists, like Kwame Nkrumah and Jomo Kenyatta. However, this centralized development planning failed to generate enough revenue to build the planned and regulated African neighborhoods. Furthermore, the ability of Africans to travel and settle where they wanted brought explosive African population growth in the cities and prevented the neighborhoods from materializing as envisioned by colonial rule.

CHAPTER 4

Housing, 1940–1952

HOUSING TO IMPROVE SLUM CONDITIONS, ADDRESS ACCOMMODATION SHORTAGES, and ultimately achieve some parity in the saniscape bound up sanitation to development. While embarking on housing projects, officials and planning experts integrated the neighborhood unit. This urban unit, first developed in New York a decade earlier and later adopted in Europe, aimed to provide amenities such as schools, libraries, recreational facilities, and healthcare centers to improve the quality of urban life for Africans and enable them to enhance their living standards.[1] For colonial planners, housing and neighborhood units became a means of addressing various pressures from rapid urban demographic growth, modeling and stabilizing what was considered appropriate urban behavior, and providing controlled social and political avenues for Africans.[2] African housing in communities equipped with social amenities sanctioned class-based residential segregation and tried to repudiate racialized housing, shifting from the "sanitation syndrome" of the early twentieth century to the "development syndrome."[3] Nazi Germany had exposed the evil implications of racism, and racial discrimination was becoming a political liability in the empire, especially when the loyalty of colonial subjects was crucial to winning the war and preserving the empire.[4] Class became more prominent in urban politics as Western-educated and wealthy Africans became increasingly crucial to colonial rule. Examining housing and its components, including toilets and baths, demonstrates that better sanitation was both an imagined and physical marker of class. Private and communal toilets and baths inscribed class in the saniscape.

Housing in Accra and Nairobi is part and parcel of the broader politics of development in the British Empire. Despite colonial planning, as elsewhere, changes only occurred with widespread pressure from African urban residents. Political pressure exerted by urban residents and labor pushed imperial planners and colonial officials to begin paying attention to the housing needs of subject populations neglected for decades. Within the British Empire, Trinidadians expressed their pent-up grievances through festivals, street carnivals, singing, riots, and calypso, compelling a chain of official reactions to address underinvestment and inadequate housing needs in the 1930s.[5] Because of the common challenges cities across the empire faced, the Colonial Office (CO) transferred the Trinidadian model of addressing housing problems to other cities. This initiative, partly funded by British taxpayers' money through the Colonial Development and Welfare Act of 1940, led to the establishment of mass housing and new towns. The empire-wide current in housing influenced developments in Accra and Nairobi, where most African urban residents lived in congested and overcrowded neighborhoods with inadequate and absent sanitation infrastructure and services. In Nairobi, for example, Africans disliked the barrack-like housing that had caused unrest in Trinidad. For that reason, the CO recommended that the settler state replace them with family housing within three years.[6] Inadequate housing critically fueled urban discontent, leading the CO to declare the importance of mass housing.[7] But the housing initiatives were insufficient and came too late. Growing urban discontent during wartime and the postwar era continued to feed mass anti-colonial sentiments and set the stage for movements and party politics, blowing the winds of change in government and replacing British colonial officials with African nationalist leaders in the 1950s and 1960s.[8]

Mass Housing, Opportunities, and Development in the British Empire

As a social intervention, mass housing was not just about providing a roof over the head. The Fabian Colonial Bureau and Arthur Creech Jones, member of Parliament and later secretary of state for the Colonies, promoted housing as a strategic opportunity to use local building materials. As seen in previous chapters, by conflating local building materials and slum-like conditions in African communities, technocrats and officials encouraged using imported materials to benefit British industries, urban growth, and employment opportunities for the metropole while discouraging African building materials. This housing project would shift colonial policy from a reliance on imported iron, cement, timber, and other building materials from Britain to African building resources, with significant implications for the local economy, the development of local industries, and the preservation of imperialism and colonial rule.[9] Creech Jones asserted, "It was certainly a great mistake that more use was not made of local raw materials for building before the war," creating the disadvantageous situation where "local building materials were not developed."[10] The challenges with production and shipping during World War II brought about a crushing reckoning. Additionally, imperial and colonial agents believed that utilizing local materials would build local industries, create jobs for urban residents, and earn the loyalty of colonial subjects. Mass housing could improve poor sanitation conditions in the interwar years by reducing urban poverty and living standards.[11]

Mass housing initiatives in the Gold Coast and Kenya cast a fresh imperial and colonial gaze on local building resources, including timber, stones, and clay, as potential raw materials for projected wood, tile, and brick industries. While a novel development agenda, the project could not magically correct the massive dire housing shortages and decades of colonial underinvestment. Having discredited the foreign occupation that colonial rule was, housing shortages opened an opportunity for anti-colonial nationalists to criticize the colonial state and make claims of being better suited to provide redress for colonial underdevelopment. This colonial moment had far-reaching consequences for the development conundrum beyond formal decolonization.[12] Officials and experts from the United Nations and the colonial metropole encouraged residents to build houses. Support schemes, including loans, land grants, and relaxed municipal building codes in specific neighborhoods, were among the many initiatives intended to encourage residents to build houses and relieve officials of public housing schemes.[13]

Logically, the housing schemes in Accra and Nairobi took different trajectories due to the various settlement histories. The colonial state aimed to rehouse earthquake victims, reduce housing shortages by selling houses, and provide for-rent compound houses at Sabon Zongo for its laborers. On the opposite side of the continent, the settler state aimed to improve the living conditions and infrastructure of African residents in Nairobi through housing and amenities in local communities. While providing housing to alleviate shortages and "slums," the officials and the municipality hoped to "stabilize" Africans in Nairobi as permanent families. Stabilization, especially in Nairobi, was a clear policy shift from trusteeship to development, representing a social vision for an African middle class characterized by homeownership and family values.[14]

Politics of Housing in Accra and Nairobi

In 1948, an African boycott of cotton textiles, canned meat, flour, spirits, and other European, Syrian, and Lebanese merchandise in Accra was followed by a demonstration of veterans who had returned from World War II to find living conditions difficult. When the veterans mobilized to present their grievances to colonial officials on February 28, 1948, and many Accra residents joined them, the police shot at the crowd, killing two and wounding many. By then, looting and burning of European, Syrian, and Lebanese stores were underway. Shooting at the crowd of petitioners worsened the chaos and compelled the colonial administration to declare an emergency. By the time officials restored order, many residents had lost their lives, and others sustained injuries. Over £2,000,000 worth of property was damaged.[15] The Watson Commission, which investigated the 1948 disturbances in Accra, underscored the connection between housing shortages and the uprising. It noted racial discrimination in housing against African government employees. Echoing the Colonial Office in the Trinidadian case, the commission urged officials to make an "effort on African working class houses," cautioning that "nothing contribute[d] more to social unrest than the shortage of houses for the people."[16] The commission confirmed previous African concerns of racism that European civil servants' housing took precedence over their African counterparts.[17] Six years ago, Creech Jones predicted that veterans would likely be unhappy due to insufficient and unavailable housing:

> The question of the demobilization of men from colonial territories now serving in the forces, attention was drawn to the need to take into account the higher standard of living to which many of them will have become accustomed during

> their service. This change of outlook may be expected to lead many of them to look for housing of a better type than that with which they were previously content.[18]

In addition to African civil servants facing racialized housing discrimination, veterans required adequate housing equal to the standards they became accustomed to during their service in the war. Housing shortages were undoubtedly a serious urban concern with prominent class and race implications.

Similar urban unrest marked housing shortages in Nairobi. In 1950, a general strike by Kenyan labor leaders disrupted public services and businesses in Nairobi. After the strike, two thousand Kikuyu lost their jobs. They became part of the increasing number of unemployed and landless Kikuyu who had migrated to Nairobi's crowded and underserved African neighborhoods in Pumwani, its Eastlands environs, and the city's outskirts. The neighborhoods were the destinations of white Highland squatters, whom settlers evicted to obtain more land to meet wartime expanded demand for agricultural production. These African migrants moved into Nairobi, already plagued by severe housing shortages, low wages, and worsening living standards. The neighborhoods would be the fertile grounds for mobilizing anti-colonial and anti-settler sentiments as many residents identified with the Kikuyu organizers of the Land Freedom movement, Mau Mau. Two years after the strike, the Kenyan government declared the Mau Mau an emergency, mainly a Kikuyu rebellion against the colonial settler order. Before the emergency ended, there were numerous deaths of Africans and Europeans. The state detained many suspected Mau Mau subversives, including Jomo Kenyatta, without trial. Colonial heavy-handed rule and the official response to urban revolt provided common ground for Western-educated African elites and their numerous urban allies to unite against a repressive alien system.[19]

Kenya's colonial state and the municipal council knew about the link between housing shortages and uprisings in urban areas. They had expressed fears of the likely spread of rioting from Mombasa caused by the "lack of proper housing."[20] As the Mau Mau emergency approached, the *Standard* published an article that included a quote from Alderman G. A. Tyson, chairman of Nairobi's Town Planning Committee, noting that there was "ample evidence to prove that crime incidence increases with a poor type of housing [and that] the worse the type of housing, the worse crime incidence."[21] Tyson continued that Nairobi was "steadily but surely driving into a position where [it would] have to face a social menace of unimaginable proportions."[22] Unsurprisingly, the state declared the Mau Mau emergency in October 1952, the month Tyson's quote appeared in the paper. The Kenya African Union (KAU), which championed Kenya's independence under Jomo Kenyatta's leadership, explained the causes of Mau Mau in a memorandum to Oliver Lyttleton, member of Parliament and secretary of state for the Colonies. Mau Mau was the product of a housing shortage and an increase in rents by the municipal council, contrary to relief measures proposed by the colonial state to improve the inadequacies.[23] The union further noted:

> The attitude of the Municipality to shantytowns is another source of grave dissatisfaction to Africans. In the absence of any housing accommodation many Africans have been forced, at their own expense and labor, to erect huts which would at least offer them shelter from cold and rain. One fine morning, several months after the houses have been built, a batch of Askaris arrive and commence demolition of the huts. No compensation is paid to the owners, nor are they offered alternative accommodation.[24]

The statement reinforces the argument that mass demolition was not just sanitation-driven but a mechanism to enforce white settler dominance and racialized housing segregation. It also explains why housing shortages worsened the situation for African Nairobians and contributed to the growth of Mau Mau supporters.

Post-Earthquake Reconstruction in Accra

Rehousing Scheme

Colonial officials launched the Accra Rehousing Scheme after the June 1939 earthquake to construct homes for displaced residents. A committee and subcommittees comprising colonial officials and African lawyers oversaw the state-funded rehousing scheme. They established the first large-scale housing estates in Accra, initially consisting of 1,251 two-room houses in Northwest Korle Gonno, Korle Gonno, Chorkor, Abosse Okai, Kaneshi, and Christiansborg.[25] The two-room houses provided free temporary accommodation for disaster victims for a year. The following year the committee would begin the second phase, converting the two-room houses into permanent Grade I, II, III, and IV houses. A Grade I houses was the most advanced and expensive, whereas Grade IV was economical and the least sophisticated. The committees allowed adequate land near each house and estate to accommodate later construction works. Before the second phase began,

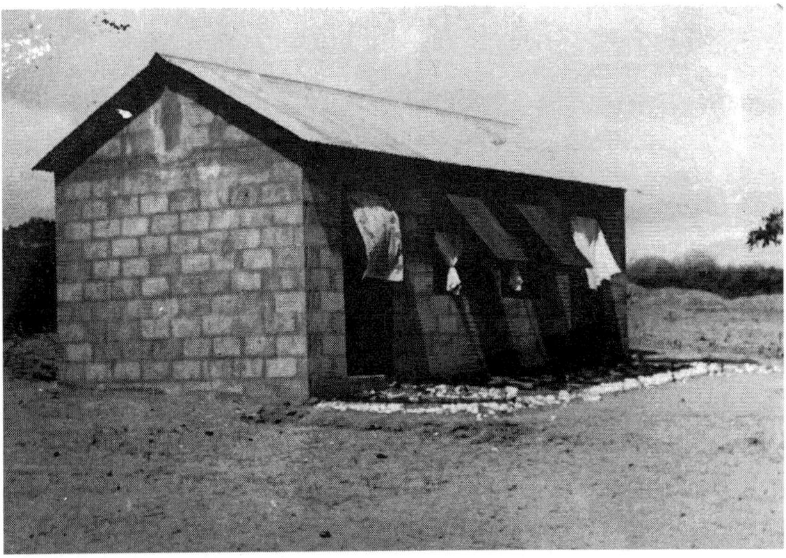

FIGURE 7. *Top*: Two-Room Temporary Housing for Earthquake Relief. SOURCE: PRO/CO/1069/46, EARTHQUAKE REHOUSING SCHEME, 1939.

FIGURE 8. *Bottom*: Model layout fishermen's compound housing as built in West Korle Gonno. SOURCE: PRO/CO/1069/46, EARTHQUAKE REHOUSING SCHEME, 1939.

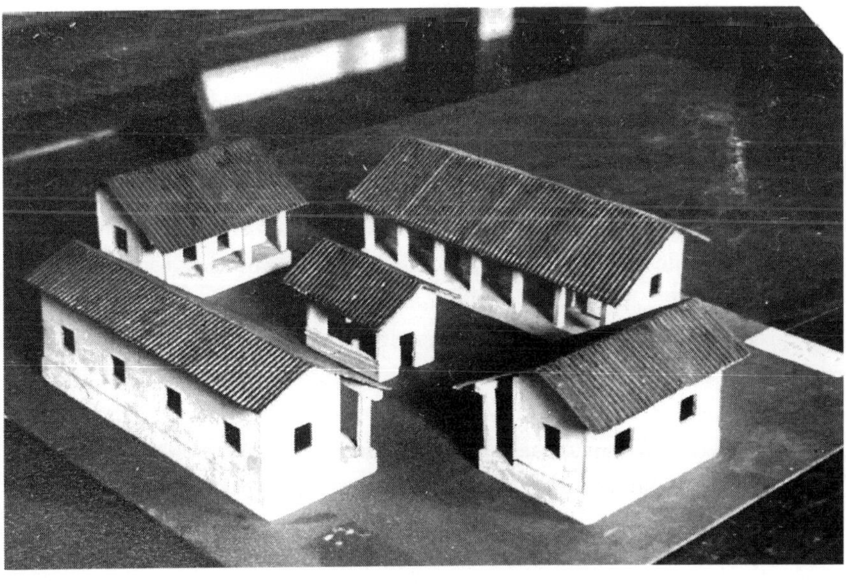

an occupant declared an intention to buy the home and indicated the grade to which the house was to be converted.[26] The permanent houses would distinguish the socioeconomic status of the buyers. The committees further designed separate and exclusive compound houses for the low-income and poor Ga and migrant communities in Korle Gonno and Sabon Zongo.[27] With a clear intent to maintain a separation of Accra's wealthy and less wealthy, the committee expressed "the desirability of planning approach roads to better-class areas so that they did not traverse the poorer districts."[28] This deliberate planning strategy underscores the intentional nature of segregation by class.

Land acquisition from the Ga by the colonial state was one of many challenges the committee and subcommittee encountered, ultimately leaving the rehousing scheme incomplete. The Ga owned land communally. They entrusted it to the custodianship of family and lineage heads and chiefs. During colonial rule, the meanings of this traditional land tenure transformed, complicating the process of land alienation for urban development.[29] Following the rehousing plan, the efforts of the committee and subcommittees to negotiate the alienation of substantial portions of land in Accra and its surroundings failed. Some African landowners even refused to engage with them.[30] The report of the Rehousing Committee on the land acquisition problems noted:

> But a multiplicity of claims by stools, families, and individuals presented many difficulties for the adoption of the same procedures by which Government obtained possession of lands in the other Estates. No other step had been taken to acquire this area, and it may be unnecessary in the future for the sub-committee to reopen the matter.[31]

They reported their inability to secure plots of land along the Accra-Nsawam and the Accra-Dodowa roads due to multiple claims of individuals, families, and lineages. As a result, they deemed it impossible to continue negotiations, reducing the extent of the scheme. Colonial incapacity to implement its envisioned development fits into a broader pattern of urban projects, highlighting the limitations of colonial power and the ambiguity of modernization.[32]

When the custodians formally transferred land for the rehousing scheme, it was under stringent conditions that fulfilled the original purpose of providing relief for the Ga who lost their houses because of the earthquake. In the Deed of Conveyance, which outlined the terms of land transfer, the committees could grant freehold rights to a respective community member interested in buying a house. However, buyers who were considered strangers, non-subjects of the Ga State, were allowed leasehold titles for only sixty years, after which the committee was to reconvey freehold rights back to landowners. There were other requirements to meet before strangers could become homeowners, including paying the custodians a mandatory £5.10 ground-rent fee.[33] Apparently, the terms were not the first but a watered-down version of an earlier deed that specified that houses were to be sold to members of the Ga community. A stranger required approval from the custodians to make a purchase, and a stranger would pay a customary fee of £5.10. Additional dictates of the earlier comparatively hardline version included a return of undeveloped land to appropriate custodians and the offer of unsold houses to the respective landowning stools, individuals, and families.[34] Although the custodians grudgingly hammered out agreeable terms with the committees, individual Ga would show their discontent over the alienation of land and the sale of houses.[35]

Besides land problems, some of the people to whom the committee aimed to sell the houses also posed another challenge to the scheme. Grade I houses, for example, targeted a class of Syrians and African businesspeople, lawyers, and physicians, but only a handful of them were interested. Instead, they preferred to build their own homes to suit their taste outside the planned area farther north of Accra.[36] However, the major blow came from the Ga community, which originally resided in the African seaside communities, where the earthquake hit the hardest. The high cost of the houses discouraged them from purchasing homes. The fisherfolk, for instance, made their money mainly from fishing; how much they made depended on the seasonal catch that the "head fisherman" (or fisherwoman), who likely owned the boat and fishing net, distributed among the boat crew after taking a portion. The fish reached the market for sale through a middle person, often the wife of the head fisherman, who also had a share in the profit.[37] The committee revised the policy for the fisherfolk, deciding to sell the compound houses or rent a unit for three shillings and six pence per month. In 1942, when rent was due, two-thirds of the fisherfolk left their rooms and returned to their original neighborhoods, confusing the entire Accra renewal plan. They

> crowded into large rooms, live[d] on open ground-level verandahs, occup[ied] shacks of few sheets of corrugated iron or rent[ed] small rooms—almost cupboards—in old swish buildings. In fact, they live[d] in the greatest state of poverty and squalor.[38]

The refusal to stay in the Korle Gonno disrupted the colonial state's fiscal and physical plan, which sought to reinvest the rent proceeds and rearrange Accra's built environment based on residents' socioeconomic status and the infrastructural needs of the port city. It reinscribed Ga urbanism into the saniscape east of Korle Gonno, where colonial officials had long aimed to develop into what they imagined as fitting for the modern British capital of the Gold Coast.

Yet there was another way the departure of most Ga people from Korle Gonno forced the scaling back of the rehousing plan. The previous chapter showed that the young fisherfolk generation was a vanguard against land alienation for colonial development in the post-disaster reconstruction plan. The colonial state hoped to use the rehousing scheme to mediate intergenerational tensions over land alienation. By making them rent payers to the head fisherman and older members of the communities to whom the committee and subcommittees would sell the fisherfolk's compounds, officials attempted to reign them in through the older generation. Under the scheme, Ga buyers of the fisherfolk compounds would allocate rooms in each compound house to the young fisherfolk in their boat crew.[39] The planned housing and tenancy arrangement for older and younger fisherfolk could immobilize the younger generation from any reaction to land further alienation since their elders and the colonial state own the very roof under which they lived. However, the deep generational gap, especially over illicit land sales, was hard to resolve. The committee and the state's attempt to use the compound houses and tenancy arrangements to control the young fisherfolk backfired as most Ga departed and restored the close-knit settlement pattern along the coast east of the lagoon, a pattern the colonial state had long sought to eliminate.[40]

Unexpectedly executed, the move by the fisherfolk was more significant than a mere setback to the rehousing scheme. Colonial power hinged on controlling the capital city, which was the pivot of power and commerce. Houses covered a large portion of the cityscape. Their inability to make the fisherfolk stay in Korle Gonno shows the incompleteness of colonial power and urban projects.[41] The one-third who remained in the compound houses were mostly Ga women. These women, some head fisherfolk, had direct and sustained access to the colonial cash economy from retailing. The women cultivated the practice of saving money from their trade and invested in boats and nets, which they rented to the fishing crew. Through their active participation in the rehousing scheme, the women provided the committee and officials with a direct channel to reap from colonial investment and plow the money back into the rehousing scheme.[42] This mechanism, facilitated by the women, was instrumental in maintaining and reproducing the scheme, no matter how limited, showing the women's intricate role in sustaining the post-earthquake rehousing scheme.

Neighborhood Unit in Accra

The original blueprint for the Accra Rehousing Scheme positioned the estates and houses along class lines. Housing for the poor residents was to the west of the seaside African communities of James Town and Ussher Town. The fisher community and migrant laborers' estates were at the littoral of Korle Gonno to the west and Sabon Zongo to the northwest. As mentioned, the rehousing committees considered it essential to reinforce the separation of the fishing community and laborers from the rest of Accra's estates by designing and constructing roads to "better-class areas" so that they did "not traverse the poorer districts."[43] Besides using roads as barriers, the committee promoted using plants and trees to fence off communities. To that end, it appointed one of its members to oversee a Department of Aboriculture and Horticulture that would handle planting grass verges and trees along the roads to bolster the division.[44] Again, problems with land tenure, building materials, labor, budgeting, and specialists impeded the realization of the overall road construction plan.

As the colonial state struggled with the rising cost of building materials and labor, completing the homes and infrastructure dragged out, allowing homeowners, the rehousing committee, and officials of the social work department to take the initiative and make additional adjustments over time. Until the end of colonialism, the scheme managers worked with occupants to convert temporary buildings into permanent houses. The neighborhood pressure group, the Christiansborg Estate Council, continually petitioned the governor to convert their temporary accommodations. They stated that only 58 of 369 houses in the estate were completed by 1945. While they waited for the committee, occupants, demonstrating their resourcefulness and adaptability, adjusted their homes to provide sanitary accommodations and protect them from cold and warm temperatures, rains, and burglaries.[45]

The pressing need for technical expertise, driven by the severe housing shortages, "slum clearance," and the complex task of city planning, led to the appointment of Emmanuel Maxwell Fry for the four West African British territorial possessions in 1943. At his appointment, Fry served with the Army Royal Engineers in West Africa. The colonial state sourced his payment from the crucial Colonial Development and Welfare Fund. Before commencing his duties, Fry embarked on a study trip to the United States to further his knowledge of city planning.[46] An "architect with a global reputation," Fry was an attaché and adviser to Noel F. Hall, the resident minister of West Africa, whose office was in Accra.[47] Like earlier commentators of the contrast in Accra's built environment, Fry noted the city's uneven saniscape, which constituted open spaces dividing African neighborhoods with poor sanitation and well-laid-out and serviced European segregated areas.[48]

With the help of T. S. Clark, an African urban planning expert from the Gold Coast, Fry merged the neighborhood unit urban planning concept with the post-disaster rehousing in Accra and completed and submitted what became the first "overall plan for Accra" in 1947.[49] The work of these experts reveals the transfer of Western ideas of the neighborhood unit overseas. The crux of the plan was that "the needs of the family expressed first in the dwelling itself" before being extended "in terms of paths and roads, markets, shops, recreation."[50] The neighborhood unit's core idea was prioritizing housing needs, which included sanitary infrastructure, before extending to the thoroughfare, markets, shops, and recreational facilities. Integrating housing and amenities was crucial to fulfilling social and development needs. The activities and functions of cities, "however large and complicated," were "directly related to the needs and capacities of family units."[51] The experts spatialized development through physical planning, envisioning affluent and less affluent residential areas as self-contained neighborhoods. They envisioned the colonial government using urban planning to promote social progress and welfare for Accra's residents by providing amenities and infrastructure near homes within the next ten to fifteen years.[52]

Social work officials came to play a significant role in this imagined development of urban Africans. They collaborated with engineers and planning experts to construct economic neighborhood units with social services.[53] Fry's neighborhood unit plan redesigned the seaside Ga communities to make space for community centers and open areas, but that required land in the closely-knit communities. Implemented according to plan, some residents would need to lose their land or home to make way for amenities. That meant displacement. It would have added land contestation to ongoing ones linked to the colonial state's post-earthquake reconstruction plan.[54] Although the neighborhood unit witnessed many challenges, some of which included land and wartime-related shortages, including building materials and labor, they brought together urban residents who did not previously know each other into communities. For their social development, the residents mobilized into pressure groups to take advantage of the "development syndrome."[55] In 1945, the Christiansborg Estate Council, representing over two hundred residents of the new Christiansborg neighborhood, demanded concrete drains, streets, and a host of other services and infrastructure so that they could "settle peacefully and adjust themselves" for "social development."[56] A newly constituted Department of Social Welfare and Housing took direct responsibility for the rehousing scheme and government housing policy in 1946.[57]

Amenities for social development also depended on the availability of unbuilt plots. The social work department considered Christiansborg Estate for a new community center because it was an up-and-coming affluent neighborhood where the state controlled land tenure. A discussion of establishing the center in the Accra Town Council reveals a reason for lagging development in the seaside African communities. To an African councilor, James Town and Ussher Town, where many Africans resided, would benefit more from the center since it provided a meeting place to exchange thoughts and ideas and improve social standards. He reminded the council that "once the Christiansborg center was built, it would be some years before consideration would be given to the needs of the greater population at James Town or Ussher Town."[58] However, to the colonial state, Christiansborg was ideal for the community center because of the availability of suitable land and the crucial role of neighborhood unit model in social development. In general, the council president expressed official frustration with the difficulty with land for building in infrastructure where Africans controlled land tenure that "there was not an inch of land on the Gold Coast which did not belong to somebody" even if it was a refuse dump or a dustbin site.[59] Thus, amenities embedded in the neighborhood unit for social development benefited the wealthy neighborhood.

Individual financial predicaments and unforeseen circumstances within and outside the colony shaped the rehousing scheme and accompanying infrastructure and amenities, (re)configuring the original housing scheme. Despite this incompleteness, the rehousing scheme produced elements of the neighborhood unit. Many residents were upset about the rising cost of houses, which led to higher monthly payments. In 1948, the price of two-room houses increased from £120 to £250, Grade III houses went from £190 to £396, and Grade II houses went up from £386 to £500. The committee redesigned Grade I houses for superior five-room accommodations, but the selling price remained at £570. Partly due to price inflation, some residents defaulted, others vacated, and the committee transferred their mortgages to people on the waitlist. Completed homes depended heavily on the budget allocated to residents able to pay their mortgages. Occupants with the means further made gardens and built and maintained live fences of Madras thorns around their houses. The amenities of each estate, such as market sheds, shops, estate offices, playgrounds, and social centers, were factored into the cost of houses, reflecting the affluence of each estate. The colonial state funded post offices and police stations and designated undeveloped land for various purposes, such as schools and churches. It sold 450 vacant plots for £60 to the public to build their homes.[60]

Housing as a social development program was the most challenging legacy the colonial state would bequeath to the African nationalists in the buildup to formal decolonization in the 1950s. T. M. Kodwo-Mercer, commissioner for the Gold Coast, opened an address to a joint meeting of the Royal African Society and Royal Empire Society that planning and housing, among other things, were embodied in the Gold Coast Development Program, which aimed at fulfilling "the age-long will of the people; the will to raise their standard of living."[61] Kodwo-Mercer might have aggrandized the people's will, stretching it as far back as the Fante Confederation of the nineteenth century. Still, he aptly illustrated how Kwame Nkrumah's politics struck a chord with the masses who looked to the developmental state to remedy the decades of neglect, swept his party to victory in 1951, and paved the way to the formal end of colonial rule. Kodwo-Mercer described housing as a "hydra-headed problem," which the Nkrumah government attempted to grapple with.[62] It enmeshed the nationalists in the so-called developmentalist state even before they acquired full power.[63]

Infrastructures and Class

Sanitation amenities were also critical markers of socioeconomic status. Accra's geographical expansion with the rehousing scheme presented challenges in providing adequate sanitation infrastructure and services. It had a senior building inspector and a European inspector to assist him in covering the newly expanded city of forty square miles. The city's engineer had two assistants who needed engineering training.[64] The thinly stretched experts and assistants could not keep up with the sanitation needed by ensuring that communal and private toilets throughout the city were in good physical order and conformed to municipal building regulations. Residents had constructed about two thousand private corrugated-iron toilets to avoid the public ones. The town engineer, health officers, and their respective assistants marked some for demolition. The idea of demolishing the toilets became an intense issue in the Accra Town Council. One of the African councilors' toilet was also marked, and under pressure from their various constituencies, the other African councilors joined him in requesting the council president stop the town engineer from the planned mass demolition. They argued that because of wartime shortages in imported building materials from Britain, residents could not build their private toilets per the municipal regulations.[65]

Also, the public toilets were too few to accommodate the population densities in the overcrowded African neighborhoods. The evidence of inadequacy was the long lines of people waiting for their turn to enter the toilets in the mornings. Again, land acquisition for public toilets partly explains the few public toilets. The process through which the state acquired land and leased it to the council to build the toilet was complicated, as seen in the rehousing scheme. Despite the shortages, the president approved the demolition request for 250 corrugated-iron private toilets.[66] A month later, the council debated open defecation on the beach, in drains, and at street corners because of the severe shortage of toilets and the inconvenience of municipal-provided public toilets, compelling a renewed discourse on sewers in Accra and a requirement for toilets and septic tanks in building blueprints.[67] The unauthorized public toilets throughout Accra, including in James Town and Ussher Town, which the colonial state targeted for renewal, reinforce the incomplete execution of the rehousing scheme.

Where baths and toilets were positioned and the number of people sharing them geographically mapped class on the cityscape. The shared sanitation facilities were the most distinctive features of the compound houses for the Ga fishing and migrant communities. The facilities were part of each rectangular compound house located at accessible places for all residents. Households in compound houses of twenty-four and twelve rooms shared a set of these facilities.[68] Ione Acquah, the spouse of an African civil servant in the Gold Coast, conducted a social survey of Accra from 1953 to 1956, which showed that communal toilets and bathhouses were often in disrepair and inadequate. The persistent problems compelled most residents to use public toilets and bathhouses.[69] The public toilets served two-room residents as well. These were individual houses, each consisting of a verandah, kitchen, bathroom, and store. Acquah's survey revealed that 68 percent and 41 percent of households did not have access to private toilets and baths and had to rely on public facilities. Due to the limited number of toilets compared to bathrooms, public restrooms were under significant strain and often exceeded their capacity. In Sabon Zongo, for instance, the toilets frequently became dirty and occasionally emitted offensive odors.[70] By creating nuisance and health threats for most urban residents, the communal facilities undermined the social advancement promoted by the neighborhood unit.

On the other hand, the expensive houses in Accra contained private toilets and baths. The compartments of Grade III houses were similar to the two-room buildings except for adding a medium-size sitting room and an indoor toilet and bath. The committee upgraded some of the houses to Grade II, with two large bedrooms, a second verandah, and a toilet and bath. In place of grade I, they redesigned some houses to superior ones with five bedrooms and sanitation facilities. Except for the few wealthy households fitting their property with running water for flushing their toilets and for other domestic use, most occupants of Grades II, III, and superior houses equipped their residences with pan toilets. Others carried buckets of water from outside pipes to flush and bathe.[71]

African Housing in Nairobi

A Race to House the Growing African Nairobian Population

In the 1940s, the high wartime prices of agricultural produce led to an unprecedented economic boom in Kenya's economy. This boom accelerated investment in Nairobi's development, which also received funding from colonial grants, loans, and London's money market. Investing in developing Nairobi's physical infrastructure began to position the city as a regional commercial center, inspiring settler optimism in playing a dominant role in East Africa. During this time, there were some improvements in African housing.[72] However, it was becoming clear that officials and the municipality alone could not handle the decades-old backlog of the housing deficit. As housing demand ballooned, officials and settlers prodded private employers to help alleviate the housing shortages by fulfilling their obligation of providing accommodation for their respective employees.[73] The 1940s witnessed the completion of African housing, some of which were in Makongeni (Kaloleni), Starehe, Ziwani, and Bondeni. For example, in 1945, the state began an ambitious African housing project in Makongeni (Kaloleni) and Starehe that it completed in 1947.[74] However, the housing backlog in Nairobi was staggering, underscoring the severity of the acute shortages. In their decision-making, officials failed to recognize that 15,000 out of 40,000 Africans desperately needed accommodation. This was particularly challenging as African Nairobians chose to avoid the census, which officials used as a tool for punitive measures. African wariness led to conservative estimates of their housing needs.[75] The municipality's temporary housing in Marurani, projected to be demolished in five years and replaced with permanent housing, aimed to alleviate the shortages. However, resorting to that desperate solution was a stark testament to waste and gross underestimation of the shortages.[76] Even with this temporary measure, there was still a significant need to accommodate the growing African "desire to reside in Nairobi."[77]

Unlike the Accra rehousing scheme, which emerged directly from the earthquake, African housing in Nairobi has been a subject of intense debate since the city's founding. Stopgap projects cropped up, but the state, municipality, and private employers avoided bearing the high cost of a mass housing project. African housing in Nairobi was different also because it integrated the neighborhood concept of planning earlier in the process. In the minds of the committees, architects, and officials in charge, their "experience and knowledge of the African's requirements" informed the design and construction of the units.[78] The units were self-contained, each comprising communal buildings, shops, schools, health centers, and other facilities that the state and the municipality thought would boost the self-image of Africans who had long endured health risks and repelling sites of poor sanitation conditions.[79] The buildings were single houses arranged in blocks of two to four, intended to accommodate three to seven people. According to the initial plan, a neighborhood would accommodate 65 to 120 Africans, depending on the plot size. The Ziwani project yielded twenty-two houses per acre, and monthly rents varied from ten to thirty-five shillings. There were three basic types of houses: room, living, and bedroom; living and two-bedroom houses of semi-detached buildings; and blocks of four units.[80] The Ziwani project included experimental houses for "wealthier Africans," but officials later abandoned it because of the high rent of thirty-five shillings and Africans' lack of interest in them.[81] Rapid population growth and overcrowding would soon worsen the neighborhoods' deterioration.

It was not the African residents whose presence set the initial downturn of the neighborhoods but the official decision to build at a poorly drained site. The names Makongeni and Ziwani depict the site's bad environmental quality. As seen at the beginning of Nairobi's founding, the unsuitability of the environment was what precipitated the debate to relocate the entire city. The soil was moist black cotton. Ziwani, for example, means "by the marsh," indicating the waterlogged black cotton soil. Makongeni was at the old sisal plantation near Nairobi African Stadium.[82] Making the site buildable involved an extra layer of work draining the soil of moisture. After removing moist topsoil, the building foundations had to be laid on a level floor of concrete, cement, sand, and ballast. Without this initial construction work, water would stagnate and eventually collapse the buildings.[83] However, that incurred added costs and consumed much-needed money to be channeled into further housing to alleviate the desperate shortages. The estimated total cost of the Ziwani project was £30,000, but the actual expense ballooned to £100,000 at completion.[84] The Makongeni project involved 612 houses and cost £150,000. It was the most expensive African housing project. The decision to build at the site, despite the prohibitive cost and waste, was significantly influenced by racial residential segregation. Officials and the settler-dominated municipality strategically chose the site to align with the earlier vision of a segregationist blueprint for the so-called healthy development of the city.[85]

The high cost of developing the site for residential purposes scared off private employers of African labor obligated by the Master and Servant Ordinance to build houses there for their employees. Driven to make profits, the firms, owned by Europeans and South Asians, found the prerequisite of draining the site a waste of money. Thus, the need to house their employees exacerbated the housing shortages. Racial residential segregation "compelled [them] to build upon land which can be used for other purpose than the residence of Africans, a restrictive factor should [they] at any time be compelled to realize [the] investment."[86] Additionally, the nature of the location made it difficult to sell the property because few investors were willing to develop property there.[87] For these reasons, many South Asian and European private employers left their African employees to meet their accommodation needs in unplanned peri-urban and already congested African locations. By not contributing their housing quota to alleviate the shortages, the employers contributed to the poor sanitation conditions in which Africans lived. In April 1948, just after completing Ziwani and Makongeni, a survey revealed the neighborhood units were overcrowded.[88]

In the postwar period, African housing in Nairobi continued to receive funding from Colonial Development money. Half of the projects between 1945 and 1952 depended on funds that officials and the municipality continued to mismanage in their relentless vision for a divided Nairobi based on racial residential areas.[89] Still, the rate of housing was "not fast enough to permit the abolition of grossly unsatisfactory housing conditions . . . nor [did] it allow the improvement of housing owned by government, council, and private employers."[90] In 1952, the Nairobi City African Affairs officer estimated that ten thousand of the eighty thousand Africans in Nairobi did not have houses and had to share accommodation with others.[91] This estimate was two years after the new Bahati and Gorofani African housing projects completed and absorbed more Africans.[92] Benefiting from hindsight, Ernest Vasey observed that the site had:

> Not been suitable for building and close development, a fact which has added to the cost of African housing and services. Areas set aside for African housing are likely to be more intensely developed than other residential areas and it is important, therefore, that wherever possible a good type of land should be chosen, suitable for easy drainage, etc., and not necessitating expensive foundations for houses to be built.[93]

Vasey had gained a reputation for advocating for Africans. He was a businessman, president of the Nairobi Rotary Club between 1949 and 1950, twice Nairobi's mayor, and two years later, the financial minister. He noted how the decision to build on those sites made sanitation worse. His advocacy for better African houses helped to change official and municipal policy on African housing in the 1950s and 1960s.[94]

Besides Vasey, Western-educated and skilled Africans also found the poor environmental conditions in the new neighborhoods unacceptable. Their needs, too, were critical in shaping later African housing policy. Most of the houses in Makongeni and Ziwani were for different groups of employees.[95] Some were two-room residences for married and "more senior class" Africans and single-room buildings for bachelors and lower-paid workers with families.[96] This class of Africans, including barristers, laboratory technologists, and biochemists, earned enough income to rent and purchase houses in exclusive European and South Asian residential areas. To officials sympathetic to their plight, Western education had "taught them . . . [to] despise" the poor sanitation in the neighborhoods and to distance themselves from other Africans.[97] Later, in the Ministry of Works, European officials attempted to secure housing for their African coworkers. However, discriminatory housing practices by South Asian and European landlords seeking to preserve racial residential segregation stonewalled the efforts.[98] Meanwhile, African demand for better housing compelled a shift in official thinking about constructing upscale African estates. A conference on African housing in Nairobi in 1955 emphasized the need for separate housing for the "more self-respecting members of the community" to physically and socially distance them from the African urban masses.[99] From the 1950s, the colonial state, the municipality, and private employers pooled resources and built self-contained flats for high-income residents at subsidized rates.[100]

Neighborhood Unit in Nairobi

How the colonial state and the settler community envisioned Nairobi in terms of its dominant regional role manifested in the city's 1948 master plan. L. W. Thornton

White, P. R. Anderson, and L. Silberman from South Africa made the master plan reinforcing the neighborhood unit for African housing. In July 1945, the experts made three working visits to Nairobi and submitted a twenty-five-year development strategy the following year. This strategy revised Walton Jameson's city plans two decades ago. Like the Jameson Nairobi plan, the master plan followed urban models in settler South Africa. It aimed for the social integration of multiethnic African urban residents through a spatial "design that incorporate[d] effectively the principles of social organization in a neighborhood unit."[101] Silberman's contribution as a sociologist in the Department of Social Studies at the University of Witwatersrand was significant due to the imperial and colonial shift in policy toward social progress and welfare.[102] White, the chair of the Department of Architecture at the University of Cape Town, collaborated with Anderson, a civil engineer based in Johannesburg, on the physical design and planning.[103] The experts adhered "to the principles of planning that take their measure on the human and technical needs . . . such as privacy, open space, education, protection from through-traffic supplies, etc."[104] The leaders of government and municipal departments and private enterprises in Nairobi's European and South Asian communities met with the three experts and expressed their interest in developing a master plan reinforcing separation.[105] It was just a matter of incorporating even sanitation and social amenities in all newly planned residential areas.

When White, Anderson, and Silberman visited Nairobi in the 1940s to develop the master plan, the city was racially divided. Class-based residential segregation was also evident. To the east of the railway yards along Doonholm Road was Eastlands, with a high African population density. It was an overcrowded and congested close-quarters development on black cotton soil likely to flood during heavy rains. The ground held large pools of stagnant water suitable for mosquito breeding. Additional environmental dangers to the residences were the railway tracks dividing the location and the planned industrial zone to the south. In contrast, to the north and west of the central business district, European housing was situated on large plots surrounded by gardens on higher ground with red, quickly drained soil that was less likely to flood. Wealthy South Asians moved to the relatively more spacious residential area of Parklands to the north, while poor classes were overcrowded across the Nairobi River and commercial areas.[106] This uneven saniscape had not transformed significantly when King George's order declared Nairobi a city and the colonial state declared the Mau Mau emergency in the 1950s.[107]

Infrastructures and Class

Some Africans lived in relatively more comfortable and spacious conditions in Nairobi's neighborhood units, like Makongeni and Ziwani. They were self-contained communities with shops, post offices, police stations, superintendent's offices, welfare clinics, social centers, schools, open spaces, and gardening plots. The residents included long-term laborers and Western-educated and well-paid African employees with families.[108] In general, the housing designed for various groups of employees included two-room residences for married and "more senior class" Africans and single-room buildings for lower-paid workers with families and bachelors. By providing amenities and family accommodations, the colonial state and municipality aimed to encourage an improved standard of living and the permanent residency of Africans in Nairobi. To allocate housing, officials and the municipality prioritized the timeline of applications, family status, duration of residency in Nairobi, and formal income. Some African Nairobians had multiple streams of income.[109] The chairman of the Housing Board noted the rarity of better housing:

> Even the Africans working for the Railway administration which generally speaking have always been well to the fore with improved housing and labor conditions, cannot expect to obtain family housing before their ninth year of service. With other employers, the position must be much worse.[110]

For African employees to obtain family housing and bring their spouses and children to Nairobi, they had to work for roughly a decade and earn sufficient income. Beginners with less money could only afford bed spaces in single rooms (dormitories). The fact that the design of houses allowed for the accommodation of single employees, however, did not prevent laborers from bringing their families. Continued overcrowding in the bachelor houses and the constant demand for additional accommodation for unattached laborers compelled officials to convert the few family accommodations into single and bed-space residences.[111]

In the 1940s and 1950s, communal toilets and bathrooms were the sanitary facilities used by laborers and other impoverished residents of Nairobi. These facilities were in separate blocks in accessible areas within Makongeni, Ziwani, Starehe, Ghorofani, and Bahati.[112] As in Accra, the sanitation amenities in Nairobi were unpopular among residents. They were often in unkempt conditions. Additionally, the toilets and bathrooms were in open locations and often in disrepair, exposing users to the public gaze. African residents, public health and social workers, and some government officials called for their replacement with individual and private family facilities. At the conference of African housing in Nairobi in 1955, participants did not just reveal that more "self-respecting members of the community [were] penalized by the misuse of the latrines by the ignorant." They also noted the "embarrassment [they] caused by unwise placing of latrines."[113] The communal toilets were a blight on the neighborhood units, providing a reason for Western-educated, high-income African residents to press for improved housing, with private toilets and baths befitting their status.[114]

Eventually, the municipal council built flats with flush toilets and showers for Western-educated and well-paid Africans. The earlier flats came to Ziwani. They comprised a living room, two bedrooms, a kitchen, and front and back verandahs. They rented each unit at thirty-five shillings. The low purchasing power of most African residents led to a decline in municipal interest in further pursuing the project.[115] Most Africans could not afford the high rent, although they showed interest in them. However, housing committees, commissions, officials, and individual Nairobi residents encouraged the municipality to return to the scheme. As a result, the municipality, government, and private employers pooled their resources and built self-contained flats for high-income residents at subsidized rates. By 1958, flats with advanced amenities were ready for African civil servants at Doonholm II and Mayfair housing estates. Each flat contained a bathroom and flush toilet. The rent for the Mayfair Estate (Old Racecourse) flats costs seventy shillings per month to senior African civil servants. They comprised a living room, kitchen, food store, three bedrooms, bathroom, separate water closet, and a back verandah fitted with laundry facilities. Each house at Doonholm II Estate (Doonholm Road), consisting of a living room, two bedrooms, kitchen, combined shower and water closet, and a balcony, was rented to government servants at fifty shillings per month. Other self-contained houses with private bathrooms and toilets followed these estates.[116]

Conclusion: Inadequate Housing, Urban Discontent and Development

Frederick Cooper's description of colonial rule in the 1930s and 1940s is apt. Imperial and colonial agents "choked on the narrowness of the pathways" they created for urban and urbanizing Africans.[117] The colonial state and experts favored Europeans

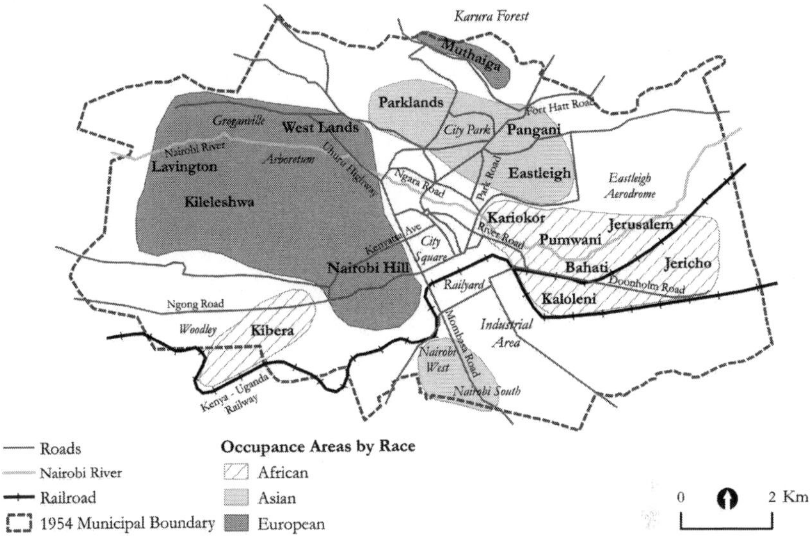

FIGURE 9. Nairobi Map after the 1950s. It shows the racialized residential areas of Africans and South Asians. The map also shows the locations of some of the new African estates.
SOURCE: MCVICAR, "TWILIGHT OF AN EAST AFRICAN SLUM," 61.

in housing and health in Accra despite objections from Western-educated elite Africans. With more Africans seeking urban opportunities and population explosions, imperial and colonial agents could no longer ignore housing shortages and the narrow pathways for them in the cities. Inadequate African housing and its contribution to urban discontent in Accra demonstrates that the city's residents added to the mounting pressure on imperial and colonial rule to address shortages and slum-like conditions. The extant historiography has marked this moment as a turning point in the Gold Coast's drive to political independence.[118] The Nairobi strike and Mau Mau in the 1950s also have roots in housing shortages. More than a decade ago, the gathering of the Nairobi Rotary Club and Associated Chamber of Commerce, high-profile colonial officials, including the governor, and the press (see chapter 2) noted the potential for urban discontent and mass uprising because of housing shortages. A group of entrepreneurial Africans in Pumwani petitioned the municipal council during the interwar period, claiming that tenants-at-will excluded Africans from the urban economy and partly caused housing shortages and "slums." On the eve of Mau Mau, a similar observation from European settlers and the KAU reinforced the importance of housing to urban stability. Like the Gold Coast, the historiography of Kenya has marked the postwar moment in Nairobi as a critical juncture on the road to independence.[119]

Urban housing as a pathway to socioeconomic reforms was essential to the empire at its weakest moment to win the loyalty of the subject populations and keep foreign occupation viable. If only colonial rule had promoted local building materials instead of favoring imported ones from industrial Britain, it would have created employment opportunities for urban Africans to afford decent housing and amenities, ultimately leading to improved living standards. Robert Home, however, shows that this colonial development mindset emerged only as a matter of practicality.[120] It provided an opportunity that African nationalists could and did latch onto to rally urban masses seeking housing and development, a need that colonial rule did not address. Kwame Nkrumah and Jomo Kenyatta were exposed to this developmental way of thinking in Britain. Emmanuel Akyeampong argues that these nationalists adapted this thinking as a pathway to improving the socioeconomic conditions of Africans.[121] This developmentalism had far-reaching consequences beyond colonial rule.[122]

Among numerous experts, urban planners and social workers played a vital role in the development agenda, following the example set by medical and sanitation experts like Simpson that technocrats could utilize their expertise to address social issues. However noble the concept of arranging the urban built environment into neighborhood units seemed, it could only tackle some of the aspirations of African urban residents. The Christiansborg Estate Council in Accra was able to mobilize and make claims for the colonial state to complete their houses and provide facilities for their social development. It made it to the priority list of the Department of Social Welfare for a new community center. Western-educated Nairobi Africans, who could afford housing in the better-serviced European and South Asian residential areas, disliked inadequate sanitation in the African locations. They requested the settler state, municipal council, and private employers to provide flats in upscale neighborhoods. The aspiration of this class of Africans gradually transformed Accra's and Nairobi's saniscape as colonial officials separated their housing from the mass of African residents while, at the same time, continuing to shield Europeans from unwanted proximity to their African neighbors. Colonial rule recognized the importance of educated and well-to-do Africans to the workings of the colonial state and increasingly focalized their interests. The uneven saniscape along class lines crystalized during this period.

The land tenure problem was the most difficult, challenging the transformation of the cityscape by class. For various reasons, the Ga, who owned most of Accra's land, limited the project because of their well-founded suspicion of the colonial motives. From experience, colonial rule made little accommodation in its development plans for Africans. Most of the Ga who had taken temporary shelter in the two-room relief housing returned to their earthquake-devastated neighborhood as a preferred place to continue their livelihoods. On the other hand, the colonial state and settlers controlled land in Nairobi, but "stabilizing" Africans through housing and development was far from complete because of a host of reasons, such as settler determination to consolidate racialized residential segregation and a mismanagement of African housing funds. Anderson has demonstrated how corruption in the Nairobi City Council has detrimentally impacted African housing.[123]

Seen from the perspective of sanitation, the neighborhood unit housing schemes envisioned by the experts to provide for the needs of families were incomplete. Sanitation infrastructure was the most visible deficiency in the housing project. Wartime material shortages, rising labor costs, and population growth left the housing scheme wanting. The residents of Accra could not have to wait for a "reasonable" time to construct their basic needs for convenience, as demonstrated by the widespread number of toilets in the city. Bill Marshall's *Bukom* fictionalizes the meanings of self-help with constructing private toilets for self-improvement and development in the African seaside communities.[124] As a way of seeking self-advancement, improvement, and moving forward, development gained expression among African urban residents in many ways similar to Marshall's portrayal in the novel. African self-help in making their places of convenience in a period of adversity and dislike for colonial communal toilets was more comprehensive than European and expert fixation on the aesthetic appearance of the city.[125] Communal sanitation infrastructures continued to be the primary features of the neighborhood units in Nairobi's African locations, which most Western-educated Africans saw as unfitting for their status. Since they could afford European and South Asian standard housing, they sought out accommodation there, unsuccessfully, and compelled upscale neighborhoods with private family toilets and baths. Interest in Western hygienic standards on the cityscape correlated with social class, similar to Ruth Rogaski's observations.[126] Despite the failure of housing projects to achieve their intended outcomes, they did contribute to establishing sanitation infrastructure within the built environment based on social class.

The next chapter focuses on waste in the cities' final decade of colonial rule. It continues the thread of sanitation infrastructure, explaining how it enabled the removal and stagnation of garbage and sewage in different residential communities.

CHAPTER 5

Waste, 1952–1963

WASTE WAS AN UNWANTED MATTER THAT ENDED UP IN THOROUGHFARES, DUSTBINS, sewers, drains, and other open areas in the city. It included household garbage, sewage, ashes, and scraps. While control of urban waste depended on various technologies, waste outflow from different neighborhoods was manual and relied on laborers. The challenges of this manual system coalesced into accumulated, stagnant, and scattered waste, with the African residential locations bearing the brunt. This system brought sanitation to the brink during urban emergencies, such as riots and strikes. However, such a crisis also enabled and reinforced urban waste politics. The infrastructures required to cleanse the cities of accumulated and stagnated waste became aspirations of urban residents, local government, and the state in a moment of development within the colonies and empire in the 1950s. Although this chapter starts in this decade, the experiences of urban waste problems predate the period. Therefore, it stretches back to the previous decade to foreground a continued persistence of unequal waste clearing in the various residential areas of Accra and Nairobi. It first discusses refuse and sewage in Accra in two sections before similarly turning to those same themes in Nairobi. While some infrastructural improvements occurred and improved the saniscapes of both cities, they had less impact on the densely populated African communities that had been the target of colonial slum discourse, demolition, and housing. The saniscapes continued to manifest unevenness in distributing infrastructure to cleanse waste.

Tensions over Uncleared Refuse and Shift in the Politics of "Slum Clearance" in Accra

How the colonial system prevented littering and enforced modern waste-disposal practices through prosecutions had unintended consequences. The *Daily Graphic* depicted sanitation inspectors as "terrorists" and "unnecessary bullies" and fueled widespread negative perceptions of the colonial order. Because of the fines and prosecutions for various sanitation offenses, this repressive image stirred up fear and rebellion.[1] The *Daily Graphic* described the commonplace spectacle of "housewives after seeing them [sanitary inspectors] run helter-skelter in fear and lock themselves up or quit the residence, leaving behind the squalor for inspection."[2] For individuals prosecuted and charged with sanitation offenses, it felt like they carried the entire "burden" of a repressive colonial sanitation system, creating a negative image not only of sanitation inspectors and their municipal employers but also of the colonial order as a whole.[3] A heavy penalty of four shillings strained the relationship between extended family members if one of them, who was in good financial standing, failed to contribute to the payment of the fine.[4] This public image of colonial rule did not bode well for cultivating loyal subjects, giving nationalists additional rallying issues against the colonial state. To achieve an Accra clean from littering and scattering, the Ministry of Health under the Nkrumah-led government, which was preparing to take over government from British officials in the 1950s, petitioned sanitary inspectors to establish rapport with residents by educating them, rather than issuing summons, prosecutions, and fines.[5]

Nkrumah arrived on the Gold Coast scene in 1947, when the cost of living in Accra had multiplied more than twofold since the prewar period. In these harsh socioeconomic realities, the newly formed United Gold Coast Convention (UGCC) invited Nkrumah from Britain to serve as its general secretary. Inflation in prices of imported and locally produced goods continued and caused widespread discontent, which peaked in a month-long African boycott of European, Syrian, and Lebanese firms in January and February 1948. It was at the boycott's end that veterans marched to present the petition to the governor, and as seen in chapter 4, the police shot into the crowd, and chaos followed in the city. Within this context, Nkrumah attracted the support of a diverse group of people with his movement for "Self Government Now." Nkrumah's message would lead to his break from the UGCC and the formation of the Convention People's Party (CPP) under his leadership in 1949. The powerful collective effort of his supporters, including veterans, women, farmers, youth, and other groups, united behind his national movement. Their votes in the popular elections in 1951, 1954, and 1956 paved the way for the Gold Coast's formal independence in 1957 and its eventual transformation into the Republic of Ghana in 1960.[6] Toward formal independence, the Minister of Health, Imoro Egala, sought to transform the repressive image of inspectors by encouraging them to endeavor "to be powerful health educators as well as good inspectors" in 1954.[7] Egala's statement captured a broader agenda of rebranding how local sanitation authorities enforced sanitation. Three months after Egala's statement, officials introduced "the first practical measure towards introducing a health week, to be held yearly" and redeploying the colonial idea of "slum clearance" not as demolishing and remaking James Town, Ussher Town, and Christiansborg, but as clearing refuse and promoting hygiene.[8]

In the 1950s, not much had changed in clearing refuse in these African communities compared to well-off European residential areas in the previous decade. In the European areas, sufficient municipal services prevented waste buildup and stagnation, overcrowded and less prosperous neighborhoods, primarily inhabited by African residents, often faced prolonged periods of uncleared waste. A string of correspondence between Christiansborg (Osu) residents and the Accra Town Council indicates this uneven saniscape. Led by J. Quist-Therson, who was an African barrister-at-law and one of the core founders of the UGCC, Christiansborg residents drew the Council's attention to the "situation in which some parts of this city [were] kept in a tolerable condition while other parts [were] allowed to go completely to the dogs."[9] In this instance, Quist-Therson referred to the practice of leaving "plenty of rubbish" uncleared in Christiansborg. This incident of uncleared waste in the community was a regular subject of discussion in the Accra Town Council meetings. In one such meeting in 1946, Councilor Dinah N. Quist highlighted sanitary segregation, like what Quist-Therson raised about four years earlier, when she brought up the idea of clearing waste regularly along similar lines in European residential areas and some parts of Adabraka, built in the aftermath of the plague outbreak described in chapter 1, where wealthy Africans, Syrians, and

Lebanese resided.[10] The issue of uncleared and accumulated waste remained a persistent challenge in most African neighborhoods, constantly reminding them of the state's neglect of their communities.

Uncleared waste, such as household garbage, left in and around bins for more than a week in Accra's African communities, prompted an urgent meeting of members of the Accra Town Council on October 23, 1945. The waste overflowed dustbins, spilling onto thoroughfares, unleashing unbearable smells and attracting an army of flies known to spread pathogenic microbes like vibrio cholera, in human populations. When unregulated and delayed, the uncleared waste attracted stray dogs and scavengers, contributing to the scattering. The potential health crisis was a significant concern. In the heated discussions that ensued during the meeting, it became apparent to the council members and officials in the Health Department and the Public Health and Town Planning committees that some residents routinely left their garbage outside on the ground in specific neighborhoods even when the bins were not completely full, making clearing tedious.[11] Other reasons for the uncleared waste surfaced, including broken garbage trucks, inadequate garbage trucks, and a shortage of laborers. With this in mind, the medical officer of health and others in the meeting requested the council to increase the sanitation budget. In pressing his case, the officer argued that more money was crucial to employ more laborers, purchase and maintain necessary garbage trucks, and improve sanitation technologies, including dustbins. However, some council members expressed opposition, advocating for stricter supervision and control of the laborers. For those supporting this view, the "increase in expenditure year in and year out" did not effectively address the dire refuse stagnation, leaving sanitation as the "worse and the most criticized" service of the Accra Town Council among Accra's African residents.[12] Although the sanitation budget increased annually in the preceding twelve years, the council continued to experience challenges meeting the waste burden of a demographically and spatially expanded Accra.[13]

Advocating close supervision of laborers as a viable solution to the trash problem was persuasive to the African councilors. The laborers, some of whom were Kroo migrants from Liberia, swept public places and emptied the contents of bins. They cleared and transported truckloads of refuse to the city incinerator near Korle Lagoon, worked the municipality's sanitation trucks operated the incinerator, and filled swamps with ashes from the incinerator.[14] Their daily interactions with residents gave them a unique position to impact public attitudes toward waste disposal and management. Daily interaction with laborers predisposed residents to listen to and follow the directives of laborers rather than sanitary inspectors, who, the council and educated Africans ironically wanted to provide education on hygiene. In fact, throughout the British Empire, lower-ranking employees of the colonial government and municipalities, like the laborers, influenced daily sanitation practices and public health policy.[15] In an inquiry into the uncleared waste crisis, residents told Councilor Vernon L. Buckle that laborers instructed the public not to put refuse into the dustbins but to place it around the bins.[16] The laborers' directive to scatter waste was not a straightforward "weapon of the weak" strategy elsewhere.[17] The laborers had difficulty loading "refuse from inside the dustbins," especially in the rainy seasons when water soaked the bin contents, making them heavy to load.[18] Scattered and stagnant waste did not result solely from poorly motivated laborers but also from the failure of sanitation technologies. The ecology of refuse collection could have compelled more innovative water-resistant technologies to prevent rain from soaking the waste. Also, the soaked refuse could not burn in the municipal incinerator, hence the need to spread and dry it on the ground.[19] The lack of appropriate technology and adequate labor supervision, coupled with the "unpleasant nature" of waste work, relatively low wages compared to Accra's high cost of living, and poor housing of laborers contributed to the trash problem in the capital city, which, in theory, was supposed to uphold strict sanitation standards.[20]

However, the most fraught aspect of Accra's refuse challenges was not the uncleared refuse scattered in and around the bins. It was the trash on domestic and private premises. The municipal council required residents to remove household garbage and put it in bins at various neighborhood locations. Sanitation inspectors, who had gained notoriety for indiscriminately issuing summons, causing arrests, and bringing litigations and fines for minor infringements, were responsible for enforcing the council's requirement. As a resident noted, because of the fear the inspectors instigated and their unpopular methods, they spoiled the "good cause" of hygiene they were supposed to teach and instill in residents.[21] As a result, the inspectors likely contributed to the scattered waste. While some residents adopted a "rebellious attitude towards" sanitation and littered drains, thoroughfares, and other public places managed by the Sanitary Department attached to the Accra Town Council, others avoided encounters with the inspectors. In avoiding the inspectors, residents missed receiving proper hygiene guidance to counterbalance the laborers asking them to put trash around the bin rather than inside.[22] In such circumstances, sanitary inspectors forfeited the opportunity to establish rapport and obtain valuable feedback for improving Accra's sanitation. Ashes, scraps, and domestic refuse from homes, scattered in public spaces around dustbins and on thoroughfares, could not be solely because of subversion but proof that the means through which colonial rule sought to instill a sanitary order among urban residents were unpopular and counterproductive. Shifted from domestic and private premises to public places, misplaced and accumulated waste was as much the fault of the council and colonial officials, who often and spontaneously blamed the unsanitary nature of Accra on the attitude of Africans. Colonial disciplinary measures, like summons and fines, meant to alter African waste disposal and management practices and to cleanse Accra exacerbated the unsanitary conditions.

Piled-up and misplaced waste widened the cracks within the Accra Town Council. The African councilors blamed the city's trash problems on incompetence within the Health Department. For an extended period, the councilors and officials of the Health Department were at each other's throats. At the same time, medical officers persistently called out the Public Works Department and the colonial bureaucratic hierarchy for poor sanitary infrastructure, including access roads to waste bins. At the emergency waste meeting, Councilor S. E. Odamtten struck a chord by suggesting that the council was not without blame for the crisis. Odamtten observed that the answer to Accra's waste problem lies with the council properly supervising and controlling the Medical Officer of Health and his assistants.[23] In 1947, Councilor Richard Akwei strongly condemned what he considered "the slipshod manner" of the medical officer in reporting sanitation details. The councilor criticized the president of the Accra Town Council for consistently blocking a reproach to the medical officer.[24] African councilors had detected shortfalls in the medical officer's reports, contributing to inaccurate estimates of Accra's sanitary needs. Persistent reporting faults caused financial losses and growing tension between the council and the Health Department. The tension was just a microcosm of an empire-wide situation involving professional rivalries.[25]

The Medical Officer of Health had distanced himself from the Accra Town Council, which he perceived to be predominantly composed of inquisitive African members. The officer frequently missed meetings and relayed information to the members through the council's European president. Some councilors viewed the officer's habitual absence as a sign of disrespect for their authority. Councilor

Akwei expressed dissatisfaction with the officer's failure to attend meetings to address concerns about uncollected waste:

> The attitude of the Medical Officer of Health . . . [was] indifferent or had no regard for the Council. He pointed out that the services of the Medical Officer of Health were not gratuitous as stated by the President at the last meeting, Council being responsible for the payment of half his salary and was therefore a servant of the Council . . . [and] under obligation to attend meetings.[26]

Despite fully funding the Sanitary Department, the underfunded Accra Town Council only had half the budget to cover the cost of a full-time resident medical officer. The council relied on the colonial state's Health Department, specifically the medical officer of health, to manage the department. Consequently, the medical officer felt more accountable to the colonial state than the council. However, the African councilors demanded accountability, as the council paid half his salary.[27] This tense relationship continued to escalate due to widespread uncleared, stagnant, and scattered waste.

Even with an adequate budget, good sanitation still required diplomatic coordination between the council and the state and the goodwill of residents and laborers. However, the colonial sanitation system was empty of these attributes. Tensions over noncooperation between the colonial state and the Council mounted after the February 1948 riots, when Accra's sanitation reached the "verge of absolute collapse."[28] The colonial state imposed a curfew from 7 p.m. to 6 a.m. in response to the disturbances, which disrupted refuse removal between nightfall and dawn. Although the Council adjusted its services, the African members considered the official decision to impose the curfew without consultation as contempt for their position as local authorities, demonstrating a lack of foresight on the part of the colonial state regarding the implications of stagnant waste on the health of most Africans in the city.[29] Things reached a head when the director of medical services threatened to withdraw his medical officers from the Sanitary Department if the Accra Town Council did not follow certain practices:

> Fall in line with modern practice and establish a Cleansing Department separately from Health Work and expressed grave concern at the "retrograde attitude" adopted by the council . . . he was no longer prepared to assist the Council with the part-time services of qualified health staff if that staff was not to be utilized in administration of conservancy and scavenging services and unless arrangements

> were made without delay to relieve those officers of such duties he would be compelled to instruct them to cease carrying them out.[30]

The director of medical service took exception to the Council's habit of pressuring his medical officers to supervise waste removal in the African neighborhoods.

Meanwhile, the colonial state enlisted African chiefs and traditional officeholders to help police and prosecute residents for littering and scattering trash. It did little to decrease the city's waste problem. Concerned residents frequently published their observations about heaps of garbage continuing to pile up even where "native authority" was directly exercised. In the "hidden and open places" of James Town, Ussher Town, and Christiansborg, "hideous and ugly sites" made headlines in newspapers because of "nothing else but dirt and rubbish."[31] The accumulation of uncleared waste sparked public demands for neighborhood demolition and renewal.[32] An article in the *Daily Graphic* expressed disappointment:

> Nothing has happened to remove the rotten heart to Accra and to rebuild it as the worthy nucleus of the capital of an all-but-independent nation not of course to speak of alleviating the disgraceful conditions of its inhabitants or the odors of putrefaction which continue to surround them.[33]

The unremoved and accumulated waste provided grounds for residents of Accra and newspapers to justify the demolition of Accra's "slums." The lag in sanitation justified demolition of neighborhoods with persistent stagnant waste, and in the mind of advocates, would, in turn, bring about the renewal of the places into clean, spacious, and impressive construction.

When uncleared and stagnant waste in African communities caused tension between the colonial state, African representatives in the council, and residents of Accra, whether through demolition or prosecution and fines, the resulting widespread resentment created an opening to rally urban residents to the nationalists' cause. During the intense nationalist rallies in the late colonial period, the term "slum clearance," which imperial and colonial agents had used as a basis to justify the mass demolition of congested African neighborhoods, became recalibrated by nationalists as a refuse cleanup campaign in the very areas that colonial rule targeted in the interwar period. The goal of the "slum clearance" campaign was to convince Ga voters, who had significant influence and lived in the congested areas, that the incoming African-led government would be less invasive of their space and livelihoods. "Slum clearance" sought to use schoolchildren for cleanup campaigns to demonstrate how to clean their homes and surroundings. It also involved film shows to educate residents on hygiene.[34] Adopting this comprehensive sensitization strategy of cleansing the capital, the nationalist government distanced itself from depictions of authoritarianism and foreignness often associated with colonial rule to forge close relationships with residents in overcrowded African neighborhoods at the center of Accra.

Sewage and Sewers in Accra

Removing sewage was also labor-intensive and faced similar challenges as clearing refuse from the city. For decades, officials, the council, and experts proposed installing a waterborne sewer system to reduce the reliance on poorly paid laborers with methods and technologies that were a nuisance and threat to public health. However, the significant expenditure and requirement of abundant water supply discouraged the project. Official and expert discussions on a sewer system in Accra reached a high point in the Hugh Clifford governorship.[35] The colonial state shelved the project, citing the distraction and lack of resources during the war and the Depression. The city relied on a patchwork of drains, pits, and septic tanks without a proper sewer system. These were far from ideal, as buckets (pan latrines) collected a mixture of waste materials like sullage, excreta, and urine, posing significant health risks. Laborers manually and precariously removed and conveyed the waste, maintaining the colonial metabolic order.

In the 1940s and 1950s, when the city's population and size expanded significantly, the visibility of sewage reignited public calls for a sewer system. The calls were often crystallized in visions for city development worthy of the capital of the modern nation.[36] In James Town, Ussher Town, and Christiansborg, installing sewers was challenging due to the lack of space and inadequate water supply for Accra residents.[37] When Quist-Therson petitioned the council and government about the nuisance and health threat of unremoved buckets containing excrement at Christiansborg, the president of the Accra Town Council referred to

> a comprehensive scheme of drainage, sewage, and slum clearance . . . for Accra. Each of these undertakings has engaged the attention of Government and the Council. A start was made in their execution, but the lack of materials no less than the absence of supervisory staff, has necessitated a postponement for the duration of the war.[38]

This response, citing the war and lack of materials, was similar to earlier excuses for the colonial state's inability to sewer the city before and during the interwar period. It deflected part of the blame on the African neighborhoods, referring to the need for a facelift of the built environment by constructing drains, sewers, and "slum clearance."[39] But the councilor maintained that the need to sewer and drain the city was "staring the authorities in the face years before the war," so the absence of the needed infrastructure was evidence of "official neglect and inadequacy."[40] Global catastrophes and disruptions were a convenient excuse for the lag.

Ioné Acquah's social survey of Accra contrasted the uneven saniscape of sewage removal in the African and European communities in the 1950s. Acquah noted that all European bungalows and their servants' quarters in "government residential areas were adequately supplied."[41] At the same time, communal toilets in "the town center and in Sabon Zongo became dirty and, at times, offensive."[42] The bungalows in sparsely populated government residential areas like Victoriaborg and Ridge, had septic tanks and received adequate municipal service. At the same time, overcrowded and congested neighborhoods such as Korle Gonno, Abose Okai, Sabon Zongo, and Labadi used communal toilets. Maxwell Fry, the architect and urban landscape designer who produced the first plan for Accra, also documented this unevenness. European bungalows, the newly constructed government estates, and privately owned African houses had "private water-borne sewage systems running into their own septic tanks," which were of "improved type," offering "excellent services" to residents.[43] He reported an "objectionable" smell emanating from frequently uncleared excreta in communal toilets in the less affluent African residential communities.[44]

Repeated delays and commonplace incidents of non-removal of excreta trapped the African residential areas in a perpetual state of inefficacious sanitation. Because of the health threats and nuisance of uncleared waste, some residents objected to the city engineers' blueprints to construct communal toilets and urinals near their homes, further exacerbating the shortages. For ratepayers living in the communities, this vicious cycle of uncleared waste and scarcity of adequate places of convenience was unacceptable. In 1944, ten residents submitted a petition to the colonial secretary to oppose the construction of a public toilet near their homes by the Health Department and Council.[45] Led by J. Quist-Therson, the petitioners emphasized the concerns to the secretary:

> There is only one spot suitable for a sanitary site in the neighborhood and I find it rather difficult to understand why the Authorities have studiously avoided it. It is a large open space north of Ashanti Street and south of the large drains running off Lokko Street up to the beach. A latrine or other sanitary structure on that piece

of land would be accessible to the public, would be at a reasonable distance from the nearest dwelling houses.[46]

When the residents near the newly designed communal toilets and baths heard of the engineer's plan, they petitioned against it being in the location despite knowing that the facilities were crucial. The issue was not with the toilet per se but "arraying latrine pans full of human excreta" in the open, non-removal, and the nuisance from the waste. Since the petition was well-grounded in colonial public health and aesthetic sensibilities, officials and the council negotiated another sanitary site for the toilet, which had to be approved by the Central Board of Health.[47]

Tackling lagging sanitation and stagnant waste (re)configured Accra's built environment and saniscape in particular ways. In 1948, representatives of the residents of Agbogboloshie and from different sections of Accra complained about habitual poor municipal cleansing of toilets in their neighborhood. Councilor Akwei brought the issue up during the monthly meetings.[48] It generated a keen interest among residents in blueprints and the potential sites for sanitation infrastructure. In one instance, residents of Pagan Road mobilized against a yet-to-be-constructed toilet because of the disreputable culture of non-clearance of sewage and the smells, even though the facility was essential for a planned parking lot on the site. This pushback gained traction because of the site's proximity to a mosque. The protest drew overwhelming support from members of the Accra Town Council and compelled the president, together with some members of the council, the town clerk, and the town engineer to reinspect the site. After the tour, the president withdrew the project and submitted a redesign to the Accra Planning Committee and the Public Health Committee in 1949 for approval and incorporation into the city's overall plan.[49] In that very year, the Medical Department also authorized the demolition of a public toilet on Castle Road after the American Consul complained about the "stench emanating" from it. The toilet served quite a sizeable African population because of the location. Still, officials had to demolish it because of its troubling smell from poor service.[50] The disruptive nature of waste spurred a collective effort by urban residents, officials, the council, and other urban constituencies mobilizing to reshape the arrangement of the built environment.

Another feature that made the manual removal of sewage from African communities revulsive was the technology. The buckets that collected sewage were leaky and rusted. Waste seeped out of them and smeared on the bodies of laborers during removal and transport. The laborers often complained to the Accra Town Council and its engineers about the leaky and rusted technologies.[51] It explains why sometimes laborers left buckets filled with waste unattended. These buckets had no top cover, exposing the content to public sight. These buckets were the cause of public outcry. When the laborers eventually transported the leaky and uncovered buckets by conservancy trucks through the bumpy streets of the African neighborhoods, the waste splashed and spread on the rough access roads, causing a nuisance in the communities.[52] By 1950, approximately twenty-five trucks transported over four million gallons of waste from toilets used by more than 106,000 Accra residents.[53] Demographic growth in African communities put a further strain on manual removal, which increasingly became unsatisfactory. Cheap things were costlier. When put together, manual waste removal required adequate access roads, laborers, conservancy fleet, and supervision to maintain a satisfactory urban metabolism. Waste removal was unsatisfactory and unpredictable especially because a fault with any element within the interconnected sanitation conduit infrastructure was a problem, making sanitation one of the most criticized features of the Accra Town Council and colonial state functions.

Septic tanks seemed like a more reliable technology. It could make waste relatively contactless compared to the bucket system. However, the technology had its challenges. Because the water table over most of Accra was high, contamination from seepage of sewage from septic tanks into the subsoil and underground water supply posed a potential epidemiological issue. Broadly, the challenge with the septic tank was part of a broader waste ecology that made Accra unsuitable for a large population density. Also, waste on the beaches of Accra was a constant urban health threat. Accra's surface drains, which laborers flushed with seawater, had a network of channels connecting them to the sewage plant near Korle Lagoon. The plant consisted of tanks with a pipe powered by electricity that pumped untreated sludge of sullage, excrement, and other waste materials from drains into the Atlantic Ocean. However, the ocean washed a significant amount of the sludge back onto the beach, leaving officials with no choice other than to continuously employ a thinly stretched labor force to sweep and remove to ease the nuisance, smells, and houseflies. These challenges explain why Accra's first two waste disposal plans were unsuitable for the capital and dangerous to urban health.[54] Fry's plan stated that a "water-borne sewage system [was] urgently needed in Accra, installed first in the most crowded districts and then gradually extended to other parts of the town."[55] At the same time, another plan after Fry's, published just after independence, noted: "The early introduction of water-borne sewage disposal system is of the utmost importance, particularly in the heavily developed areas."[56] Both plans prioritized the "slums" and overcrowded African neighborhoods because of the chronic waste removal problem.

Having delayed sewering the city for decades, the colonial state bequeathed the project to the emerging African government. It was a necessary monumental project that the government added to plans for draining the modern capital city to promote health, social progress, and economic development. Through the Ministry of Works, the government employed the services of Messrs. David Balfour & Sons, a Britain-based firm that submitted recommendations for sewers in 1955. However, the infrastructure cost was high for a city primarily developed for colonial benefit. The Balfour report proposed the installation in phases aligned to the city's topography and drainage area. The estimated cost for the project, together with one sea outfall near Korle Gonno, was £6,000,000. At the time of the survey, Accra's population was 250,000, representing a 57 percent increase over seven years.[57] Balfour's report also prioritized installing the system in "the areas of congestion and unsanitary conditions" because of the chronic stagnant waste problems in African neighborhoods.[58] Phase I of the Balfour Scheme included neighborhoods listed as Drainage Areas 1, 2, and parts of 3, with an estimated cost of £3,000,000. Unlike other phases of the scheme, the budget for the priority areas also covered branch sewers.[59] However, when the council discussed Balfour's recommendations, it decided:

> Owing to the financial implications, Council could not, without the help of the Central Government, undertake this enormous task. In addition it was appreciated that in order to ensure success for any scheme of this nature, legislation might be necessary to make it compulsory for properties within a certain distance of a sewer to be connected thereto and also perhaps, for a special rate to be levied.[60]

In addition to the high cost the council alone could not bear, there was a need for legislative powers to compel property owners to connect their buildings to sewers and to levy maintenance rates to maintain it.

Due to a lack of money and legislative power, the Accra Town Council delayed the construction of sewers and drains, which were projected to enhance the flow of stagnant sewage away from Accra's African neighborhoods. Pending government financial assistance and a legislative instrument, the council directed the town engineer and its consultants to collaboratively work with the director of public works to design a main sewer connecting Hotel Ambassador to the plant near Korle Lagoon "with a view to the immediate construction of the portion."[61] The estimated infrastructure cost was £50,000, pre-finance with the Accra improvement fund. A sewer in this section of Accra held "some immediate importance."[62] What could be more critical than the precariousness of a potential epidemic? It was the image of Accra. With independence fast approaching and international visitors frequenting Accra, the infrastructure would showcase a sewer line as a sanitation technology befitting the modern capital. The council's action was also of practical importance. The council planned to raise funds from wealthy property owners, including those of Kingsway stores. In return, it would connect their property to the sewer line. The urgent need for sewers and drains in heavily developed and congested areas in the postwar era of development and social progress notwithstanding, and despite the recommendation of Messrs. David Balfour & Sons, whose services came about because of the critical waste problems in these priority areas, the economic and social class determined the areas to sewer. The council's priority agenda confined the underserviced communities to a perpetual cycle of neglect and sanitary inefficacy from the colonial to the eve of independence.

Colonial officials' failure to ensure equity in healthy urban waste outflows for all city sections passed on to the emerging postcolonial governments whose priority list for providing waste infrastructure privileged wealthy districts. However, as a public health technology to clear urban waste in the postwar era, waterborne sewage and how officials grappled with the absence of infrastructure continued to hold great significance for state-driven social and economic development. Sewer line construction epitomized a continuation of the so-called colonial civilizing mission premised on transforming Africa through science, technology, and medicine.[63] Six years after Balfour's report, Nkrumah's government still needed help starting Phase I of the sewage and drainage scheme. The government needed to reassess the cost due to significant changes in the city's demographics and infrastructure since Balfour's report in 1955. Rising wages and the cost of building materials were also contributing factors. A review by the same firm revealed that its previous proposal for a single sea outfall near Korle Lagoon needed updating forestall the public health risk posed to the neighboring African communities of Korle Gonno, James Town, and Ussher Town, which faced the risk of contamination from sewage pumped to the outfall. By the time sewage from around a now expanded Accra reached the outfall, having traveled a mile, it would have become septic. Another sea outfall east of Christiansborg would discharge the sewage from the eastern part of Accra early enough to prevent contamination. Additionally, increasing the water supply in Accra and connecting buildings to the water pipes, instead of residents drawing water from communal standpipes, was crucial to ensure the infrastructure's proper functioning.[64]

The revised Phase I project encompasses a larger area, including Drainage Area 10 of Korle Gonno. Additionally, the firm incorporated parts of Drainage Area 4, including the Ministry, State House precincts, and Osu Estate, into the updated Phase I. The changes correspondingly increased the cost of the scheme to £4,025,000. Considered mainly a social development project with no direct and immediate economic returns, the government looked to Group One Limited and Taylor Woodrow Limited, prepared to pre-finance the scheme under stringent credit terms. The complex sewage network also drew legal, engineering, urban design, environmental, and other expertise from the United Nations. By June 1961, officials still explored cheaper means to pre-finance Phase I, and streams of international experts visited to examine Accra's need for the infrastructure. The African communities became more exposed to the global community's gaze than ever before, and the persistent waste problem, a direct consequence of decades of neglect, became a glaring issue that could no longer be ignored.[65] To make water flow into homes and excrement, urine, and sullage to wash away, the colonial state and council needed to finance and maintain a functioning network of sewer and water connections. That required a range of activities, including plumbing works in individual buildings, the installation of pipes to connect buildings to sewer networks and pipe mains and onto pumps, energy, and sea outfalls, among other appurtenances. However, that massive and ambitious infrastructure could cost the new nations in political and economic terms. It infringed on the property and domesticity of everyday residents and entangled new African leaders in global expertise, politics, economies, and other aspects of colonial rule that had just formally ended, providing insights into early dependency, growing indebtedness, and the widespread pessimism among African citizens trapped in a cycle of perpetual borrowing, underdevelopment, and poverty.

Nairobi's Uncleared Waste and Counterinsurgency

During the Mau Mau Emergency, the violent anti-colonial protest that set the stage for Kenya's decolonization, accumulated waste pushed Nairobi to the brink of a sanitation breakdown. Through "Operation Anvil," the colonial state conducted counterinsurgent raids in African neighborhoods, leading to the arrest, exile, and prohibition of Kikuyu and their Meru, Embu, and other African Mau Mau sympathizers.[66] Since Africans were the primary labor providers, the Mau Mau period witnessed a general shortage in sanitation service. Regarding sanitation labor, the Kikuyu comprised the majority.[67] As expected, the African locations bore the brunt as waste bins were filled beyond capacity. Also, officials thought that residents scattered refuse around the bins. In an inspection, the medical officer observed:

> Another factor which constantly operates in making the locations look dirty and that is the inhabitants do not bother to put refuse in the bins, but scatter it around them, and in any case half-full bins are ransacked by urchins and the contents scattered around. . . . Probably some of the scattered refuse may be caused by passers-by and not by tenant in the houses in the area.[68]

In one breath, the officer implied that subversives were responsible for misplaced waste incidents. Waste infrastructure, such as the bins meant to keep neighborhoods clean, was the physical representation of the colonial state and the settler-dominated council in Africans' everyday lives. As evident in Nairobi's spatial development, the council used accumulated and stagnant waste as an excuse to demolish African neighborhoods and disrupt their lives. However, in another breath, the officer mentioned a culture of misplacing waste before the Mau Mau movement.

Compared to European and South Asian locations, refuse clearing services in the African neighborhoods for which the municipality's Cleansing Department was responsible had "never been entirely satisfactory and . . . been the subject of repeated representations to the City Council for a number of years."[69] Refuse accumulation in African locations had been a cause for official and municipal condemnations. Based on repeated non-clearance of refuse and resultant accumulations, the medical officer ranked Pumwani and the other African locations in Nairobi as most likely to cause and be susceptible to epidemics. South Asian quarters followed in the pecking order, with European neighborhoods classified as less likely. The officer made this ranking during World War II, when there was a plague outbreak in Nairobi and most of its victims came from Pumwani. The officer observed that uncleared and accumulated refuse created ideal conditions for rats and fleas to thrive, leading to plague transmission to humans. He stated that as long as African neighborhoods like Pumwani were not demolished, epidemics would continue to recur.[70] Waste accumulation over time and the precarious state of African health were the result of racialized segregation and unequal sanitation services, as detailed in the preceding chapters.

The colonial state questioned the municipal Cleansing Department's inability to handle the waste menace in the rapidly growing population in the locations. This doubt propelled a solution-oriented discussion of decoupling sanitation from the colonial state's Medical Department. The director of medical services suggested a change in the running of the Cleansing Department, which oversaw the uneven municipal services in Nairobi for years. Being responsible for "advising on sanitation and simultaneously being "the Executive Officer responsible over the service," the medical officer's power to decide the sections of Nairobi on which to concentrate municipal services was far-reaching. The director recommended employing a cleansing officer to carry out the executive functions involving the implementation of sanitation proposals while the medical role remained advisory.[71]

The municipality, on its part, unfairly blamed Africans for what it thought to be the inherent nature of Africans to make their location dirty.[72] The inconvenience of mass demolition and relocation because of stagnant waste caused worry in the African communities. It was disruptive to lives and livelihoods. Illustrating the waste-demolition connection and its disruption, the Executive Committee of Kenya African Union (KAU) stated:

> The attitude of the Municipality to shantytowns [is a] . . . source of grave dissatisfaction to Africans. In the absence of any housing accommodation many Africans have been forced, at their own expense and labor, to erect huts which would at least offer them shelter from cold and rain. One fine morning several months after the houses have been built, a batch of Askaris arrive and commerce demolition the huts. No compensation is paid to the owners, nor are they offered alternative accommodation. It is, of course, easy for authorities to wax eloquent on "the reeking stench, the murky hovels, the slimy lanes," etc.[73]

The statement expressed KAU's complaint against the council for frequently using demolition as their usual method for cleaning up piles of trash in certain areas labeled as dirty, slum-like, and breeding grounds for diseases such as plague, typhus, malaria, and other sanitation-related illnesses.

How the settler state handled these disruptions in waste removal from European residential areas reinforces unequal sanitation dynamics in the city. The fear of an epidemic compelled swift measures during the general strike when African laborers took to a "go-slow policy" on cleansing services and the Mau Mau emergency. The medical officer of health appealed to European residents to discard their refuse rather than wait for city authorities to assign workers to clean their premises.[74] The council and state initiated scores of measures, including surveillance and screening, to ensure the laborers "contaminated" with Mau Mau did not enter the segregated European neighborhoods. Since Anvil ensured Kikuyu laborers were no longer available, the council and state diversified sanitary laborers to avoid the "periodic crisis" whereby waste clearance came to "a standstill" whenever members of the same ethnic group were on strike.[75] Africans who passed the security clearance received wage increases for the grim working conditions associated with sanitation.[76]

While putting protective measures in place for Europeans, the African locations where residents who were not loyal to the Mau Mau cause remained vulnerable to attacks by infectious diseases. The municipality imposing fines and evicting residents as a direct approach to deter littering could hardly alleviate the problem. As the Accra case showed, fines were counterproductive. They could make waste a site for subversion. Evictions without stringent surveillance shifted overcrowding and waste problems to other parts of Nairobi.[77] The health outcome was staggering. Infant mortality rates of Africans rose from 150 to 299 per 1,000, and reports of an imminent outbreak of an epidemic surfaced.[78] As the medical officer of health reported,

> Prior to "Operation Anvil" the low sanitary standard of the locations undoubtedly lowered the standard of general health amongst the dwellers there especially in the cases of children, but no epidemic disease was known to have occurred. . . . Since the Emergency and particularly "Operation Anvil," Typhoid has been some anxiety, and since January 1st, 1954, 217 cases have been notified in Africans.[79]

The comment emphasizes the long-standing disparity in municipal services in African neighborhoods and its impact on health conditions. Mau Mau and other disruptive events worsened unhygienic conditions in African areas that had long been segregated. Uneven waste-removal practices led to high illness and death rates in underserved African neighborhoods.

Another way the state and council thought could resolve the waste problems was by constructing enclosures, including concrete walls, wire fencing, and hedges. Barriers served security functions and, in this case, an added advantage of stopping the entry of nonresidents, who officials thought were littering and contributing to overflowing waste bins and overstretching sanitation infrastructure. Besides being a mechanism for keeping neighborhoods refuse-free, they thought barriers would help individualized sanitation in neighborhoods by making private residents responsible for sweeping and disposing of waste within and outside their fences. The approach reduced the municipality's role in cleaning African locations by making residents accountable for their refuse. The director of medical services doubled down on the doubt about the municipality's ability to cleanse the African location:

> The wisdom of the present arrangements for the layouts of houses whereby large open spaces exist which have to be maintained by the city council. These constitute a vast area which will involve the city council in an increasingly large commitment for maintenance. I believe that the only way to maintain these locations in a clean condition is for these areas to be maintained in a proper state by individual responsibility or by the collective responsibility of those living in the compound. I was shown one very new housing estate which is already in danger of becoming slum. The grass was uncut and rubbish was lying about all over the compound. . . . I would recommend therefore that every plot, and this applies particularly to plots allocated to Africans for individual building, should be surrounded either by a fence or a low hedge so that individual responsibility can be clearly demarcated.[80]

The installation of barriers shifted the responsibility for waste management from the municipality to the residents. The director mentioned the effective waste management systems in other African colonial cities and stated that the residents must keep their compounds or backyards clean. The municipality would then be solely responsible for maintaining roads and drains.[81] The barriers served purposes beyond regulating the entry and exit of neighborhoods during the counterinsurgency. Medical experts believed they would promote privatized cleaning, discourage littering, and mitigate the impact of inconsistent municipal services.

Sewage, Infrastructure Vandalism, and Sanitation Security in Nairobi

As in Accra, sewage clearance in Nairobi was manual, and the bucket toilet technologies were a public nuisance. Any delays in clearing the waste and non-clearance caused much inconvenience. The use of bucket toilets expanded in conjunction with the construction of communal toilets for Africans in the 1940s and 1950s. The municipality's Cleansing Department supervised sweepers, most of whom were the Kikuyu. They removed sewage from African, European, and Indian neighborhoods. Ox-drawn carts were the primary means of transporting waste-filled buckets, but since the end of the war, trucks gradually replaced the beasts of burden.[82] The department required the laborers to do everything manually, from removing waste in the neighborhoods to discharging it at the Eastleigh sewage works.[83] Using laborers seemed cheaper on the surface. However, as seen in the case of Accra, manual labor was costly considering the support infrastructure and technologies required, including good access roads, maintenance and replacement of buckets, trucks and spare parts, and attractive incentives for laborers. Without the laborers in the event of a strike, the entire system would shut down. However, the realities of the work were harsh. Manual waste removal was intimate, intricate, and took a long time to complete. Like their Kroo counterparts in Accra, the Kikuyu sweepers were often subjected to deplorable conditions and forced to transport leaky and uncovered buckets, which left them smeared with foul sewage and smells. Yet the faulty buckets were only part of the distasteful sanitary system in the white settler capital. With population growth and disruptions, laborers had to contend with buckets overflowing their capacity. At times, laborers were frustrated with these conditions that they "dumped in open, [the] dilapidated and improvised containers" containing human excreta uncovered at the side of the road allowing "ready access to flies" and further providing thriving conditions for diseases and stocking settler condemnation and scapegoating.[84]

The African Women's League, recognizing these "revolting" sanitary labor conditions, questioned the very basis of colonial rule as a legitimate civilizing agent.[85] The absence of a "modern sewer system" provided the league a reason to confront Kenya's colonial state. In a 1946 memorandum to the secretary of state for the Colonies, the league questioned the idea of transforming colonies through technology when manual labor was the primary means of moving sewage from Nairobi's neighborhoods.[86] Officials considered the league's memorandum necessary, as it was "the first time that African women in Kenya . . . submitted agreed representations on matters of concern to them" and conceived that the "council is well aware of the need for the modern sewage system."[87] In the postwar developmentalist era, the league's appeal was influential. Its underlying objective was improving and uplifting women's conditions.[88] In this case, the league played a pivotal role in advocating for the spouses of Nairobi's sanitary laborers. As the league eloquently asserted, "We are left in the room allotted to our husbands when men goes [*sic*] to duty at night. Upon their return we recognize them at the distance by smell from human excretion collected from latrines throughout the city."[89] Smells strong enough to detect from a distance resulted from the manual removal of waste, which exposed laborers to waste for an extended period and made their bodies intimate with other peoples' excrement. Two years after the league presented the memorandum, officials authorized a probe into the living conditions of laborers and other municipal African employees. The laborers' housing in Kariokor and Sweepers Lhandies were the least satisfactory in Nairobi. They were "dark, dirty, and overcrowded . . . and [could] hardly be called desirable or hygienic."[90] This description reflects housing and sanitation in segregated African residential areas. In 1954, the director of medical services also observed the "revolting" leaky and rusty toilet buckets seeping sticky waste and smell onto bodies about which the league had raised concerns eight years earlier.[91]

Even in segregated European areas, where officials and white residents had African servant quarters on the property, the sanitation infrastructure for Africans was mainly the standard bucket toilets. While European houses connected their flushed toilets to septic tanks, they had bucket toilet systems in their African servants' quarters. Most European houses generally had waterborne toilets connected to septic tanks, and most Indian buildings lacked the facility. Fewer African houses in the locations and railway quarters had waterborne sanitation.[92] By 1951, a radius of about 1.2 square miles from the subcommissioner's office had been served with waterborne toilets, an area corresponding to Nairobi's original size in its foundational phase. Nairobi had then expanded to an area of 32.1 square miles.[93] Thus, in the 1950s, developing waterborne sanitation, including septic tanks and sewers, in Nairobi reflected social stratification, with class playing a more significant role than race. While officials considered installing waterborne toilets in African servants' quarters in the European segregated areas, they continued to expand the bucket technologies. By 1955, the municipality had purchased more buckets from South Africa, increasing the number by 200 percent.[94]

With European and South Asian residential areas relying on laborers for waste removal, the potential for disruption of sanitation during civil action was a significant concern. During the strike and Mau Mau, officials regarded installing waterborne sanitation in the servants' quarters at European residential areas as necessary to regulate the frequency and numbers of Africans crossing segregated boundaries. In a future emergency, waste would flow away from European residential areas with fixed and concrete sanitary infrastructures rather than the conventional manual labor serving as conduits. In response to the strike, the district commissioner for Nairobi stated it "became clear . . . that the weakest link in the Emergency organization is the clearance of night soil from bucket latrines."[95] Manual waste labor had given Africans leverage, and the permanent way out was to convert the toilet bucket system in servants' quarters to waterborne sanitation. Also, the acting chief secretary declared:

> Consideration is being given to the question of replacing buckets by water-borne sanitation in all Government African quarters, as the clearance of night soil proved to be a major problem during the recent [May 1950] Nairobi strike. The conversion would concern existing quarters, as it is the policy to include water-borne sanitation for servants [*sic*] quarters in all new buildings.[96]

The council adopted a new policy of providing waterborne sanitation infrastructure for existing and new African servants' quarters, reducing the number of Africans going to European residential communities to clear sewage.

European fear of Africans compromising sanitation systems stems from reports of infrastructure vandalism in African locations. With comparatively less colonial security and surveillance in the locations, the perceived sabotage of sanitation fittings gained expression in thoughts of Mau Mau subversives' excessive befouling of the surroundings of communal toilets. It was as though sanitation became the site where some Africans resisted the colonial order to the extent of instigating an imagined guerilla germ warfare against settlers during the emergency.[97] While Africans rejected settler broad-brush negative representation and demanded the political space to air their views openly without fear of retribution, settlers did not consider it far-fetched that subversives might have used sanitation sites for pushback on state repression.[98] The sanitation regulations, services, and physical infrastructure were arguably the most palpable ways African Nairobians experienced the settler order daily. The state and municipality often designate African neighborhoods as slums because of inadequate infrastructure and municipal services to prevent stagnant waste.[99] As covered in chapters 2 and 3, colonial slum discourse suggested waste-laden neighborhoods where epidemics of plague, typhus, malaria, and other sanitary-related contagions could erupt and spread. The discourse strategically provided grounds for demolition and allowed the municipality and state to exploit stagnant waste and an absent and broken sanitary system, effectively disrupting the African urban experiences. Logically, the disruption of sanitation in the locations caught the attention of the state and municipality. Both the sanitation problems and the response of the settler order was a nuisance to the African residents. Unsurprisingly, the official response to sanitation disruption was unequal, with the African locations bearing the brunt. European communities received layers of security in the form of sewers and septic tanks to prevent a potential attack from African sanitation laborers, waste stagnation, and public health emergencies.[100]

While the state and municipal council implemented sanitation security to prevent Mau Mau sympathizers from entering European residential areas, they explored funding for an extensive waterborne system. The infrastructure would cost the prohibitive sum of £3,000,000. In pursuit of this sort of capital-intensive project like waterborne sanitation, the Nairobi City Council looked to borrowing money from beyond Kenya, even London. This decision was not just a financial strategy but a statement of Nairobi's global outlook. The council argued that Nairobi's loan requirements should not be tied to Kenya alone.[101] In the meantime, the War Council, in charge of security during Mau Mau, was responsible for vetting and recruiting sanitary laborers for the European residential areas. The War Council undertook a rigorous screening process, particularly for the Embu and other ethnicities, to ease settler fear that the Kikuyu had not "contaminated" them with Mau Mau. The War Council strongly advised the municipality that while the laborers were "vouched for," it was imperative that they wore distinctive uniforms for easy identification and housed in a location "less corrupt and dangerous than Kariokor" to facilitate effective policing. Switching laborers' ethnicities and enforcing strict measures temporarily solved sanitary insecurity. The potential implications could be catastrophic if a sanitary breakdown were to occur due to an African strike or mass refusals.[102] The gravity of the situation prompted Deputy Governor F. Crawford to put forth a significant proposal in August 1955, envisioning a solution for Nairobi's sanitary future:

> The only solution, at any rate for the non-African residential areas, including their domestic servants [*sic*] quarters—the chief danger point as regards subversive activities—is to force as far as is possible all non-African householders to install individual septic tank systems.[103]

During the Mau Mau uprising, the absence of septic tanks and flush toilets posed security risks because the sanitary laborers, who served as alternative infrastructure, had the potential to become guerrillas and attack settler families. Settlers without septic tanks and flush toilets on their property had to install them in both the main buildings and servant's quarters.

In 1959, Crawford's proposal to replace bucket toilets with flush toilets, septic tanks, and sewer lines remarkably improved Nairobi's built environment. However, much of the spatial transformation was nonetheless restricted to European and

South Asian communities in the Hill, Parklands, and Westlands neighborhoods. The new upper-class African residential areas of Mbotela and Ofafa Estates in the Doonholm neighborhood also included sewer and drain installations. The residents received "direct or indirect assistance from the government and private employers" to afford flats.[104] In the same year, the medical officer of health at the Nairobi City Council noted:

> The installation of sewers in the Parklands/Westlands, Hill and Eastleigh areas has meant that the service of notices on all owners of properties in the areas affected, and the supervision and testing of all new drainage systems installed. The 178 premises connected to these sewers during the year represents only a small proportion of those involved, but when the conversions have been completed a great step will have been taken towards removing the nuisances inevitably associated with bucket latrines, conservancy tanks, and sullage pits. In spite of the heavy costs involved, the response to the notices has been good, and it seems likely that only in very few instances will court action be necessary to enforce the Council's requirements.[105]

While determined to take court action to compel non-compliant European and South Asian property owners to install the sanitation infrastructure, the medical officer celebrated the positive response to Crawford's proposal. By 1960, the installations significantly reduced bucket toilets from 5,004 to 3,785 officially, marking a significant step toward making sewage removal less dependent on manual labor.[106]

Despite recognizing the security benefits, some property owners could not afford sewer connections or septic tanks. Seeing that prosecution alone could not compel settlers to individually bear the cost of installing waterborne sanitation, officials took a decisive step by passing legislation that empowered the council to construct the infrastructure and recovered the cost. This move would profoundly impact the settler part of the saniscape over time.[107] The sewage disposal plant at Eastleigh collected waste from a network of sewers. Municipal trucks also emptied septic tank contents into the plant. The plant treated the sewage and discharged it into the Nairobi River, which joined the Athi River at a distance. The overloading of the plant, which resulted in partially treated sewage, meant health risks to the South Asian and African communities living nearby. To compound matters, these communities lacked the concrete infrastructures needed to improve waste outflow from their neighborhoods. [108]

> The laying of drains and construction of septic tanks and conservancy tanks in black cotton areas has always been a serious problem—so serious that not until the

> red soil and murrum plots has been fully developed was any large-scale building on such sites considered.[109]

The Eastlands part of Nairobi's saniscape did not receive municipal and state infrastructure support, although the need was dire. The medical officer gave the excuse that the black cotton soil made it too expensive to install the infrastructure. In the calculation, layers of reinforced waterproof concrete in the soil would add extra cost to drains' and septic tanks' floors, walls, and roofs. The city believed another hurdle to be increasing Nairobi's water supply and connecting individual buildings to pipes. These excuses gave officials and the council reason to hold up further development in the African locations.[110]

Delays in remaking Eastlands to enable the installation of drains, septic tanks, and other waterborne infrastructure meant the lack of universal sanitation services and infrastructure. It left Nairobi a divided saniscape with densely populated and unsanitary neighborhoods in close proximity to the central business district, which had modern sewers and drains. In Pumwani, for example, the lack of infrastructure allowing for stagnant waste in the community made experts discuss why "conditions remained virtually unchanged."[111] The location had been earmarked for demolition by the council during the war, but the government halted the action due to the shortage of accommodation for Africans. This decision, driven by the council's desire to demolish Pumwani, not only contributed to the neglect of sanitary services and infrastructure but also laid bare the stark reality of the divided city that racialized residential segregation had produced.[112] Health experts "wonder[ed] how long this slum [could] remain without giving rise to a serious epidemic."[113] Black cotton soil not only was unsuitable for building houses but proved a conducive environment for vectors and disease transmission. As conditions deteriorated in the 1960s, the medical officer of health warned the council and residents about the dire public health risk Pumwani posed. The lack of improvement and the "continued insanitary conditions" were not just abstract concepts but real threats to the health and well-being of the city.[114]

Conclusion: Stagnant Waste and Uneven Sanitation

By focusing on waste as a lens through which to see the processes driving Accra's and Nairobi's changing saniscapes in the 1950s and 1960s, the chapter reveals the crucial role of sanitation laborers in the network of waste infrastructures in turning on and off the trash and sewage outflows. Although laborers relied on the cooperation from residents, well-maintained access roads, functional incinerators, trucks, and technologies such as waste bins and scores of others, without the laborers, the sanitation system could shut down, making the cities an eyesore, smelly, and vulnerable to epidemics. Ryan Johnson and Amna Khalid argue that these laborers were among a broad category of lower-level employees who enormously influenced public health policies and practices during colonial rule.[115] Despite the different postcolonial dynamics in Rosalind Fredericks's scholarship, laborers within a complex network of urban residents and materials constituted a "vital infrastructure" in cleaning the city's trash.[116] Despite this crucial role of laborers, uncleared, stagnant, and scattered waste was the cause of technological failure and colonial hierarchies of sanitation. In Accra, all these factors coalesced in the influence of laborers on residents to spread out their garbage to enable easy transport and burning in the incinerator, contributing to the persisting waste menace in the African residential areas. Labor shortage during the Nairobi strike and Mau Mau brought about widespread trash accumulation and littering because of inadequate sanitation security. It compelled the privatization of household refuse management and brought Europeans closer to their waste.

Accumulated and scattered waste had significant political implications. Brian Larkin's work is constructive in framing uncleared waste as affective and intensely political.[117] And Colin McFarlane shows that waste makes waste management infrastructures critical to urban governance and sets in motion "fraught and contentious processes of socio-material engineering."[118] The accumulation of uncleared waste in African residential areas in Accra led to heavy court fines for families and strained relations within the extended family due to some members not contributing to defraying the fees. The uncleared garbage sparked intense arguments within the Accra Town Council, with racial undertones. African representatives felt that the president was siding with the European health officer, preventing them from holding the officer accountable for repeated instances of uncleared waste in African communities. On a national level, Nkrumah's health minister and the government rebranded the unpopular colonial "slum clearance" schemes as a refuse cleanup campaign rather than mass demolition, relocation, and renewal of African neighborhoods. This shift in policy presented African leaders seeking decolonization and political office as more sensitive to urban residents in providing sanitation. In the context of a strike and Mau Mau in Nairobi, pileups and littering dynamics differed from Accra. Although some European officials sympathetic to the plight of African locations sought bureaucratic changes to address the repeated waste stagnation, the settler system defaulted to the discussions of prior anemic settler control systems to enhance control barriers to African movements, thinking it would alleviate pileups and deliberate littering in the African locations. The official idea of fencing individual African houses to make each household responsible for their sanitation, instead of the municipality council, was another way medical experts and officials thought they could alleviate pileups and scattering. African women of the league were particularly passionate about the smells of their husbands from removing waste, and they petitioned the Colonial Office, expressing their dissatisfaction with the "uncivilized" attribute of Nairobi's sanitation technologies and poor maintenance culture.

As a political material, waste became entangled in developmentalism during the buildup to formal independence with far-reaching consequences. Cleaning accumulated and stagnant waste in the city using modern infrastructure and technology became part of the discourse of progress. In this sense, Sophia Stamatopoulou-Robbin's discussion of waste as "infrastructural" and "enabler" evokes what governing bodies and residents did to mitigate accumulated and stagnant refuse and sewage.[119] As one of the nagging problems of urbanization, uncleared and scattered waste and the infrastructure for mitigating them were a focal point for the development-minded state. Because of the poor maintenance of Accra's "shitscape," including buckets and communal toilets, and the delayed removal of waste, residents organized to negotiate the proximity of these facilities to residential areas, mosques, and workplaces so as not to suffer the resulting nuisance and smells.[120] Following the logic of Brenda Chalfin's overarching argument, this sort of grassroots act, seeking an effective and civilized approach to urban waste management and shaping the arrangement of the built environment, was political.[121] Nate Plageman has also noted this political engagement in the *Daily Graphic*, demonstrating how the writers connected waste infrastructure with the progress and development of Accra.[122] Government-led sewer projects, for example, were crucial in addressing the shortcomings of manual sewage removal and showcasing the Gold Coast as a modern nation. However, the focus on modernizing Accra diverted attention from the urgent sanitation needs of its populated areas. African women of the league indicated the importance of a sewage system in Nairobi as a progressive, modern, developed city. But the development of Nairobi's "shitscape" did not come about following the women's appeal but for security to reduce the number of Africans frequenting European residential areas. These residential areas changed significantly as the settler system promoted extensive septic tanks and sewer construction to replace bucket toilets and reduce manual waste removal. Officials and the municipal council postponed providing these waste infrastructures in Nairobi's African locations, which urgently needed them.

Thus, in both cities, the densely populated African neighborhoods continued to manifest lagging sanitation systems and waste problems in contrast to the residential locations of Europeans and well-to-do Africans. The production of these saniscapes fits into McFarlane's argument about sanitation as discursive and constructed infrastructures, making a vulnerable and dysfunctional "cyborg city."[123] Sanitation infrastructures, services, and regulations varied. Neighborhoods that lagged in these essential urban features experienced chronic waste stagnation and pileups, provoking the public and government discourse of slums, demolition, and housing. How urban residents continued to experience these challenges even after colonial rule is the subject of the epilogue. It explains the persistent sanitation disparity in the cities as the outcome of urban policies and practices tackled in this and previous chapters.

Epilogue

Everything Old Is New Again

Looking at Rendeavour's Appolonia City and Tatu City projects in Accra and Nairobi, one can see the continued flow of global capital into these cities in a neoliberal form rather than under imperial control. As a transnational company and the largest private developer of African cities, Rendeavour's investors hail from the United States, Norway, Britain, and New Zealand. It would seem that Rendeavour's management, experts, investors, and partners are embarking on a novel urban development endeavor. However, Rendeavour's construction of new cities due to housing shortages and sanitation challenges in established ones brings the past into the present. It echoes the (re)production of colonial saniscapes. The Appolonia and Tatu projects raise critical questions about making cities livable for a section of urban residents and bring to mind early colonial efforts to build segregated residential communities to make the tropics healthy for Europeans. This contemporary iteration of separate residential communities also provides self-contained enclaves for wealthy urban residents who prefer not to encounter urban congestions and "slums" daily. The separate cities provide an escape from the "dysfunctional" aspects of Accra and Nairobi.[1] Since demolition and the relocation of communities would cause widespread pushback and claim-making among affected residents, as seen in Ga seaside communities and Pangani, building new residential areas in established neighborhoods has been and still is politically disastrous.

Rendeavour is developing self-contained cities reminiscent of the neighborhood units built outside Accra and Nairobi in the 1940s and 1950s by imperial experts and colonial officials. The corporation's stated vision is to drive accelerated economic growth, fulfill the aspirations of Africa's emerging middle and upper class, and further urban development by addressing issues such as congestion, housing shortages, and infrastructure deficiencies. This vision evokes colonial developmentalism and the aspirations of Fabianism and imperial agents in interwar and postwar eras. At the time, population explosion, slum-like locations, and housing shortages caused widespread concerns within and outside the colonial cities. Recalling the aspirations of African residents since the inception of colonial rule, T. M. Kwodwo Mercer, in the 1950s, stated the importance of meeting the development needs of Accra's African residents through housing and sanitation.[2] The lines of connection to Nairobi during the same period are striking. Educated Africans, Kenya's officials sympathetic to Africans, and the Master Plan expressed the need for African housing with adequate sanitation.

The Rendeavour housing projects feature mixed-income dwellings, commercial and industrial areas, schools, health centers, offices, and other community facilities. In Accra, Rendeavour envisions that Appolonia City will create a seamless live-work-play satellite city with residential, retail, commercial, educational, healthcare, and recreational facilities. The planned development includes 25,000 housing units, a 200-acre light industrial park, a 120-acre central business district, and over 300 acres of public parks and gardens.[3] A similar idea underlies Rendeavour's aims to decongest Nairobi through Tatu City's "unique live, work, and play environment."[4] When completed, Tatu City would also consist of a "mixed-use development" of medical centers, a shopping district, homes, schools, offices, "nature areas, a sports & entertainment complex, and a manufacturing area for more than 250,000 residents and tens of thousands of day visitors."[5] These projects require a significant labor force to construct and maintain them. In a sense, the projects could contribute to alleviating overcrowding and improving sanitation by redirecting sections of residents and some urban activities to the satellite cities. In another sense, they provide residents wishing to escape the congested and slum conditions in Accra and Nairobi enclaves to live and work.

When building self-contained residential communities in the colonial past, the states and municipal authorities paid little attention to the housing and sanitation of African laborers who constructed and maintained them. Victoriaborg was the first of such self-contained communities. Following the advice of an African medical expert, colonial officials developed Victoriaborg, the first enclave for Europeans exclusively to distance them from the poor sanitation in the seaside African neighborhoods of Accra where they previously lived. Victoriaborg provided Europeans with adequate amenities and infrastructure, allowing them to live, work, and socialize with little interaction with the African neighborhoods. However, colonial rule had minimal plans for improving the Ga communities that hosted the laborers who built and sustained the sanitation infrastructure and services for Europeans. Similarly, in Nairobi, the settler regime had no housing for African workers until after sanitation experts successively recommended a segregated African location. Officials established Pumwani for Africans after two decades into the twentieth century. The colonial regime gradually relocated poorer South Asians and Africans from the Nairobi market (Indian Bazaar) to protect Europeans from sanitation-related diseases that had become prevalent in the market because of poor sanitation infrastructure and municipal services.

With urbanization and recurring outbreaks of transmissible diseases, officials and experts wanted to make buffer zones as an added layer of insulation for segregated European enclaves, even as they did not provide infrastructure and municipal services in neighborhoods where Africans lived. The lag in sanitation became the official excuse to repurpose the built areas of Africans as buffer zones, but because African livelihoods were at stake, colonial officials and their technocratic advisors could not make them as envisioned. They could only fully make the buffers in less developed neighborhoods with little resistance. Western-educated Africans in Accra and wealthy South Asians criticized the colonial discriminatory policy of prioritizing adequate sanitation in European residential enclaves and neglecting the African communities. The distribution of sanitation across the urban landscapes is what this book has called the saniscape. From their inception as colonial capitals, Accra and Nairobi's complex socioeconomic classes challenged a clear cut racial attribute of the saniscape, even as sanitation services, infrastructure, and regulations in different neighborhoods were unequal. These racial and class differences found expression in disputes over the expansion of Victoriaborg east toward Christiansborg and settler efforts to relocate the Nairobi market. How the struggles played out and the respective outcomes demonstrate the varying roles of Africans in shaping the urban landscapes of Nairobi and Accra.

The sanitation outcomes of subordinating the needs of Africans to those of Europeans exacerbated in the interwar years, creating slum-like conditions in the Ga seaside communities, Zongo, Pangani, and Pumwani, even as the residents were critical in reproducing the urban and colonial economies. In Accra, the Ga people utilized their longstanding skill in navigating the turbulent seas to support import and export trade, which was central to the colonial economy. They also welcomed migrant workers, providing them land and housing to settle. The workers provided the labor for roads, sanitation, and European residential areas. These migrant workers accommodated newcomers in their neighborhoods, socialized them into urban life and helped to make the harsh living conditions of the city somewhat bearable. In Nairobi, the physical appearance of the African locations of Pangani, Kibera, and Pumwani expressed not only a deficit in sanitation but also the inability of employers to adequately house their employees and preserve Nairobi as a "white city" as settlers imagined.[6] This shortage created an opening for African entrepreneurs to provide temporary housing for many laborers who also reproduced urban economies. Without success, some of these African entrepreneurs went so far as to petition the settler-dominated municipal authority, requesting land tenure to invest in landed property and alleviate housing shortages.

Widespread use of the term "slums" to describe African locations and the hostility of the colonial systems due to the sanitation lag was a distraction from residents' lives, livelihoods, aspirations, and positive contributions to reproducing the cities' essential functions. Recent ethnographies of Accra and Nairobi have argued the dynamism of Africans in forging governance structures and (re)making Old Fadama and Kaloleni, both of which have roots in British colonial rule.[7] The residents of Old Fadama and Kaloleni in the respective books of Paul Stacy and Constance Smith show a continuation of the resilience of African residents who, living under precarity of demolition and relocation, labored to improve their neighborhood hoping that it would immobilize the municipal authority.[8] Overcrowded African communities maintained urban populations, the colonial systems' lifeline, in building and maintaining the cities and facilitating commercial activity. They were the sanitation laborers crucial to public health, the employees of colonial stores and commercial enterprises, and the road and construction workers on whom the flow of wealth within the empire relied. Yet official negative depictions of "slums" deflected from how the colonial economy invented the locations and their residents as problems that needed fixing. Attracting the influx of cheap workers without matching housing and sanitation caused overcrowding, which overstretched the few municipal services and infrastructure available in African areas, leading to slum-like conditions. However, official correspondence, expert reports, and African newspapers scapegoated African cultural and extended family systems, traditional architecture, and architectural materials as the cause and components of the so-called slums.

Official and popular discourse of the term "slum" evoked mass demolition of neighborhoods. However, the extent to which demolition was successful reflects the different histories of Accra and Nairobi as the respective capital cities of non-settler and settler colonies. The Ga communities held land tenure and could frustrate colonial urban reforms, not necessarily because they disliked change, but because the colonial regime and the Accra Town Council, controlled by colonial appointees, had repeatedly demonstrated that officials did not have the interest of Africans at heart in their plans to develop the city. Officially designating African neighborhoods as "slums" to justify demolishing them and rebuilding the city to fit into the colonial imagination of a modern capital city served the interest of a few African entrepreneurs, expatriates, and the regime. Even Western-educated Africans, who also were in favor of transforming Accra along the lines of European cities, criticized officials when they demolished African houses without providing them with alternative ones. Unlike the Ga in Accra, Pangani residents could not prevent demolishing and relocating their neighborhood despite making their property hygienic to disable municipal action. However, they demonstrated to the municipal council, which liked to think of Nairobi as a European city, that they also had rights. Contrary to the desire and expectation of the settlers in the municipality, the residents prosecuted their case for the illegal demolition of their property and received higher compensation for damages. Demolition in both cities shifted and spread the sanitation problems from one place to another, as seen in Korle Gonno and Pumwani, reinforcing the argument that colonial rule invented "slums" in the cities.

The presence of "slums" indicated housing shortages. They provide context for imperial and colonial housing initiatives during and after World War II. It is crucial to underscore the fact that the initiatives were also a testament to the determination of Accra and Nairobi residents to improve their living conditions. They refused to accept the slum-like surroundings and neglect of sanitation, which they had endured for decades, joining the empire-wide push for better living conditions across cities in colonial territories. The Watson Commission, which investigated the pivotal disturbances in Accra in 1948, gathered testimonies from African civil servants who reported experiencing racial discrimination in colonial housing policies vis-à-vis their European counterparts. Around the same period, Nairobi officials expressed concerns about severe shortages in African housing, which had echoes in interwar settler calls to properly house Africans to avoid a revolution and an upset of the colonial order.

However, housing went beyond providing a roof over people's heads. Colonial officials incorporated housing into development, relying on experts, such as urban planners and social workers, to improve living standards, drive social progress, and secure the loyalty of Africans. In other words, the housing policies spatialized development by providing educational facilities, recreational amenities, post offices, and other infrastructure in neighborhood units. They were borne out of practicality to ease widespread urban disturbances and meet local and international concerns about the desperate conditions in the cities. However, the development initiatives were too little to resolve the decades of backlog in housing needs. As a result, these grand plans did not materialize as envisioned. In Accra, Ga land tenure and determination to preserve the right to their ancestral home reduced the scale of the project. In Nairobi, settlers mismanaged housing funds in their determination to keep the city divided along racial lines. There were shortages of building materials, and construction and labor costs increased. Despite these challenges, the housing project inscribed the contours of social class into the saniscape. In both cities, communal toilets and baths increasingly became the mark of poor neighborhoods. Western-educated Africans expressed interest in and obtained self-contained residential areas with private toilets and baths.

One defining attribute of the cities' uneven saniscape was how long waste could delay, pile up, and stagnate in different residential districts. Both cities depended on manual labor and a network of material infrastructure to remove refuse and sewers from residential areas. Throughout the colonial period, African communities received minor municipal services to clear waste and maintain hygiene, stoking official and public discourse of slums threatening public health and offending sight and smell. Amid the urban protests and crisis after World War II, the accumulated refuse and stagnant sewer enabled politics of waste within the politics of anti-colonial sentiments and nationalism. Kwame Nkrumah's health minister and Accra's residents believed Africans were not at fault for the municipal and colonial neglect of removing waste from their neighborhoods and providing mass education on hygiene. After all, Accra was a city that colonial officials had claimed as their capital and the people as their subjects. Therefore, penalizing the residents through lawsuits, fines, demolitions of their neighborhoods, and forced relocation from the city center was unjust. The discourse of "slum clearance" took on a new meaning, not as demolition but as a trash cleanup exercise to educate residents on managing domestic waste and proper hygienic practices. This urban approach to sanitation casts the incoming African government as benign and better suited to deliver the development of urban residents through public health education. Accumulated waste also enabled official and public discussions of and moves to construct and add waste infrastructures in the built form of Accra to manage the sewage and smell problems the city faced. The idea of adding a sewer to Accra's built form showcased the city as the modern capital of independent Ghana.

Lack of funds, planning, and the practicality of installing sanitation infrastructure in densely developed and populated sections of Accra, and the fixation on showing the world how modern the city was posed a severe challenge and distracted the government from the dire need for a network of sewers, drains, and pipelines to clear waste in the Ga seaside neighborhoods. Thus, removing waste in these overcrowded core areas continued to challenge the city. Because waste disposal, adequate housing, and water supply remained problematic, diseases such as dysentery, enteric fever, trypanosomiasis, bilharzia, hookworm, and roundworm continued to afflict residents despite new vaccines, drugs, and insecticides controlling the incidents of malaria, tuberculosis, and yellow fever since the 1950s.[9] After independence, the population influx concentrated in these neighborhoods, and the newcomers, most of whom work in the "informal" sector near the Makola market and its environs, added to the waste challenges.[10] Less than ten years after colonial rule, the *Canberra Times* described Accra as having "gleaming new skyscrapers rise next to rusty roof hovels, beautiful residences, and stench-filled slums."[11] This description of the divided city recalls depiction of Accra by Henry Morton Stanley before it became the capital and by Simpson in the interwar period. Problems with removing waste, especially in the "stench-filled slums," persisted and have become the municipal authority's most "dysfunctional" function, opening it to the most severe criticisms of residents, the media, and international agencies.[12]

Nairobi's waste crises brought the city's sanitation system to the brink because most of the laborers were Kikuyu, who the settler state accused of causing Mau Mau. The accumulation of stagnant waste, which laborers would have cleared in less disruptive times, alerted settlers to the potential of guerilla attacks on Europeans when laborers were in the residential areas for waste removal. Mau Mau was not the first time sanitation laborers disrupted service. Harry Thuku recalls one such disruption after a mass protest in Nairobi, causing his arrest and exile.[13] The Nairobi strike of the 1950s was another event that disrupted waste removal. Ngũgĩ wa Thiong'o fictionalizes the strikes as the attempt of Africans to show the settler state that they wanted freedom.[14] Realizing the need for sanitation security enabled a municipal-wide call for Europeans to construct concrete sanitation infrastructures, such as septic tanks and sewers, to reduce manual waste removal. While encouraging Europeans to construct water-borne sanitation infrastructure in their residential locations, the state and municipal authority vetted laborers and required them to wear a distinctive uniform when clearing refuse and sewage in the segregated areas. For the African locations, officials instead encouraged barriers to prevent Mau Mau subversives, who they imagined as committing acts of sanitation vandalism and possibly engaging in guerrilla waste and germ warfare. After a few years, the constructed sanitation infrastructure transformed the saniscape of the segregated European residential areas. The physical changes were uneven compared to the African locations in Eastlands, which bore the brunt of the disruption in sanitation. Like the African seaside neighborhoods in Accra, Eastlands desperately needed these sanitation infrastructures.

Poor sanitation is a significant factor that theorists and experts consider when analyzing urbanization trends in Africa. In the second decade of the twentieth century, covered in chapter 1, about four million Africans lived in the continent's cities. By 2008, the United Nations announced a significant global shift, with 50 percent of people living in cities globally. Over 373 million Africans were part of this urban population. While more people lived in urban areas in Europe and the Americas, Africa and Asia drove this urban transition. As Laurent Fourchard has noted, the explosion in the population of cities reveals recent crucial unique urbanization processes in world history, even if there are doubts in projections that 770 million Africans will be urban residents by 2030.[15] Scholars and experts working for governments and nongovernmental organizations within and outside the continent have described this rapid urban growth in Africa as unrestrained, distinct from other urbanization processes, and pathological because of the inability of the urban economy to reduce poverty, most visible in slum-like locations. The locations prompt criticisms of African cities as pathological and dystopian. Because slum-like conditions are development issues, seemingly showing the government's inability to implement social intervention policies to alleviate them and effectively regulate the populations residing in the communities, scholars and experts have called African states "failed states" and the cities ungovernable and in crisis.[16] They became the subject of African novelists depicting corruption, pessimism, and underdevelopment based on their analysis of the urban scene in the immediate decades of the postcolonial era.[17] As detailed in the preceding chapters, sanitation and slum-like conditions in Accra and Nairobi stretch back to the colonial period. While arguing the guilt of inequity in British colonial rule's urban health policies and practices and the constraints of global economic and political order in the postcolonial period, it is crucial to acknowledge the possibilities opened to African governments at independence and after.[18]

Frankie Freeman, a recent journalism graduate at Stanford University and the Overseas Press Club's 2010 Theo Wilson scholar, witnessed a fight about to break out at the entrance to a public toilet in Ashiaman, near Accra. A man who seemed better off attempted to jump a line to use the toilet but retreated to his original position after a brief scuffle. The people ahead of him refused to allow him to use the toilet before them despite him explaining that he would be late for the office and incur the wrath of his supervisor. The man correctly asserted that waiting to use the toilet would have been a massive problem if he had diarrhea. As Freeman correctly notes, queuing to use a toilet for about twenty minutes may seem odd to many Western readers, but it is a regular occurrence in overcrowded and congested communities in Accra. Besides the humiliation in the queue, people disliked that the toilets were gender insensitive, poorly serviced, and smelled terrible.[19] Under such living conditions, the man in the scuffle to use the toilet would relocate to a high-income neighborhood with a private toilet if he could afford it. Not only would he be escaping the humiliating incident at the communal toilet and improving his standard of life, but he would also be reducing the chances of cholera infections and other sanitation-related diseases, especially in the event of flooding. In fact, people moving from overcrowded and congested neighborhoods to less dense middle-class neighborhoods after landing a better job and improved income was and still is a trend in my experience living in Accra. African discontent with urban sanitation created the market for real estate organizations like Rendeavour.

My conversation with the young, promising city planners and engineers in the Nairobi City Council reveals this discontent with poor sanitation and an aspiration for better residential infrastructure. As I mentioned, the planners and engineers disapproved of my visit to Kibera, repeating settlers' negative depictions of African locations as slums and evoking colonial justifications for demolitions. While the experts did not explicitly mention demolition as a solution, they gave me a little talk, as a foreigner, about the importance of avoiding Nairobi's "slums," like Kibera. They cited crime, diseases, congestion, and overcrowding, among other reasons, for avoiding these communities. These reasons are the sort of things that appeal to people who can afford to live in Tatu City. Although they are technocrats, the jobs of my interlocutors depend on politicians who now know that the demolition of "slums" is political suicide. During anti-colonial nationalism, African elites like Jomo Kenyatta mobilized the support of the residents of these neighborhoods toward the struggle for independence. This role of "slum" dwellers in propelling Kenyatta and his co-nationalists to power is a subject of Thomas Akare's fiction. Akare went so far as to invite readers to imagine the lives of government ministers who once were residents in the "slums" of Nairobi.[20] Kenya's politicians have turned to them for votes during elections since independence.[21] Because the complete demolition of the neighborhoods could negatively impact the political future, private developers like Rendeavour have a better prospect of seeking political support to build Tatu City in a less established and populated area outside Nairobi.

While providing jobs and helping to alleviate urban unemployment, Rendeavour's city development projects in Accra and Nairobi make housing accommodations for a small percentage of affluent urban residents who can afford their property. This book has shown how past urban developments in the two cities drew in laborers and ancillary populations but made little provision for them, leading to housing and sanitation pressures on nearby neighborhoods. In a matter of time, those neighborhoods accommodating the laborers and the accompanying populations reinvented the cycle of severe housing shortages and dreadful sanitation conditions urban theorists characterize as slums. It is worth recalling Patrick Geddes's and W. J. R. Simpson's observations about wealthy districts amid slum-like areas in cities, which this book has called the urban saniscape.

Notes

PREFACE

1. However, the research into sanitation reforms in the tropics, within which Accra and Nairobi were located, benefitted science and medicine, improving lives beyond Africa. See Helen Tilley, *Africa as a Living Laboratory: Empire, Development, and the Problem of Scientific Knowledge, 1870–1950* (Chicago: University of Chicago Press, 2011). Edward Said also makes a similar point about how Europeans drew from other parts of the world despite their perceived superiority over the "other." See *Orientalism* (New York: Vintage Books, 1979); *Culture and Imperialism* (New York: Knopf, 1993).
2. Thomas S. Gale, "The Struggle against Disease in the Gold Coast: Early Attempts at Urban Sanitary Reform," *Transactions of the Historical Society of Ghana* 16, no. 2 (January 1995): 186; Robert Home, *Of Planting and Planning: The Making of British Colonial Cities*, 2nd ed. (London: Routledge, 2013), 133–34; Colin McFarlane, "Governing the Contaminated City: Infrastructure and Sanitation in Colonial and Postcolonial Bombay." *International Journal of Urban and Regional Research* 32, no. 2 (June 2008): 415–35.
3. David Harvey, *Paris, Capital of Modernity* (New York: Routledge, 2003), 248–60; Khaled Fahmy, "Modernizing Cairo: A Revisionist Narrative," in *Making Cairo Medieval*, ed. Nezar AlSayyad, Irene A. Bierman, and Nasser Rabbat (New York: Lexington Books, 2005); Khaled Fahmy, "An Olfactory Tale of Two Cities," in *Historians in Cairo: Essays in Honor of George Scalon*, ed. Jill Edwards (Cairo: The American University Press, 2002). Reformers in New York also called for similar changes to New York during the same period. See

David M. Scobey, *Empire City: The Making and Meaning of New York City Landscape* (Philadelphia: Temple University Press, 2002).

4. Home, *Of Planting*; David Arnold, *Colonizing the Body: State Medicine and Epidemic Disease in Nineteenth-Century India* (Berkeley: University of California Press, 1993).
5. Jennifer Hart, *Making an African City: Technopolitics and the Infrastructure of Everyday Life in Colonial Accra* (Bloomington: Indiana University Press, 2024), 37.
6. Naaborko Sackeyfio-Lenoch, *The Politics of Chieftaincy: Authority and Property in Colonial Ghana, 1900–1950* (Rochester, NY: University of Rochester Press, 2014), 49–61.
7. John Parker, *Making the Town: Ga State and Society in Early Colonial Accra* (Portsmouth, NH: Heinemann, 2000), 195–201.
8. Thomas S. Gale, "Official Medical Policy in British West Africa, 1870–1930" (Unpublished PhD thesis, University of London, 1972), 66–71.
9. Herbert H. Werlin, *Governing an African City: A Study of Nairobi* (New York: Africana Publishing Co., 1974), 39–41.
10. Werlin, *Governing an African City*, 39–43; Timothy H. Parsons, "Jumping Tribal Boundaries: Space, Mobility, and Identity in Kenya," in *Mapping Migration, Identity, and Space*, ed. Tebea Linhard and Timothy H. Parsons (Cham, Germany: Palgrave Macmillan, 2019).
11. The Ga arrived in Accra at different times in bands of extended family from Ayawaso, their original capital. Ayawaso was about eleven miles northwest of Accra. When the Ga arrived, they met groups of Guans already established in the territory. As refugees, the Ga fled from a defeat in a war with the Akwamu. See Frank E. K. Amoah, "Accra: A Study of the Development of a West African City" (Unpublished MA thesis, University of Ghana, 1964), 9–25; Parker, *Making the Town*, xvii, 1–12; Sackeyfio-Lenoch, *The Politics of Chieftaincy*, 23–5; Hart, *Making an African City*, 3–9.
12. Richard R. Brand, "A Geographical Interpretation of the European Influence on Accra, Ghana since 1877" (Unpublished PhD thesis, Columbia University, 1972), 30–31.
13. Sackeyfio-Lenoch, *The Politics of Chieftaincy*, 1–2; Brand, "A Geographical Interpretation," 30–32.
14. Gale, "The Struggle," 188–89, 185–203; Sackeyfio-Lenoch, *The Politics of Chieftaincy*, 2; Parker, *Making the Town*, 97–98.
15. Parker, *Making the Town*, 100.
16. Gale, "The Struggle," 188–94; Parker, *Making the Town*, 99; Brand, "A Geographical Interpretation," 34.
17. Gale, "The Struggle," 194.
18. Parker, *Making the Town*, 141–46; Gale, "The Struggle," 196; K. David Patterson, "Health

in Urban Ghana: The Case of Accra 1900–1940." *Social Science and Medicine* 13B (1979): 251–68.

19. A Liverpool School of Tropical Medicine observer quoted in Patterson, "Health in Urban Ghana," 252.
20. Terry Hirst, *The Struggle for Nairobi* (Nairobi: Mazingira Institute, 1994), 4–13.
21. Werlin, *Governing an African City*, 37; James Smart, *A Jubilee History of Nairobi* (Nairobi: East African Standard, 1950), 13.
22. Godwin R. Murunga, "'Inherently Unhygienic Races': Plague and the Origins of Settler Dominance in Nairobi, 1899–1907," in *African Urban Spaces in Historical Perspective*, ed. Steven J. Salm and Toyin Falola (Rochester: University of Rochester Press, 2005), 104–9; Hirst, *The Struggle*, 41–45; Werlin, *Governing an African City*, 39.
23. Murunga, "'Inherently Unhygienic Races,'" 102–6; Smart, *A Jubilee History*, 13–19; Werlin, *Governing an African City*, 38.
24. Smart, *A Jubilee History*, 17; Murunga, "'Inherently Unhygienic Races,'" 108.
25. Milcah Amolo Achola, "Colonial Policy and Urban Health: The Case of Colonial Nairobi," in *The Urban Experience in Eastern Africa c. 1750–2000* Azania Special Volume XXXVI–XXXVII, ed. Andrew Burton (Nairobi: British Institute in Eastern Africa, 2002), 120; Smart, *A Jubilee History*, 17; Murunga, "'Inherently Unhygienic Races,'" 108–9; Werlin, *Governing an African City*, 40–1.
26. Achola, "Colonial Policy and Urban Health," 122; Murunga, "'Inherently Unhygienic Races,'" 105–6.
27. Kefa M. Otiso, "Colonial Urbanization and Urban Management in Kenya," in *African Urban Spaces in Historical Perspective*, ed. Steven J. Salm and Toyin Falola (Rochester, NY: University of Rochester Press, 2005), 83; British East Africa Protectorate, "Report on the Sanitation of Nairobi," 1913; Murunga, "'Inherently Unhygienic Races,'" 105–7.
28. David M. Anderson, "Corruption at the City Hall: African Housing and Urban Development in Colonial Nairobi," *Azania: Archaeological Research in Africa* 36–37, no. 1 (2010): 138–54, 140–41; Achola, "Colonial Policy and Urban Health," 122.
29. Home, *Of Planting*; Nightingale, *Segregation*.
30. Jackson and Uduku, "Sub-Saharan Africa," 407–8.
31. Ato Quayson, *Oxford Street Accra: City Life and the Itineraries of Transnationalism* (Durham, NC: Duke University Press, 2014); Anthony D. King, *Urbanism, Colonialism, and the World-Economy: Cultural and Spatial Foundations of the World Urban System* (London: Routledge, 1990). Paul Wheatley, *City as Symbol* (London: University College, 1969); Janet Abu-Lughod, "Tale of Two Cities: The Origins of Modern Cairo." *Comparative Studies in Society and History*, 7 (1965), 429–57.

32. Kwasi Kwarteng, *Ghosts of Empire: Britain's Legacies in the Modern World* (London: Bloomsbury, 2011), 3.
33. Raymond E. Dumett, "The Campaign against Malaria and the Expansion of Scientific Medical and Sanitary Services in British West Africa 1898–1910," *African Historical Studies* 1, no. 2 (1968), 166.
34. Stephanie Newell, *Histories of Dirt: Media and Urban Life in Colonial and Postcolonial Lagos* (Durham, NC: Duke University Press, 2020), 20.
35. Rob Nixon, *Slow Violence and the Environmentalism of the Poor* (Cambridge, MA: Harvard University Press, 2011).
36. Liora Bigon, *French Colonial Dakar: The Morphogenesis of an African Regional Capital* (Manchester: Manchester University Press, 2016), 1–3.
37. AbdouMaliq Simone, *For the City Yet to Come: Changing African Life in Four Cities* (Durham, NC: Duke University Press, 2004), 214.
38. Gale, "Official Medical Policy," 417–18.
39. David E. Apter, *Ghana in Transition* (New York: Atheneum, 1963), 65.
40. Samuel S. Quarcoopome, "Political Activities in Accra: 1924–1945" (unpublished MA thesis, University of Ghana, 1980), 70–9.
41. Kwame Nkrumah, *Ghana: The Autobiography of Kwame Nkrumah* (London: Panaf Books, 1957), 94.
42. Gale, "Official Medical Policy," 8–9.
43. Hirst, *The Struggle*, 84.
44. Harry Thuku, *Harry Thuku: An Autobiography with the Assistance of Kenneth King* (Nairobi: Oxford University Press, 1970), 45–6.
45. Bill Marshall, *Bukom* (London: Longman, 1979).
46. Thomas Akare, *The Slums* (Oxford: Heinemann, 1981).

INTRODUCTION

1. Gale, "Official Medical Policy," 108–10; Brand, "A Geographical Interpretation," 41–2.
2. Gale, The Struggle," 192; Richard R. Brand, "A Geographical Interpretation," 78–80; Amoah, "Accra," 71–2.
3. Gale, The Struggle," 197.
4. British East Africa Protectorate, *Report*, 12.
5. Werlin, *Governing an African City*, 37–67; R. W. Walmsley, *Nairobi: The Geography of a New City* (Kampala, Uganda: East African Literature Bureau, 1957), 22–31; Alan Gilbert, "The Return of the Slum: Does Language Matter?" *International Journal of Urban and*

Regional Research 31, no. 4 (December 2007): 697–713.

6. Jonathan Roberts, *Sharing the Burden of Sickness: A History of Healing and Medicine in Accra* (Bloomington: Indiana University Press, 2021), 116–17.
7. David Anderson, *Histories of the Hanged: The Dirty War in Kenya and the End of Empire* (New York: W. W. Norton & Company, 2005), 181–82.
8. David Harvey, "Labour, Capital, and Class Struggle around the Built Environment in Advanced Capitalist Society," in *Classes, Power, and Conflict: Classical and Contemporary Debates*, ed. Anthony Giddens and David Held (Basingstoke, UK: Macmillan, 1982), 545.
9. Janet Abu-Lughod, "Tale of Two Cities: The Origins of Modern Cairo." *Comparative Studies in Society and History* 7, no. 4 (July 1965), 429–57; Janet Abu-Lughod, *Cairo: 1001: Years of the City Victorious* (Princeton, NJ: Princeton University Press, 1971). Bissel notes that the dual city was a projection of colonial racial and cultural ideology with little basis in urban society. See William Cunningham Bissell, *Urban Design, Chaos, and Colonial Power in Zanzibar* (Bloomington: Indiana University Press, 2011), 180–81.
10. See both Khaled Fahmy's chapters on Cairo: "Modernizing Cairo" and "An Olfactory Tale."
11. Home, *Of Planting*, 133–34; McFarlane, "Governing the Contaminated City," 416.
12. Fahmy, "Modernizing Cairo"; Fahmy, "An Olfactory Tale."
13. On the role of the Industrial Revolution on public health and city planning, see Home, *Of Planting*; Ambe J. Njoh, *Urban Planning and Public Health in Africa: Historical, Theoretical, and Practical Dimensions of a Continent's Water and Sanitation Problematic* (Farnham: Ashgate, 2012).
14. Daniel R. Headrick, *The Tools of Empire: Technology and European Imperialism in the Nineteenth Century* (New York: Oxford University Press, 1981), 3–12.
15. Headrick, *The Tools of Empire*, 63–201; For the literature on the threat of diseases to Europeans, the colonial enterprise, and the measures, see Philip D. Curtin, "Medical Knowledge and Urban Planning in Tropical Africa." *The American Historical Review* 90, no. 3 (June 1985): 594–613; Raymond E. Dumett, "The Campaign against Malaria and the Expansion of Scientific Medical and Sanitary Services in British West Africa 1898–1910," *African Historical Studies* 1, no. 2 (1968): 153–97; George Oduor Ndege, *Health State and Society in Kenya* (Rochester, NY: University of Rochester Press, 2001); Kalala Ngalamulume, *Colonial Pathologies Environment and Western Medicine in Saint-Louis-du-Senegal 1867–1920* (New York: Peter Lang, 2012); Kalala Ngalamulume, "Keeping the City Totally Clean: Yellow Fever and the Politics of Prevention in Colonial Saint-Louis-du-Sénégal 1850–1914." *The Journal of African History* 45, no. 2 (2004): 183–202; Philip D. Curtin, "'The White Man's Grave:' Image and Reality, 1780–1850." *Journal of British Studies* 1 no. 1 (November 1961): 94–110; Philip D. Curtin, "The End

of the 'White Man's Grave?' Nineteen-Century Mortality in West Africa." *Journal of Interdisciplinary History* 21, no. 1 (Summer 1990): 63–88; David Arnold, "Medicine and Colonialism," in *Companion Encyclopedia of the History of Medicine*, Vol. 2, ed. W. F. Bynum and Roy Porter (London: Routledge, 1993), 1393–1415; Gale, "The Struggle."

16. Meredith Turshen, *The Political Ecology of Disease in Tanzan*ia (New Brunswick, NJ: Rutgers University Press, 1984); Randall M. Packard, *White Plague, Black Labor: Tuberculosis and the Political Economy of Health and Disease in South Africa* (Berkeley: University of California Press, 1989). For additional scholarship on the political economy of health in Africa, see James W. Brown, "Increased Intercommunication and Epidemic in Early Colonial Ashanti," in *Disease in African History: An Introductory Survey and Case Studies*, ed. Gerald W. Hartwig and K. David Patterson (Durham, NC: Duke University Press, 1978), 180–206; Benjamin Talton, "'Kill Rats and Stop Plague': Race, Space, and Public Health in Postconquest Kumasi." *Ghana Studies* 22 (2019): 95–113; Elizabeth A. Eldredge, "Drought, Famine and Disease in Nineteenth-Century Lesotho." *African Economic History*, no. 16 (1987): 61–93; Maryine Lyons, *The Colonial Disease: A Social History of Sleeping Sickness in Northern Zaire, 1900–1940* (Cambridge: Cambridge University Press, 1992); Achola, "Colonial Policy and Urban Health."
17. Thomas S. Gale, Lagos: The History of British Colonial Neglect of Traditional African Cities." *African Urban Studies*, 5 (Fall 1979), 11–24; Achola, "Colonial Policy and Urban Health"; Packard, *White Plague*; Patterson, "Health in Urban Ghana."
18. Gwendolyn Wright, "Ambiguous Modernisms of African Cities," in *The Short Century: Independence and Liberation 1945–1994*, ed. Okwul Enwezor (Munich: Prestel, 2001), 225–26.
19. Curtin, "Medical Knowledge," 594–613.
20. Thomas S. Gale, "Lagos: The History of British Colonial Neglect of Traditional African Cities," *African Urban Studies*, no. 5 (Fall 1979): 11–24; Thomas S. Gale, "Segregation in British West Africa (La Ségrégation en Afrique Occidentale Britannique)," *Cahiers d'Études Africaines* 20, no. 80 (1980): 495–507; Gale, "The Struggle," 185–203. See also Raymond E. Dumett, whose paper Curtin draws on: "The Campaign against Malaria," 153–97.
21. Maynard W. Swanson, "The Sanitation Syndrome: Bubonic Plague and Urban Native Policy 1900–1909," The *Journal of African History* 18, no. 3 (1977): 387–410.
22. Swanson, "The Sanitation Syndrome," 387–410. Swanson's other works further explain the relationship between urban sanitation, race, and disease. See Maynard W. Swanson, "'The Asiatic Menace:' Creating Segregation in Durban 1870–1900," *The International Journal of African Historical Studies* 16, no. 3 (1983): 401–21; Maynard

W. Swanson, "Urban Origins of Separate Development." *Race* x, no. 1 (1968): 31–40. Kalala Ngalamulume has expanded on this line of research, investigating how officials addressed diseases stemming from poor sanitation. See Ngalamulume, *Colonial Pathologies*; Ngalamulume, "Keeping the City," 183–202; Ambe J. Njoh also compares colonial administrative philosophies and how they influenced racialized planning policies: Ambe J. Njoh, "Colonial Philosophies, Urban Space, and Racial Segregation in British and French Colonial Africa," *Journal of Black Studies* 38, no. 4 (March 2008): 579–99; Ambe J. Njoh, *Planning Power: Social Control and Planning in Colonial Africa* (London: UCL Press, 2007).

23. For a discussion of how discourse works in a colonial society, see Timothy Burke, *Lifebuoy Lux Women: Commodification, Consumption, and Cleanliness in Modern Zimbabwe* (Durham, NC: Duke University Press, 1996), 1–36.
24. British historical epidemiologist Thomas Mckeown argues that people lived longer because of better living standards than medicine. For this Mckeown thesis, see Nancy Leys Stepan, *Eradication: Ridding the World of Diseases Forever?* (Ithaca, NY: Cornell University Press, 2011), 24–7; Thomas Mckeown, *The Modern Rise of Population* (London: Edward Arnold, 1977).
25. Roberts, *Sharing the Burden*, 135–77; Spencer H. Brown, "A Tool of Empire: The British Medical Establishment in Lagos, 1861–1905," *The International Journal of African Historical Studies* 37, no. 2 (2004): 309–43; Mari Webel, "Medical Auxiliaries and the Negotiation of Public Health in Colonial North-Western Tanzania," *The Journal of African History* 54, no. 3 (November 2013): 393–416; Arnold, "Medicine and Colonialism," 1400–1401; Iain Jackson and Ola Uduku, "Sub-Saharan Africa," in *Architecture and Urbanism in the British Empire*, The Oxford History of the British Empire Companion Series (Oxford: Oxford University Press, 2016), 407.
26. Packard, *White Plague*; Patterson, "Health in Urban Ghana."
27. Roberts, *Sharing the Burden*; John Parker, *In My Time of Dying: A History of Death and the Dead in West Africa* (Princeton: Princeton University Press, 2021); Ndege, *Health, State, and Society*. Jomo Kenyatta, *Facing Mount Kenya: The Tribal Life of Gikuyu* (New York: Vintage Books, 1965).
28. Roberts, *Sharing the Burden*.
29. Ruth Rogaski, *Hygienic Modernity: Meanings of Health and Disease in Treaty-Port China* (Berkeley: University of California Press, 2004), 2–3.
30. Rogaski, *Hygienic Modernity*, 193–224.
31. Stephanie Newell, *Histories of Dirt: Media and Urban Life in Colonial and Postcolonial Lagos* (Durham, NC: Duke University Press, 2020), 34–38.

32. Newell, *Histories of Dirt*, 54–55.
33. The following selected literature discusses racial residential segregation in African cities. See Gale, "Segregation," 495–507; Odile Goerg, "From Hill Station (Freetown) to Downtown Conakry (First Ward): Comparing French and British Approaches to Segregation in Colonial Cities at the Beginning of the Twentieth Century," *Canadian Journal of African Studies / Revue Canadienne des Études Africaines* 32, no. 1 (1998): 1–31; John W. Cell, "Anglo-Indian Medical Theory and the Origins of Segregation in West Africa," *The American Historical Review* 91, no. 2 (April 1986): 307–35; Carl H. Nightingale, *Segregation: A Global History of Divided Cities* (Chicago: University of Chicago Press, 2012); Njoh, "Colonial Philosophies," 579–99; Njoh, *Planning Power*; Susan Parnell, "Creating Racial Privilege: The Origins of South African Public Health and Town Planning Legislation," *Journal of Southern African Studies* 19, no. 3 (September 1993): 471–88.
34. Nate Plageman, "'Accra Is Changing, Isn't It?': Urban Infrastructure, Independence, and Nation in the Gold Coast's 'Daily Graphic,' 1954–57," *The International Journal of African Historical Studies* 43, no. 1 (2010): 137–59; Stephanie Newell, *The Power to Name: A History of Anonymity in Colonial West Africa* (Athens: Ohio University Press, 2013).
35. Jennifer Robinson, "A Perfect System of Control? State Power and 'Native Locations' in South Africa," *Environment and Planning* 8, no. 2 (1990): 135–62; Timothy Mitchell, *Colonizing Egypt* (Berkeley: University of California Press, 1988); Timothy Mitchell, *Rule of Experts: Egypt, Techno-Politics, Modernity* (Berkeley: University of California Press, 2002); Gwendolyn Wright, *The Politics of Design in French Colonial Urbanism* (Chicago: University of Chicago Press, 1991); Wright, "Ambiguous Modernisms"; Andrew Burton, *African Underclass: Urbanisation Crime & Colonial Order in Dar es Salaam* (Nairobi: The British Institute on East Africa, 2005); Bissell, *Urban Design*.
36. Wright, *The Politics of Design*; Bissell, *Urban Design*.
37. Burton, *African Underclass*.
38. Hart, *Making an African City*, 12.
39. Luise White, *The Comforts of Home: Prostitution in Colonial Nairobi* (Chicago: University of Chicago Press, 1990).
40. Recent scholarship on development embraces African notions of socioeconomic progress before the 1940s, pushing its chronological and conceptual boundaries beyond the colonial and technocratic ambit. See Joshua Grace, *African Motors: Technology, Gender, and the History of Development* (Durham, NC: Duke University Press, 2021); Corrie Decker and Elisabeth McMahon, *The Idea of Development in Africa: A History* (Cambridge: Cambridge University Press, 2021); Emmanuel Akyeampong, "African

Socialism; Or the Search for an Indigenous Model of Economic Development?" African Economic History Working Paper Series, No. 36/2017.

41. The colonial depictions of African residential areas as disordered from the early articulations to contemporary narratives of African cities in crisis, prompt government and international interventions. Some literature aims to counter these crisis narratives by showing the resilience of the communities. See Carole Ammann and Fill Förster, eds., *African Cities and the Development Conundrum*, vol. 10 (Leiden, Netherlands: Brill, 2018); Mike Davis, *Planet of Slums* (London: Verso, 2006); John Parker, "Urbanization and Urban Cultures," in *The Oxford Handbook of Modern African History*, ed. John Parker and Richard Reid (Oxford: Oxford University Press, 2013), 359–77.
42. Mitchell, *Rule of Experts*, 15. See Myers for a similar line of thought. Garth Andrew Myers, *Verandahs of Power: Colonialism and Space in Urban Africa* (New York: Syracuse University Press, 2003); Bissell, *Urban Design.*
43. Liora Bigon, *French Colonial Dakar: The Morphogenesis of an African Regional Capital* (Manchester: Manchester University Press, 2016); Laurent Fourchard, "Between World History and State Formation: New Perspectives on Africa's Cities," *The Journal of African History* 52, no. 2 (July 2011): 223–48; Brenda S. A. Yeoh, *Contesting Space: Power Relations and the Urban Built Environment in Colonial Singapore* (Kuala Lumpur, Malaysia: Oxford University Press, 1996).
44. PRO/CO533/117, Secretary to Treasury, April 28, 1913.
45. PRO/CO533/117, Secretary to Treasury, April 28, 1913.
46. Gale, "The Struggle"; Gale, "Official Medical Policy"; Gale, "Segregation."
47. Nightingale, *Segregation*, 1–16.
48. Ryan Johnson, "Mantsemei, Interpreters, and the Successful Eradication of Plague: The 1908 Plague Epidemic in Colonial Accra," in *Public Health in the British Empire: Intermediaries, Subordinates, and the Practice of Public Health, 1850–1960*, ed. Johnson and Amna Khalid (New York: Routledge, 2012), 143; Jonathan Roberts, "The Black Death in the Gold Coast: African and British Responses to the Bubonic Plague Epidemic of 1908." *Gateway* 3 (2001): 10–2; Home, *Of Planting*, 77–87; R. A. Baker and R. A. Bayliss, "William John Ritchie Simpson (1855–1931): Public Health and Tropical Medicine," *Medical History* 31 (1987): 450–65; G. H. Brown, "Sir William John Ritchie Simpson," *Lancet* IV (1931): 414.
49. William John R. Simpson, *Report of Sanitary Matters in Various West African Colonies and the Outbreak of Plague in the Gold Coast* (London: Darling and Sons Ltd., 1909).
50. Gale, "Segregation," 501–04; Dumett, "The Campaign against Malaria," 171–72.
51. PRO/CO96/528, Memorandum, 1913; KNADS/AG/4/14, W. J. Simpson, *Report on*

Sanitary Matters in the East Africa Protectorate, Uganda, and Zanzibar (London: Colonial Office, 1915); East African Protectorate, "Nairobi Sanitary Commission," 1913.

52. *West Africa Times*, "Sanitation and Housing: The Alternatives," May 9, 1931.
53. Harold Cooper, "West African Race Rapport Supplants 'Mosquito Politics,'" *African News* 1, no. 9 (November 1954): 4.
54. Cooper, "West African Race Rapport," 4.
55. Cooper, "West African Race Rapport," 4.
56. *West Africa Times*, "Sanitation and Housing."
57. Janet Abu-Lughod, "The Legitimacy of Comparisons in Comparative Urban Studies: A Theoretical Position and an Application to North African Cities," in *The City in Comparative Perspective: Cross-National Research and New Directions in Theory*, ed. John Walton and Louis H. Masotti (New York: John Wiley & Sons, 1976); Liora Bigon, "Urban Planning Colonial Doctrines and Street Naming in French Dakar and British Lagos c. 1850–1930," *Urban History* 36, no. 3 (December 2009): 426–48; Njoh, "Colonial Philosophies," 579–99; Mahmood Mamdani, *Citizen and Subject: Contemporary Africa and the Legacy of Late Colonialism* (Princeton, NJ: Princeton University Press, 1996); See also Adelaja Odutola Odukoya, "Settler and Non-Settler Colonialism in Africa," in *The Palgrave Handbook of African Politics Governance and Developmen*t, ed. Samuel Ojo Oloruntoba and Toyin Falola (New York: Palgrave Macmillan, 2018), 173–86; Mahmood Mamdani, "Beyond Settler and Native as Political Identities: Overcoming the Political Legacy of Colonialism," *Comparative Studies in Society and History* 43, no. 4 (October 2001): 651–64; Donald Denoon, "Understanding Settler Societies," *Historical Studies* 18 no. 73 (1979): 511–27. Kenneth Good, "Settler Colonialism: Economic Development and Class Formation," *The Journal of Modern African Studies* 14, no. 4 (December 1976): 597–620; Yu-ting Huang and Rebecca Weaver-Hightower, eds., *Archiving Settler Colonialism: Culture Space and Race* (London: Routledge, 2019); Dane Kennedy, *Islands of White: Settler Society and Culture in Kenya and Southern Rhodesia, 1890–1939* (Durham, NC: Duke University Press, 1987); Robert Bickers, ed., *Settlers and Expatriates: Britons over the Seas* (Oxford: Oxford University Press, 2010).
58. Mamdani, *Citizen and Subject*, 8.
59. For Accra, see Parker, *Making the Town*; Sackeyfio-Lenoch, *The Politics of Chieftaincy*; Hart, *Making an African City*; Roberts, *Sharing the Burden*. For Nairobi, see Werlin, *Governing an African City*; White, *The Comforts of Home*; Anderson, *Histories of the Hanged*; Parsons, "Jumping Tribal Boundaries"; Anja Kervanto Nevanlinna, *Interpreting Nairobi: The Cultural Study of Built Forms* (Helsinki, Finland: Bibliotheca Historica, 1996).

CHAPTER ONE. BUFFER ZONES, 1908–1920

1. Louis Pasteur (a French Scientist) and Robert Koch (a German doctor) confirmed the germ theory in the same period. The theory states that pathogenic microorganisms too small to see with the naked eye cause and spread diseases.
2. Dumett, "The Campaign against Malaria," 159–60.
3. David Scott, *Epidemic Disease in Ghana 1901–1960* (London: Oxford University Press, 1965), 28.
4. Nightingale, *Segregation*, 159–92; Bissell, *Urban Design*, 149–84.
5. Curtin, "Medical Knowledge," 239–41.
6. Gale, "Official Medical Policy," 233.
7. Gale, "Segregation," 495.
8. Patterson, "Health in Urban Ghana," 257.
9. Gale, "Segregation," 495.
10. Gale, "The Struggle," 198.
11. East Africa Protectorate, "Nairobi Sanitary Commission," 1913.
12. Smart, *A Jubilee History*, 32–34; Otiso, "Colonial Urbanization," 73–97.
13. East Africa Protectorate, "Nairobi Sanitary Commission," 1913.
14. PRO/CO533/192, A. M. Jeevanjee, Sanitation in Nairobi; A. M. Jeevanjee, Sanitation in Nairobi, A. M. Jeevanjee and Co. to the Land Officer, Nairobi, March 22, 1915; PRO/CO533/211, Telegram from the governor of the East Africa Protectorate to the secretary of state for the Colonies, June 16, 1919; East India (Indians in East Africa), *Correspondence in Regards the Position of Indians in East Africa* (*Kenya and Uganda*) (London: His Majesty's Stationery Office, 1921).
15. For a detailed analysis of the racist notion of Africans and South Asians as inherently dirty, see Murunga, "'Inherently Unhygienic Races,'" 98–100.
16. Gilbert, "The Return," 703.
17. Johnson, "*Mantsemei*," 143–4; Roberts, "The Black Death," 12–13; Gale, "Segregation," 498.
18. Simpson, *Report on Sanitary Matters*, 47.
19. PRO/CO96/520, Accra Rest House—Site for the Rest House: Segregation Zone, Government House, August 22, 1912; PRO/CO96/517, Site for Rest House, Accra, Government House, Accra, May 15, 1912; CO96/518, Government House, Accra, June 27, 1912.
20. Roberts, "The Black Death," 18–20.
21. PRO/CSO96/540, Segregation at Accra, Memorandum by W. J. Simpson, May 24, 1913.

22. Dumett. "The Campaign against Malaria," 166; Ross/46/0/27, Sanitation in West Africa, Fighting Tropical Diseases—Address by Professor Simpson, December 5, 1908. Sir Alfred Jones, president of the Liverpool Chamber of Commerce and chairman of the African Trade Section, invited him to the luncheon. Ronald Ross, who was also at the event, endorsed Simpson.
23. Home, *Of Planting*, 46; Gale, "Official Medical Policy, 288–91.
24. CO96/517, T. E. Rice to Principal Medical Officer Hopkins, May 9, 1912.
25. PRO/CSO96/540, Segregation at Accra, Memorandum by W. J. Simpson, May 24, 1913; PRO/CO96/528 Memorandum by Alexander Fiddian, April 18, 1913.
26. PRO/CSO96/540, Segregation at Accra, Memorandum by W. J. Simpson, May 24, 1913; Curtin, "Medical Knowledge," 602.
27. PRO/CSO96/540, Segregation at Accra, Memorandum by W. J. Simpson, May 24, 1913; Roberts, *Sharing the Burden*, 124–25.
28. Stephen Addae, *The Evolution of Modern Medicine in a Developing Country: Ghana 1880–1960* (Edinburgh: Durham Academic Press, 1997), 118–19.
29. PRO/CSO96/540, Segregation at Accra, Memorandum by W. J. Simpson, May 24, 1913; PRO/CO96/528 Memorandum by Alexander Fiddian, April 18, 1913.
30. PRO/CSO96/540, Segregation at Accra, Memorandum by W. J. Simpson, May 24, 1913; PRO/CO96/528 Memorandum by Alexander Fiddian, April 18, 1913.
31. CO96/528, Governor Hugh Clifford to Lewis Harcourt, March 8, 1913.
32. CO96/528, Governor Hugh Clifford to Lewis Harcourt, March 8, 1913.
33. PRO/CSO96/540, Segregation at Accra, Memorandum by W. J. Simpson, May 24, 1913; PRO/CO96/528 Memorandum by Alexander Fiddian, April 18, 1913.
34. PRO/CO96/528, Governor Hugh Clifford to Lewis Harcourt, March 8, 1913; Addae, *Evolution of Modern Medicine*, 64.
35. PRO/CO96/528, Governor Hugh Clifford to Lewis Harcourt, March 8, 1913.
36. Governor Mathew Nathan quoted in Dummet, "The Campaign against Malaria," 140.
37. See Dumett, "The Campaign against Malaria."
38. PRO/CSO96/540, Segregation at Accra, Memorandum by W. J. Simpson, May 24, 1913; PRO/CO96/528 Memorandum by Alexander Fiddian, April 18, 1913; Roberts, *Sharing the Burden*, 124–25.
39. Brand, "A Geographical Interpretation," 83–85.
40. PRO/CSO96/540, Segregation at Accra, Memorandum by W. J. Simpson, May 24, 1913; PRO/CO96/528, Memorandum by Alexander Fiddian, April 18, 1913.
41. PRO/CO96/528, Governor Hugh Clifford to Lewis Harcourt, March 8, 1913; PRO/CSO96/540, Segregation at Accra, Memorandum by W. J. Simpson, May 24, 1913; PRO/

CO96/528, Memorandum by Alexander Fiddian, April 18, 1913.

42. PRO/CSO96/540, Segregation at Accra, Memorandum by W. J. Simpson, May 24, 1913; PRO/CO96/528, Memorandum by Alexander Fiddian, April 18, 1913.
43. Widespread resistance to taxation stretches back to the Poll Tax Ordinance 1852. The reluctance to pay contradicted custom because the African chiefs, who were responsible for collecting the taxes, did not seek the consent of residents. The way they collected the taxes had loopholes that enriched the tax collectors, and most of the money collected paid the salaries of British officials. When residents of Christiansborg resisted strongly, the British bombed the town, causing severe casualties. James Town and Ussher Town barely escaped bombing because the British were able to manage the uprising. The British regime had to withdraw the Poll Tax in 1861. In the 1920s, the people of Christiansborg remembered this incident when the chief of Christiansborg told the officials that the residents did not want to die again from newly proposed taxation. The regime had turned the everyday person in Accra against taxation because of the bitter experience of death associated with it. See Quarcoopome, "Political Activities in Accra," 20–40.
44. Gale, "Official Medical Policy," 97–101.
45. Parker, *Making the Town*, 144.
46. Roberts, *Sharing the Burden*, 114. For a description of traditional ways of keeping sanitation, see Casely Hayford, *Gold Coast Native Institutions: With Thoughts upon a Healthy Imperial Policy for the Gold Coast for the Gold Coast and Ashanti* (London: Sweet and Maxwell Limited, 1903), 109–10.
47. PRO/CO96/514, Secretary of State to the Acting Governor, April 22, 1911.
48. Gale, "Official Medical Policy," 335–37.
49. PRO/CO96/528, Governor Hugh Clifford to Lewis Harcourt, March 8, 1913.
50. CO96/528, Memorandum, April 18, 1913.
51. Parker, *Making the Town*; Sackeyfio-Lenoch, *The Politics and Chieftaincy*; Hart, *Making an African City*.
52. *Gold Coast Nation*, "The Gold Coast Independent Olorun Fumi House, Station Road Accra, Saturday, August 3rd 1918: The Accra Town Council and the Town Councils Ordinance 1891" August 3, 1918; Gale, "Official Medical Policy," 252–54; Roberts, *Sharing the Burden*, 151–52.
53. *Gold Coast Leader*, "Editorial Notes," May 10, 1913.
54. Roberts, *Sharing the Burden*, 152.
55. *Gold Coast Leader*, "Editorial Notes," May 10, 1913.
56. Mitchell, *Rule of Experts*, 15; Wright, *The Politics of Design*, 7; Hart, *Making an*

African City. This experience fits into Bissell's and Wright's urban planning, design, and development analysis. See Bissell, *Urban Design*, 149–215; Wright, "Ambiguous Modernisms." 225–28.

57. There haven't been many changes to the public toilets to date. See Frankie Freeman, "Ghana: The Waste Land." *World Policy Institute* (2010), 47–53.
58. *Gold Coast Independence*, "The Public Health and Sanitation," August 26, 1922; *Gold Coast Independence*, "Proceedings of the Meeting Between the Ga Manche and the Manchemei and the Town Council," October 7, 1922; M. J. Field, *Religion and Medicine of the Ga People* (London: Oxford University Press, 1937), 112; Hart, *Making an African City*, 48–9; Gale, "Official Medical Policy," 71–74; Roberts, *Sharing the Burden*, 152–53; Addae, *The Evolution of Modern Medicine*, 139–40.
59. Roberts, *Sharing the Burden*, 163–4.
60. *Gold Coast Nation*, "The Gold Coast Independent Olorun Fumi House, Station Road Accra, Saturday, August 3rd, 1918: The Accra Town Council and the Town Councils Ordinance 1891" August 3, 1918.
61. *Gold Coast Nation*, "Notes and Comments: A New Segregation Theory, the Tables Have Turned," March 20, 1913.
62. *Gold Coast Leader*, "The Mosquito Eropaganda and Segregation," August 12–26, 1911.
63. *Gold Coast Nation*, "Notes and Comments," April 24, 1913; PRO/CO96/518, Government House Accra, June 12, 1912.
64. PRO/CO96/518, Government House Accra, June 12, 1912.
65. Fahmy, "Modernizing Cairo"; Fahmy, "An Olfactory Tale."
66. *Gold Coast Nation*, "Notes and Comments."
67. KNADS/AG/4/15, Investigation of Malaria and Other Tropical Diseases and the Establishment of Schools of Tropical Medicine, 1903, 18.
68. *Gold Coast Nation*, "Notes and Comments."
69. *Gold Coast Nation*, "Notes and Comments."
70. See Ato Quayson and Richard Grant for the spatial growth of Accra. Quayson, *Oxford Street Accra*; Richard Grant, *Globalizing City: The Urban and Economic Transformation of Accra Ghana* (Syracuse: Syracuse University Press, 2009).
71. PRO/CO96/528, Governor Hugh Clifford to Lewis Harcourt, March 8, 1913; CO96/528, Memorandum, April 18, 1913.
72. PRO/CO96/528, Governor Hugh Clifford to Lewis Harcourt, March 8, 1913.
73. PRO/CO96/528, Governor Hugh Clifford to Lewis Harcourt, March 8, 1913.
74. Murunga, "'Inherently Unhygienic Races,'" 105.
75. Smart, *A Jubilee History*, 14. Also for a description of the two places, see Murunga,

"'Inherently Unhygienic Races,'" 105–6.

76. Murunga, "'Inherently Unhygienic Races,'" 105; Smart, *A Jubilee History*, 14.
77. Murunga, "'Inherently Unhygienic Races,'" 106; Also see Zarina Patel, *Challenge to Colonialism: The Struggle of Alibhai Mulla Jeevanjee for Equal Rights in Kenya* (Nairobi: The Standard Ltd., 1997).
78. British East African Protectorate, *Sanitation of Nairobi*, 10.
79. Murunga, "'Inherently Unhygienic Races.'"
80. Murunga, "'Inherently Unhygienic Races.'"
81. KNADS/AG/4/14, Simpson, *Report on Sanitary Matters.*
82. KNADS/AG/4/14, Simpson, *Report on Sanitary Matters.*
83. PRO/CO96/520, Accra Rest House—Site for the Rest House: Segregation Zone, Government House, August 22, 1912; PRO/CO96/517, Site for Rest House, Accra, Government House, Accra, May 15, 1912; CO96/518, Government House, Accra, June 27, 1912.
84. KNADS/AG/4/14, Simpson, *Report on Sanitary Matters.*
85. KNADS/AG/4/14, Simpson, *Report on Sanitary Matters.*
86. British East African Protectorate, *Report on the Sanitation of Nairobi, Report on the Townships of Naivasha, Nakuru, and Kisumu by George Bransby Williams* (London: Waterlow and Sons, 1907); Nightingale, *Segregation*, 159–91.
87. PRO/CO533/192, Second Report by Sub-Committee on Simpson Scheme.
88. Werlin, *Governing an African City*, 43; Hirst, *The Struggle*, 44; Murunga, "'Inherently Unhygienic Races,'" 106–7; Patel, *Challenge to Colonialism.*
89. PRO/CO533/192, Nairobi Sanitation, Area for Asiatics, 1917; PRO/CO533/192, A. M. Jeevanjee, Sanitation in Nairobi, Second Report by Sub-Committee on Simpson Scheme.
90. KNADS/AG/4/14, East African Protectorate to Lewis Harcourt, February 2, 1915; Patel, *Challenge to Colonialism*, 111, 174.
91. British East African Protectorate, *Sanitation of Nairobi.*
92. PRO/CO533/192, A. M. Jeevanjee, Sanitation in Nairobi, A. M. Jeevanjee and Co. to the Land Officer, Nairobi, March 22, 1915.
93. PRO/CO533/211, Position of Indians, Segregation of Races, 1919.
94. PRO/CO533/192, Nairobi Sanitation, Area for Asiatics, 1917.
95. PRO/CO533/192, Nairobi Sanitation, Area for Asiatics, 1917; PRO/CO533/192, A. M. Jeevanjee, Sanitation in Nairobi, Second Report by Sub-Committee on Simpson Scheme.
96. East India (Indians in East Africa), *Correspondence*, 1920s; This is a central question in Patel's book *Challenge to Colonialism.*
97. East India (Indians in East Africa), *Correspondence*, 1920s; This is a central question in

Patel's book *Challenge to Colonialism.*

98. Werlin, *Governing an African City*, 71; Brand, "A Geographical Interpretation," 43–44.
99. Hirst, *The Struggle*, 51; Werlin, *Governing an African City*, 71.
100. East Africa Protectorate, "Nairobi Sanitary Commission," 1913, 12; White, *The Comforts of Home*, 66–7.
101. East Africa Protectorate, "Nairobi Sanitary Commission," 1913, 5. These were conservative figures, especially for Africans and the South Asian community.
102. Anderson, "Corruption," 141–42.
103. PRO/CO533/192, A. M. Jeevanjee, Sanitation in Nairobi; A. M. Jeevanjee, Sanitation in Nairobi, A. M. Jeevanjee and Co. to the Land Officer, Nairobi, March 22, 1915; British East African Protectorate, *Sanitation of Nairobi.*
104. East Africa Protectorate, "Nairobi Sanitary Commission," 1913.
105. KNADS/AG/4/14, East African Protectorate to Lewis Harcourt, February 2, 1915.
106. Swanson, "The Sanitation Syndrome."
107. Nightingale, *Segregation*, 159–91.
108. Jama Mohamed, "Epidemics and Public Health in Early Colonial Somaliland," *Social Science and Medicine* 48 (1999): 507–21; Murunga, "'Inherently Unhygienic Races.'" See also Brown, "Increased Intercommunication," 180–206; Myron Echenberg, *Plague Ports: The Global Urban Impact of Bubonic Plague between 1894 and 1901* (New York: New York University Press, 2007); Talton, "Kill Rats," 95–113.
109. Ngalamulume, *Colonial Pathologies*; Ngalamulume, "Keeping the City"; Ngalamulume, *Colonial Pathologies*; See also Njoh, "Colonial Philosophies"; Njoh, *Planning Power.*
110. Patel, *Challenge to Colonialism.*
111. For segregation before the twentieth century, see Nightingale, *Segregation.*
112. Bissell, *Urban Design*, 1.

CHAPTER TWO. SLUMS, 1920–1940

1. Davis, *Planet of Slums*, 21.
2. S. Martin Gaskell, ed., *Slums* (London: Leicester University Press, 1990), 1.
3. For more on the etymology on the word "slum," see H. J. Dyos, "The Slums of Victoria London," *Victorian Studies* 11, no. 1 (September 1967): 2–40; H. J. Dyos and D. A. Reeder, "Slums and Suburbs," in *The Victorian City: Images and Reality*, vol. I (London: Routledge & Kegan Paul, 1973), 362–63.
4. Dyos, "The Slums," 7–10, 2–40.
5. Patrick Geddes as noted in Dyos and Reeder, "Slums and Suburbs," 363.

6. Patrick Geddes as noted in Dyos and Reeder, "Slums and Suburbs," 360–61.
7. Gaskell, *Slums*, 3–4; Dyos and Reeder, "Slums and Suburbs," 359–86.
8. Gaskell, *Slums*, 3–5.
9. PRAAD/CSO 21/8/18, Memorandum: Labor in the Gold Coast, 1931; PRAAD/CSO11/1/212, Government House Accra, December 4, 1933; CSO20/12/20, Existing Situation, 1944–47.
10. PRAAD/CSO21/8/18, Memorandum: Labor in the Gold Coast, 1931; PRAAD/CSO21/8/18, Public Works Department, Supervision of Conditions Governing the Employment of Labor, 1936; Apter, *Ghana*, 163.
11. PRAAD/CSO21/8/42, Labor Conditions in West Africa—Report by Major G. S. T. J. Orde Brown, O. B. E; PRAAD/CSO 21/8/18, Accra, Gold Coast 29 Oct. 1937; Kwame Opare Akurang-Parry, "Colonial Forced Labor Policies for Road Building in Southern Ghana and International Anti-Forced Labor Pressures, 1900–1940." *African Economic History*, no. 28 (2000), 1–25; MSS.EMP.BRIT s. 332 Box 47, File 2 Colonial Development Schemes: Housing Conditions and the Development of Building Materials Industries, December 1943.
12. PRAAD/CSO 21/8/18, Memorandum: Labor in the Gold Coast, 1931; PRAAD/CSO11/1/212, Government House Accra, December 4, 1933; CSO20/12/20, Existing Situation, 1944–47.
13. PRAAD/CSO 21/8/18, Memorandum: Labor in the Gold Coast, 1931; Parker, *Making the Town*; Roberts, *Sharing the Burden*.
14. Gold Coast, *The Gold Coast Review, 1927–28*, 70; PRAAD/CSO 21/8/18, Memorandum: Labor in the Gold Coast, 1931; RAAD/CSO21/8/18, Accra, Gold Coast, October 29, 1937.
15. Kenneth O. Morgan, *Twentieth-Century Britain* (Oxford: Oxford University Press, 2000), 8–9, 16.
16. Brand, "A Geographical Interpretation," 100–102.
17. MSS.EMP.BRIT s. 332 Box 47, File 2, Colonial Development Schemes: Housing Conditions and the Development of Building Materials Industries, December 1943.
18. Gold Coast, *The Gold Coast Review: A Review of the Events of 1920–1926 and the Prospects of 1927–1928* (Accra, 1927), 121; Gold Coast, *Report to the Secretary of State for the Colonies on the Outbreak of Plague in the Gold Coast Colony and Ashanti by Professor Sir William Simpsons* (1925), 8.
19. Brand, "A Geographical Interpretation," 82.
20. Acquah, *Accra Survey: A Social Survey of the Capital of Ghana, formerly called the Gold Coast, Undertaken for the West African Institute of Social and Economic Research, 1953–1956 (London: University of London Press, 1958)*, 28; The Gold Coast, *The Gold*

Coast Review: A Review of the Events of 1920–1926 and the Prospects of 1927–1928, Accra, 1927, 121–38.

21. Gold Coast, *Outbreak of Plague*, 8.
22. PRAAD/CSO11/1/212, Medical and Sanitary Department Annual Report, 1932–33.
23. Nii-K Plange, "'Opportunity Cost' and Labor Migration: A Misinterpretation of Proletarianisation in Northern Ghana." *The Journal of Modern African Studies* 17, no. 4 (December 1979): 655–76; John Nabila, "Depopulation in Northern Ghana: Migration of the Frafra People," in *Interdisciplinary Approaches to Population Studies*, ed. Abrahams S. David, Ebenezer Laing, and Nelson O. Addo (Accra: University of Ghana, 1972), 70–83.
24. Parker, *Making the Town*, 195.
25. PRAAD/CSO11/1/212, Government House Accra, December 4, 1933.
26. PRAAD/CSO11/1/212, Government House Accra, December 4, 1933; Brand, "A Geographical Interpretation," 102.
27. Patterson, "Health in Urban Ghana," 265.
28. PRO/CO96752/12, Deputy Director of Health Service to Director of Medical Service: Slum Clearance and Building Schemes, June 20, 1938.
29. MSS.EMP.BRIT s. 332 Box 47, File 2 Colonial Development Schemes: Housing Conditions and the Development of Building Materials Industries, December 1943.
30. PRO/CO96/752/12, Deputy Director of Health Service to Director of Medical Service: Slum Clearance and Building Schemes, June 20, 1938; CSO20/12/20, Existing Situation, 1944–47.
31. Gold Coast, *Outbreak of Plague*, 7.
32. *The Gold Coast Independent*, "Kumasi New Layout: What About Accra, The Metropolis of the Colony," May 11, 1929.
33. Patterson, "Health in Urban Ghana," 265–66.
34. PRAAD/CSO21/8/18, Memorandum: Labor in the Gold Coast, 1931.
35. PRO/CO96/752, Government House Accra, 1938; PRO/CO96/752, For the Secretary of State's Signature, September 20, 1938.
36. Parker, *Making the Town*, 199; Officials often spoke about African communities in terms similar to discussions of how New York's potentials were stifled by Manhattan's "backwardness" in the second half of the nineteenth century. See Scobey, *Empire City*, 158–88.
37. PRAAD/CSO11/1/212, Government House, Accra, Enclosure 2, December 8, 1934.
38. *Times of West Africa*, "The Square that is Bukom: Populous and Neglected Area, Muddy Streets and Stagnant Square." May 13, 1933.
39. PRO/CO96/752, Slum Clearance and Rebuilding Schemes, 1938.

40. Apter, *Ghana in Transition*, 163.
41. PRAAD/CSO21/8/18, Memorandum: Labor in the Gold Coast, 1931; PRAAD/CSO21/8/18, Public Works Department, Supervision of Conditions Governing the Employment of Labor, 1936; Apter, *Ghana in Transition*, 163.
42. PRAAD/CSO21/8/18, Memorandum: Labor in the Gold Coast, 1931; PRAAD/CSO21/8/18, Public Works Department, Supervision of Conditions Governing the Employment of Labor, 1936.
43. PRAAD/CSO21/8/42, Labor Conditions in West Africa—Report by Major G. S. T. J. Orde Brown, O.B.E; PRAAD/CO96/752, Slum Clearance and Rebuilding Schemes, 1938.
44. PRAAD/CSO21/8/42, Labor Conditions in West Africa—Report by Major G. S. T. J. Orde Brown.
45. Hayford, *Gold Coast Native Institutions*, 109–10; *Gold Coast Independence*, "Proceedings of the Meeting"; *Gold Coast Independence*, "Public Health and Sanitation."
46. PRAAD/CSO21/8/18, Accra, Gold Coast October 29, 1937.
47. PRAAD/CSO11/1/212, Government House Accra, December 4, 1933.
48. PRAAD/CSO21/8/18, Memorandum: Labor in the Gold Coast, 1931.
49. The fishing industry was seasonal, making the income stream from the shipping companies crucial. Ibid.
50. PRO/CO96/752, Slum Clearance and Rebuilding Schemes, 1938.
51. PRAAD/CSO11/1/212, Medical and Sanitary Department Annual Report, 1932–33.
52. Roberts, *Sharing the Burden*, 163–64.
53. PRAAD/CSO21/8/18, Memorandum: Labor in the Gold Coast, 1931; Patterson, "Health in Urban Ghana," 260; See also Deborah Pellow, *Landlords and Lodgers: Socio-Spatial Organization in an Accra Community* (Westport, CT: Praeger, 2002).
54. RAAD/CSO21/8/18, Accra, Gold Coast October 29, 1937.
55. Gold Coast, *Outbreak of Plague*, 7.
56. PRAAD/CSO14/1/305, Accra Zongo Rebuilding Scheme: Record of Meeting at Government House, August 24, 1939.
57. Patterson, "Health in Urban Ghana."
58. PRAAD.CSO20/1/5, At the General Monthly Meeting of the Accra Town Council held at the Municipal Offices, Accra, Monday, January 14, 1935.
59. *Gold Coast Independent*, "Kumasi New Layout"; *Times of West Africa*, "The Square."
60. *Gold Coast Independent*, "Kumasi New Layout."
61. *Times of West Africa*, "The Square."
62. PRAAD/CSO21/8/18, Accra Gold Coast, October 29, 1937.
63. PRAAD/ADM11/943, The Constitution & Bye Laws of the Asere Conservative

Association, Accra, 1927; PRAAD/CSO11/1/212, Government House, Accra, November 9, 1935, Slum Clearance and Rehousing in Accra; PRO/CO96/752, Slum Clearance and Rebuilding Schemes, 1938.

64. *Times of West Africa*, The Congested Area Problem, February 13, 1935.
65. PRO/CO533/196, The question of Segregation as Between Black and White in the East Africa Protectorate, by the Honorable J. Ainsworth, 1908–1920.
66. Thuku, *Harry Thuku: An Autobiography*.
67. White, *The Comforts of Home*, 126–46; Luise White, "Prostitution, Identity, and Class Consciousness in Nairobi during World War II," *Signs* 11, no. 2 (winter 1986): 255–73.
68. The actual number of Africans permanent in Nairobi could be higher than the official figures. See Parsons, "Jumping Tribal Boundaries," 171.
69. Anderson, *Histories of the Hanged*, 188–90.
70. Smart, *A Jubilee History*, 39; Colony and Protectorate of Kenya, *Local Government Commission*, vol. 1. (London: The Crown Agents for the Colonies, 1927), 9, 14; KNADS/BY/46/4, Offices of the District Commissioner: Demolition of Pangani, June 1, 1931; KNADS/BY/46/4, Natives in Township. June 30, 1932.
71. Smart, *A Jubilee History*, 43.
72. Colony and Protectorate of Kenya, *Local Government Commission*, 7; Smart, *A Jubilee History*, 39–66.
73. Colony and Protectorate of Kenya, *Local Government Commission*, 7–12.
74. Colony and Protectorate of Kenya, *Local Government Commission*, 9.
75. Kenya Colony and Protectorate, *Annual Report of the Commissioner for Local Government, Lands, and Settlements, 1932* (Nairobi: The Government Printer, 1933).
76. KNADS/BN/56/12, Memorandum on Native Locations, October 23, 1928.
77. R. Mugo Gatheru, *Child of Two Worlds: A Kikuyu's Story* (New York: Frederick A. Praeger, 1964), 73.
78. KNADS/RN/1/68, Office of the Municipal Native Affairs Officer: Unemployment in Nairobi, December 3, 1937.
79. Parsons, "Jumping Tribal Boundaries," 168; Gatheru, *Child of Two Worlds*, 71–2; Harry Thuku is very upfront about how the Kipande made Africans angry. See Thuku, *Harry Thuku: An Autobiography*, 19.
80. KNADS/BY/46/4, Offices of the District Commissioner: Demolition of Pangani, June 1, 1931.
81. KNADS/RN/1/67, Extract from the Report of the Kenya Land Commission on Land Occupied by Natives in and around Nairobi Municipality, 1935; KNADS/BY/46/4, Office

of the District Commissioner, Nairobi: Settlement for Detribalised and Deruralised Natives, May 13, 1931; Mary Parker, *Political and Social Aspects of the Development of Municipal Government in Kenya with Special Reference to Nairobi* (Nairobi: The Government of Kenya, 1948), 82; White, *The Comforts of Home.*

82. These women are the subject of White's book *The Comforts of Home*, 132–36. KNADS/BY/46/4, Offices of the District Commissioner: Demolition of Pangani, June 1, 1931; KNADS/RN/1/67, Extract from the Report of the Kenya Land Commission on Land Occupied by Natives in and around Nairobi Municipality, 1935.
83. White, *The Comforts of Home.*
84. KNADS/BY/46/4, Office of the District Commissioner, Nairobi: Settlement for Detribalised and Deruralised Natives, May 13, 1931; KNADS/BY/46/4, Natives in Township, June 30, 1932.
85. BY/46/4, Office of the District Commissioner, Nairobi: Settlement for Detribalised and Deruralised Natives, May 13, 1931; KNADS/RN/1/67, Kenya Land Commission on Land Occupied by Natives in and around Nairobi Municipality, 1935; Parsons, "'Kibra is Our Blood': The Sudanese Military Legacy in Nairobi's Kibera Location, 1902–1968." *The International Journal of African Historical Studies* 30, no. 1 (1997): 88–89.
86. KAR stood for King's African Rifle. See KNADS/BY/46/4, Office of the District Commissioner, Nairobi: Settlement for Detribalised and Deruralised Natives, May 13, 1931; Parsons, "Kibra," 89.
87. KNADS/RN/1/67, The Following is an extract from the Report of the Kenya Land Commission, dealing with land occupied by Natives in and around Nairobi Municipality, 1935.
88. Parsons, "Kibra."
89. KNADS/BY/46/4, Office of the District Commissioner, Nairobi: Settlement for Detribalised and Deruralised Natives, May 13, 1931.
90. Colony and Protectorate of Kenya, *Local Government Commission*, 15.
91. Native House Owners in Pumwani to the Town Clerk Nairobi, November 4, 1935; KNADS/BN/73/2, Re: Native Property Owning in Nairobi, 1937.
92. KNADS/RN/1/68, Inauguration of a Municipal Pass System for Nairobi, n.d.; KNADS/RN/1/67, Report of the Kenya Land Commission on Land Occupied by Natives in and around Nairobi Municipality, 1935.
93. White, *The Comforts of Home.*
94. KNADS/BN/56/12, Memorandum on Native Locations, October 23, 1928.
95. KNADS/BN/56/12, Memorandum on Native Locations, October 23, 1928.

96. KNADS/BN/56/12, Memorandum on Native Locations, October 23, 1928.
97. KNADS/BN/56/12, Memorandum on Native Locations, October 23, 1928.
98. KNADS/AG/22/455, Pangani: Preparations for the Removal, May 2, 1935; KNADS/RN/1/68, Office of the Municipal Native Affairs Officer. Re: Unemployed Natives in Nairobi, 1938.
99. KNADS/RN/1/67, Extract from the Report of the Kenya Land Commission on Land Occupied by Natives in and around Nairobi Municipality, 1935.
100. KNADS/RN/1/68, Office of the Municipal Native Affairs Officer. Re: Unemployed Natives in Nairobi, 1938.
101. Colony and Protectorate of Kenya, *Local Government Commission*, 14.
102. KNADS/RN/1/67, Municipal Native Affairs Officer to Chairman of the Native Affairs Committee of the Nairobi Municipal Council, May 21, 1935; KNADS/RN/1/67, Native House owners in Pumwani to Nairobi Town Clerk, November 4, 1935; KNAD/RN/1/67, Extract from the Report of the Kenya Land Commission on Land Occupied by Natives in and around Nairobi Municipality, 1935.
103. *East African Standard*, "Responsibility for the African's Future: New and Statesmanlike Attitude Required," November 1, 1937.
104. Gilbert, "The Return," 700; Alan Mayne, *Slums: The History of a Global Injustice* (London: Reaktion Books, 2017), 8–9.
105. Davis, *Planet of Slums.*
106. Sackeyfio-Lenoch, *The Politics of Chieftaincy*; Parker, *Making the Town.*
107. Parsons, "Jumping Tribal Boundaries."
108. Parsons, "Jumping Tribal Boundaries," 171.
109. John Lonsdale, "Town Life in Colonial Kenya," in Andrew Burton, ed., *The Urban Experience in Eastern Africa c. 1750–2000* Azania Special Volume XXXVI-XXXVII (Nairobi: The British Institute in Eastern Africa, 2002), 207–22; White, *The Comforts of Home*, 11–12.
110. White, *The Comforts of Home*, 1–12.
111. Hart, *Making an African City*, 21.
112. The National Council of Churches of Kenya, *Nairobi Demolitions: What Next?* (Nairobi: Church House, 1991), 2–4.
113. Gale, "Official Medical Policy," 275–76, 417–32.
114. Parker, *Making the Town.*
115. Headrick, *The Tools of Empire.*
116. Anderson, *Histories of the Hanged.*
117. Anderson, *Histories of the Hanged*, 181–229.

CHAPTER THREE. DEMOLITION, 1920–1940

1. PRAAD/CSO20/12/7, International Housing and Town Planning Congress, 1935; PRO/CO96/752, For the Secretary of State's Signature, September 20, 1938.
2. *Times of West Africa*, "Gigantic Slum Clearance Scheme at Work in England" August 13, 1934; *Times of West Africa*, "Slum Clearance," November 22, 1934; *Gold Coast Independent*, "Government Housing Scheme: Plan for Repayment, Economic Condition of the Masses," January 27, 1940; Home, *Of Planting*, 65–91.
3. Gold Coast Colony, *Report on the Medical Department for the Year 1938* (Accra: Government Printing Department, 1939), 22.
4. *Times of West Africa*, "Slum Clearance."
5. PRAAD/ADM11/1/981, Report of Conference held in Accra Town Council Offices on Tuesday, November 15, 1927; Parker, *Making the Town*, 99–102.
6. W. J. Simpson, *Report on Plague in the Gold Coast in 1908* (London: J & C Churchill, 1909), 7; PRO/CO96/517, The Accra Improvement Committee's Report, 1912; PRO/CO96/517, The Accra Improvement Committee, Appendix II, 1912; PRAAD/ADM11/1/981, Report of Conference held in Accra Town Council Offices on Tuesday, November 15, 1927; *Gold Coast Independence*, "Mr. Jones Nelson Moves for Important Social Services," February 25, 1939; *Gold Coast Independent*, "Government Housing Scheme."
7. For more about the creation of new neighborhoods and expansion of Accra beyond the seaside neighborhoods, see Marion Kilson, *African Urban Kinsmen: The Ga of Central Accra* (New York: St. Martin's Press, 1974), 8; Emmanuel Akyeampong, "Bukom and the Social History of Boxing in Accra: Warfare and Citizenship in Precolonial Ga Society," *International Journal of African Historical Studies* 35, no. 1 (2002): 39–60.
8. Home, *Of Planting*, 83–91.
9. PRAAD/ADM11/943, Address of Welcome by Asere Conservatives Association Accra to His Excellency Sir Alexander Ransford Slater KCMGE Governor and Commander-in-Chief of the Gold Coast Colony, etc., July 1927.
10. *Gold Coast Independent*, "The New Accra: Plans for its Building," July 8, 1939.
11. Emphasis is mine. PRAAD/ADM11/943, Address of Welcome by Asere Conservatives Association Accra to His Excellency Sir Alexander Ransford Slater K. C. M. G. E. Governor and Commander-in-Chief of the Gold Coast Colony, etc., July 1927; PRAADADM11/943, The Constitution & Bye Laws of the Asere Conservative Association, Accra, 1927.
12. *Times of West Africa* "Korle Gonno Layout Insanitary Condition of Native Area," June 25, 1934; *Gold Coast Independent*, "The New Accra"; PRAAD/CSO20/12/20, Existing Situation, 1944–47.
13. *Times of West Africa* "Korle Gonno"; PRAAD/CSO20/12/20, Existing Situation, 1944–47.

14. For environmental racism, see Carl A. Zimring, *Clean and White: A History of Environmental Racism in the United States* (New York: New York University Press, 2015), 1–3; For how the smell of the city compelled the transformation of the built environment, see Fahmy, "Modernizing Cairo"; Fahmy, "An Olfactory Tale."
15. *Times of West Africa* "Korle Gonno."
16. PRAAD/CSO20/12/20, Existing Situation, 1944–47.
17. *The Gold Coast Independent*, "Rebuilding Accra: Government to Launch and Subsidize, A Campaign," July 1, 1939.
18. PRAAD/CSO14/1/283, Telegram, Governor, Accra, Important, Secretary of State, London, June 24, 1939; PRAAD/CSO14/1/283, Telegram, Governor, Accra, Important, Secretary of State, London, June 26, 1939. PRAAD/CSO14/1/283, Arnold Hodson to the Right Hon. Malcolm MacDonald, July 5, 1939.
19. PRAAD/CSO14/1/283, Telegram, Governor, Accra, Important, Secretary of State, London, June 24, 1939; PRAAD/CSO14/1/283, Telegram, Governor, Accra, Important, Secretary of State, London, June 26, 1939. PRAAD/CSO14/1/283, Arnold Hodson to the Right Hon. Malcolm MacDonald, July 5, 1939.
20. PRAAD/CSO11/1/212, Government House, Accra, April 19, 1940.
21. PRAAD/CSO14/1/283, Arnold Hodson to the Right Hon. Malcolm MacDonald, July 5, 1939.
22. PRO/CO96/760/13, Malcolm Macdonald to Governor Sir Arnold Hodson, KCMG, August 31, 1939.
23. PRAAD/CSO14/1/283, Arnold Hodson to the Right Hon. Malcolm MacDonald, P. C. M. P., & C., July 5, 1939.
24. KNADS/BN/56/12, Memorandum on Native Location by Municipal Engineer, 1928; KNADS/BN/56/1, The Hon. Colonial Secretary, 1926; KNADS/BY/13/162, Report on the Plague Situation in and around Nairobi, January 28, 1942.
25. Hirst, *The Struggle*, 43; Parker, *Political and Social Aspects*, 77–78.
26. KNADS/BN/56/12, Memorandum on Native Location by Municipal Engineer, 1928.
27. KNADS/BN/56/12, Memorandum on Native Location by Municipal Engineer, 1928; *East African Standard*, "Responsibility."
28. Colony and Protectorate of Kenya, *Report of the Local*, 15; KNADS/RN/1/67, Extract on Land Occupied by Natives in and around Nairobi Municipality, 1935; KNADS/RN/1/67, District Commissioner to the Town Clerk, July 10, 1934; KNADS/RN/1/67, Municipal Native Affairs Officer to Chairman of the Native Affairs Committee of the Nairobi Municipal Council, May 21, 1935.
29. KNADS/BN/56/12, Memorandum on Native Location by Municipal Engineer, 1928;

Nixon, *Slow Violence.*

30. KNADS/RN/1/67, Extract from the Report of the Kenya Land Commission on Land Occupied by Natives in and around Nairobi Municipality, 1935.
31. KNADS/RN/1/67, Municipal Native Affairs Officer to Chairman of the Native Affairs Committee of the Nairobi Municipal Council, May 21, 1935.
32. Home, *Of Planting*, 104–7.
33. KNADS/RN/1/67, Municipal Native Affairs Officer to Chairman of the Native Affairs Committee of the Nairobi Municipal Council, May 21, 1935; Anderson, "Corruption," 143.
34. White, *The Comforts of Home.*
35. KNADS/BN/56/12, Memorandum on Native Location by Municipal Engineer, 1928; White, *The Comforts of Home*, 132–40.
36. KNADS/BN/56/12, Memorandum on Native Location by Municipal Engineer, 1928.
37. Colony and Protectorate of Kenya, *Report of the Local*, 15; KNADS/BN/56/12, Memorandum on Native Location by Municipal Engineer, 1928; Parker, *Political and Social Aspects,* 80.
38. *East African Standard*, "Responsibility."
39. Parker, *Political and Social Aspects,* 82.
40. PRAAD/CSO14/1/283, Arnold Hodson to the Right Honourable Macolm MacDonald, July 5, 1939; *Gold Coast Independent*, "Small-Time Measure: A Good Job Once and for All," July 8, 1939.
41. Brand, "A Geographical Interpretation," 76–167.
42. Gold Coast traditional authorities and educated elites rally to protest the Crowns Lands Bill of 1896 and the Lands Bill of 1897. The Bills threatened land traditional tenure but the alliance against them was successful. See *Gold Coast Independent,* "Compulsory Land Acquisition: Arbitrary Taking over by Government, Ownership Privileges Seriously Affected," August 19, 1939; *Gold Coast Independent,* "Compulsory Land Acquisition."; Parker, *Making the Town*, 195–201; Sackeyfio-Lenoch, *The Politics of Chieftaincy*, 51–54.
43. Brand, "A Geographical Interpretation," 76–167; PRAAD/CSO14/1/283, Arnold Hodson to the Right Hon. Malcolm MacDonald, July 5, 1939; *Gold Coast Independent,* "Small-Time Measure."
44. Parker, *Making the Town*, 102–7, 169–86, 205–10; Hart, *Making an African City*, 12–29.
45. PRAAD/ADM11/1/981, Report of Conference held in Accra Town Council Offices on Tuesday, November 15, 1927; PRO/CO96/752/12, Enclosure in the Gold Coast No. 540: Slum Clearance and Rebuilding Scheme, August 12, 1938; Parker, *Making the Town*, 199.
46. The councilor referred to the plague examined at the beginning of this book as officially

declared in 1908. *Gold Coast Independence*, "Mr. Jones Nelson."

47. PRO/CO96/752/12, Enclosure in the Gold Coast No. 540 of Slum Clearance and Rebuilding Scheme, August 12, 1938.
48. PRO/CO96/752/12, Acting Governor to The Right Honorable Malcolm MacDonald, August 12, 1938.
49. PRO/CO96/752/12, Acting Governor to The Right Honorable Malcolm MacDonald, August 12, 1938.
50. *Gold Coast Independent*, "The New Accra."
51. *Gold Coast Independent,* Compulsory Land Acquisition."
52. PRO/CO96/752/12, Enclosure in the Gold Coast No. 540 of Slum Clearance and Rebuilding Scheme, August 12, 1938.
53. Parker, *Making the Town*, 117; Waseem-Ahmed Bin-Kasim, "Politics of Disaster: Earthquake, Rehousing, and Confronting Colonial Rule in Accra (Gold Coast/Ghana), 1939–45." *The Journal of African History* 64, no. 2 (2023): 292–305.
54. *Gold Coast Independent*, "The Ga Manche Broadcasts on Earthquake Disasters," July 22, 1939.
55. PRO/CO96/752/12, Enclosure in the Gold Coast No. 540 of Slum Clearance and Rebuilding Scheme, August 12, 1938; PRAAD/CSO14/1/283, Arnold Hodson to the Right Hon. Malcolm MacDonald, July 5, 1939.
56. *Gold Coast Independent*, "The New Accra."
57. *Gold Coast Independent*, "The New Accra."; *Gold Coast Independent*, "Ga Manche Broadcasts."
58. *Gold Coast Independent*, "The New Accra."
59. *Gold Coast Independent,* "Compulsory Land Acquisition."
60. The stool was the symbol of chiefly authority. *Gold Coast Independent,* "Compulsory Land Acquisition."
61. *Gold Coast Independent*, "Accra Town Council," January 27, 1940.
62. *Gold Coast Independent*, "Ga Manche Broadcasts."
63. *Gold Coast Independent*, "Fishermen Meet on Removal of Fishing industry to Chorker: Young Men Object," July 15, 1939.
64. PRO/CO96/752/12, For the Secretary of State's Signature, September 20, 1938.
65. PRO/CO96/752/12, For the Secretary of State's Signature, September 20, 1938; *Gold Coast Independent*, "Ga Manche Broadcasts."
66. *Gold Coast Independent*, "Fishermen Meet with Theodore Taylor on New Fishing Township" July 22, 1939.
67. *Gold Coast Independent*, "Fishermen Meet with Theodore."

68. *Gold Coast Independent,* "The Accra Town Council and Demolition of Houses," January 13, 1940.
69. *Gold Coast Independent,* "Neither Government nor Council is Prepared to Advance Money to House Owners to Rebuild," December 30, 1939.
70. *Gold Coast Independent,* "Accra Town Council and Demolition."
71. *Gold Coast Independent,* "Neither Government nor Council."
72. PRAAD/CSO14/1/283, Arnold Hodson to the Right Hon. Malcolm MacDonald, June 30, 1939; *Gold Coast Independent,* "Rebuilding Accra"; *Gold Coast Independent,* "Rebuilding Accra"; PRAAD/CSO14/1/283, Arnold Hodson to the Right Hon. Malcolm MacDonald, July 5, 1939.
73. *Gold Coast Independent,* "Unofficial Councilors Protests Against Indiscriminate Demolition," January 13, 1940; *Gold Coast Independent,* "Clearing Up the Areas: First Steps to Rebuild Accra, Flaws in the Scheme," January 20, 1940.
74. *Gold Coast Independent,* "Unofficial Councilors"; *Gold Coast Independent,* "Clearing Up the Areas."
75. *Gold Coast Independent,* "Clearing Up the Areas."
76. PRAAD/CSO20/1/80, Malcolm MacDonald to Governor Sir Arnold Hodson KCMG, March 30, 1940.
77. PRAAD/CSO20/12/14, Lands Department to the Honourable Colonial Secretary, Town Planning—Post-War Development, March 4, 1943.
78. PRAAD/CSO20/12/14, S. S. S. to Colonial Secretary, August 30, 1943; PRAAD/CSO20/12/14, Lands Department to the Hon. Colonial Secretary, Town Planning—Post-War Development, March 4, 1943.
79. PRAAD/CSO20/12/14, Telegram, Secretary of States for the Colonies to the Resident Minister, September 4, 1943; PRAAD/CSO20/12/14, Government House to The Right Hon. the Viscount Cranborne, May 20, 1940; PRAAD/CSO20/12/12, Slum Clearance, 1942–43.
80. PRAAD/CSO20/12/20, Existing Situation, 1944–47.
81. PRAAD/CSO20/12/14, Commissioner of Lands to the Hon. Colonial Secretary, Town Planning, January 12, 1945.
82. PRAAD/CSO20/12/20, Preface, 1944–47.
83. Colony and Protectorate of Kenya, *Report of the Local,* 15; KNADS/RN/1/67, District Commissioner to the Town Clerk, July 10, 1934; KNADS/RN/1/67, Municipal Native Affairs Officer to Chairman of the Native Affairs Committee of the Nairobi Municipal Council, May 21, 1935; KNADS/RN/1/67, Extract from Report of the Kenya Land Commission on Land Occupied by Natives in and around Nairobi Municipality, 1935.

84. The *East African Standard,* January 27, 1923 quoted in Parker, *Political and Social Aspects,* 81.
85. KNADS/AG/22/455, Pangani: Preparations for the Removal, May 2, 1935; KNADS/RN/1/67, Extract from the Report of the Kenya Land Commission on Natives in and around Nairobi Municipality, 1935.
86. KNADS/AG/22/455, Pangani—Preparation for the Removal, May 2, 1935.
87. KNADS/RN/1/67, Municipal Native Affairs Officer to Chairman of the Native Affairs Committee of the Nairobi Municipal Council, May 21, 1935; KNADS/RN/1/67, Report of Native Affairs Committee Meeting Held December 6, 1935.
88. KNADS/RN/1/67, Municipal Native Affairs Officer to Chairman of the Native Affairs Committee of the Nairobi Municipal Council, May 21, 1935; KNADS/RN/1/67, Municipal Native Affairs Officer to Chairman of the Native Affairs Committee of the Nairobi Municipal Council, May 21, 1935.
89. Parker, *Political and Social Aspects,* 82; KNADS/RN/1/67, District Commissioner to the Town Clerk, July 10, 1934; KNADS/RN/1/67, Municipal Native Affairs Officer to Chairman of the Native Affairs Committee of the Nairobi Municipal Council, May 21, 1935; KNADS/RN/1/67, Extract from the Report of the Kenya Land Commission on Natives in and around Nairobi Municipality, 1935; White, *The Comforts of Home,* 132.
90. It is unclear how Juma's Islamic faith forbade him from signing and writing a minority report; KNAD/RN/1/67, Municipal Native Affairs Officer to Chairman of the Native Affairs Committee of the Nairobi Municipal Council, May 21, 1935.
91. KNADS/RN/1/67, Municipal Native Affairs Officer to Chairman of the Native Affairs Committee of the Nairobi Municipal Council, May 21, 1935.
92. *East African Standard,* "Responsibility."
93. KNADS/RN/1/67, Municipal Native Affairs Officer to Chairman of the Native Affairs Committee of the Nairobi Municipal Council, May 21, 1935.
94. KNADS/RN/1/67, Municipal Native Affairs Officer to Chairman of the Native Affairs Committee of the Nairobi Municipal Council, May 21, 1935; KNAD/RN/1/67, Native House owners in Pumwani to Nairobi Town Clerk, November 4, 1935; KNADS/RN/1/67, Extract from the Report of the Kenya Land Commission on Land Occupied by Natives in and around Nairobi Municipality, 1935.
95. KNADS/BN/73/2, Native Purchases of Land, Nairobi Township; KNADS/RN/1/67, Dyer to The Town Clerk, Nairobi, August 24, 1935; KNAD/RN/1/67, Re: Mohamed Bin Muthiheri, August 28, 1935; KNADS/RN/1/67, Native House owners in Pumwani to Nairobi Town Clerk, November 4, 1935.
96. KNADS/RN/1/67, Native House owners in Pumwani to Nairobi Town Clerk, November 4, 1935.

97. KNAD/RN/1/67, Report of Native Affairs Committee Meeting Held, December 6, 1935.
98. KNADS/RN/1/67, Extract from the Report of the Kenya Land Commission on Land Occupied by Natives in and around Nairobi Municipality, 1935.
99. Parker, *Political and Social Aspects*, 80.
100. KNADS/RN/1/67, Municipal Native Affairs Officer to Chairman of the Native Affairs Committee of the Nairobi Municipal Council, May 21, 1935; KNADS/RN/1/67, Report of Native Affairs Committee Meeting, December 6, 1935.
101. Parker, *Political and Social Aspects*, 87–88.
102. KNADS/RN/1/67, Extract from the Report of the Kenya Land Commission on Land Occupied by Natives in and around Nairobi Municipality, 1935; Parker, *Political and Social Aspects*, 97.
103. KNADS/AG/22/455, District Commissioner to The Hon. Attorney General Nairobi, April 11, 1935; Parker, *Political and Social Aspects*, 87–88.
104. KNADS/AG/22/455, Crown Council to the Hon. the CLG., June 7, 1939; Parker, *Political and Social Aspects*, 87–88.
105. KNADS/AG/22/455, Hon. Attorney General. 20–5–39; KNAD/AG/22/455, Extract from the Secretariat File No. LND. 7/3/4/2 III, April 13, 1939.
106. KNADS/RN/1/67, Municipal Native Affairs Officer to Chairman of the Native Affairs Committee of the Nairobi Municipal Council, May 21, 1935; Parker, *Political and Social Aspects*, 81, 87–88; White, *The Comforts of Home*, 132.
107. KNAD/HAK1/5/177, *East African Standard*, "Mayor on Nairobi's Slum Conditions: Council Prepared for any Project If Clear Policy is Laid Down,' July 28, 1943.
108. *East African Standard*, "Mayor on Nairobi's Slum."
109. *East African Standard*, "Mayor on Nairobi's Slum."
110. G. C. W. Ogilvie. *The Housing of Africans in the Urban Areas of Kenya* (Nairobi: The Kenya Information Office, 1946), 15.
111. See the preface of Ogilvie, *Housing of Africans*.
112. Ogilvie. *Housing of Africans*, 15.
113. Hart, *Making an African City*, 12.
114. Home, *Of Planting*, 66.
115. Parker, *Making the Town*; Bin-Kasim, "Politics of Disaster."
116. Burke, *Lifebuoy Men, Lux Women*, 3.
117. Murunga, "'Inherently Unhygienic Races.'"
118. Parsons, "Jumping Tribal Boundaries," 170–73.
119. Robinson, "Perfect System of Control?"; Myers, *Verandahs of Power*.
120. Gwendolyn Wright, "Ambiguous Modernisms," 225.

CHAPTER FOUR. HOUSING, 1940–1952

1. See footnote 16 in Luce Beeckmans, "The 'Development Syndrome': Building and Contesting the SICAP Housing Schemes in French Dakar (1951–1960)." *Canadian Journal of African Studies/Revue canadienne des études africaines,* 51:3 (2017), 359–88.
2. PRAAD/CSO20/12/20, Accra Town Plan, 1945; L. W. Thornton White, L. Silberman, and P. R. Anderson, *Nairobi Master Plan for a Colonial Capital: A Report Prepared for the Municipal Council of Nairobi* (London: His Majesty's Stationary Office, 1948).
3. Beeckmans, "The 'Development Syndrome'"; Andrew Burton, "Townsmen in the Making: Social Engineering and Citizenship in Dar es Salaam, c. 1945–1960," *The International Journal of African Historical Studies* 36, no. 2 (2003): 331–65; Swanson, "The Sanitation Syndrome."
4. Home, *Of Planting*, 125.
5. PRAAD/CSO20/12/14, Colonial Secretary Gold Coast to Colonial Secretary Trinidad, October 11, 1943; Peter Fryer, *Black People in the British Empire: An Introduction* (London: Pluto Press, 1988); Home, *Of Planting*, 192–93.
6. Richard Harris, "From Trusteeship to Development: How Class and Gender Complicated Kenya's Housing Policy, 1939–1963," *Journal of Historical Geography* 34 (2008): 314–27; Home, *Of Planting*, 193–212.
7. Thomas Hodgkin, *Nationalism in Colonial Africa* (New York: New York University Press, 1957), 63–83; Dennis Austin, *Politics in Ghana 1946–1960* (London: Oxford University Press, 1970), 11–13; Home, *Of Planting*, 190–91.
8. Timothy H. Parsons, *The Second British Empire: In the Crucible of the Twentieth Century* (Lanham, MD: Rowman & Littlefield, 2014), 143–95; Jean Allman, "Between the Present and History: African Nationalism and Decolonization." In *The Oxford Handbook of Modern African* History, ed. John Parker and Richard Reid, (Oxford: Oxford University Press, 2013), 224–40.
9. *Gold Coast Independent*, "Sanitary and Housing Conditions," July 13, 1929; Fabian Colonial Bureau was founded in 1940 to facilitate research and development that would inform colonial policy. MSS.EMP.BRIT s. 332 Box 47, File 2, Fabian Colonial Bureau: Colonial Development Schemes with Special Reference to Housing Conditions and the Development of Building Materials Industries, 1942.
10. *Gold Coast Independent*, "Sanitary and Housing Conditions."
11. *Gold Coast Independent*, "Sanitary and Housing Conditions."
12. The following scholarship provides a more expansive meaning of development and uses it to link colonial to postcolonial states. Frederick Cooper, *Africa Since 1940: The Past of the Present*, 2nd ed. (New York: Cambridge University Press, 2019); Akyeampong, "African

Socialism"; Ammann and Förster, *African Cities*; Decker and McMahon, *The Idea of Development.*

13. Ogilvie, *Housing of Africans*, 54; Colony and Protectorate of Kenya, *Report on African Housing in Townships and Trading Centres* by E. A. Vasey CMG (Nairobi: The Government Printer, 1950); B. D. Dorkenoo, "Real Solution to Housing Problem," *Daily Graphic*, January 20, 1955. KNAD/RN/1/96, F. A. Passells (City African Affairs Officer): African Housing in Nairobi, July 15, 1952; KNADS/RN/1/96, Memorandum to the Right Hon. Oliver Lyttleton M. P. Secretary of State for the Colonies, October 5, 1952; Ghana Information Services, *Ten Great Years* (Accra: Ghana Information Service, 1960).
14. Burton, "Townsmen in the Making," 331–65; Harris, "From Trusteeship to Development."
15. Roger S. Gocking, *The History of Ghana* (Westport, CT: Greenwood Press, 2005), 83–4; W. E. F. Ward, *A History of Ghana* (London: George Allen and Unwin Ltd., 1958), 340–42.
16. Colonial Office, *Report of the Commission of Enquiry into Disturbances in the Gold Coast 1948* (London: His Majesty's Stationery Office, 1948), 7–8, 63, 68.
17. Colonial Office, *Report of the Commission.*
18. Creech Jones made the statement before becoming Secretary of State for the Colonies; Creech Jones MSS.EMP.BRIT s. 332 Box 47, File 2, General Aspects of the Housing Problem in the Colonial Empire, January 1942.
19. John Lonsdale, "Kenya: Home County and African Frontier," in *Settlers and Expatriates: Britons over the Seas,* ed. Robert Bickers (Oxford: Oxford University Press, 2010); Anderson, *Histories of the Hanged,* 9–53, 181–229; Dave Hyde, "The Nairobi General Strike [1950]: From Protest to Insurgency," in *The Urban Experience in Eastern Africa, ed. Andrew Burton (Nairobi: British Institute in Eastern Africa, 2002*), 235–53.
20. Ogilvie, *Housing of Africans*, 15.
21. *East African Standard,* "Nairobi to Argue with Government over Housing Burden," October 30, 1952.
22. *East African Standard,* "Nairobi to Argue."
23. KNADS/RN/1/96, Memorandum to the Right Hon. Oliver Lyttleton M. P. Secretary of State for the Colonies, October 5, 1952.
24. KNADS/RN/1/96, Memorandum to the Right Hon. Oliver Lyttleton M. P. Secretary of State for the Colonies, October 5, 1952.
25. PRAAD/RG5/1/245, Gold Coast, Report of the Accra Earthquake Rehousing Committee, 1940.
26. PRAAD/RG5/1/245, Gold Coast, Report of the Accra Earthquake Rehousing Committee, 1940; PRAAD/CSO20/1/112, Untitled, Mary 4, 1942; PRAAD/CSO14/1/329, Notice: Accra Rehousing Scheme, 1940; Gold Coast, *Gold Coast Review,* 1950, 36–38; *Daily*

Graphic, "Houses will be Ready Soon," March 12, 1955; *Daily Graphic*, "161 Employees of Housing Department to be Sacked," March 12, 1955.

27. PRAAD/RG5/1/245, Gold Coast, Report of the Accra Earthquake Rehousing Committee, 1940; PRAAD/CSO20/1/112, Accra Rehousing Scheme: Progress Report—February 1944; PRAAD/CSO20/1/77, Accra Rehousing Scheme—2nd Report, Part I, Introduction, 1948.
28. PRAAD/RG5/1/245, Gold Coast, Report of the Accra Earthquake Rehousing Committee, 1940.
29. See Naaborko Sackeyfio-Lenoch for land tenure, landed property, and urban development in Accra. Naaborko Sackeyfio-Lenoch, "The Politics of Land and Urban Space in Colonial Accra," *History in Africa* 39 (2012): 293–329; Sackeyfio-Lenoch, *The Politics of Chieftaincy*.
30. PRAAD/RG5/1/245, Gold Coast, Report of the Accra Earthquake Rehousing Committee, 1940.
31. PRAAD/RG5/1/245, Gold Coast, Report of the Accra Earthquake Rehousing Committee, 1940.
32. Wright, "Ambiguous Modernisms," 225; Bissell, *Urban Design*.
33. PRAAD/CSO20/1/77, Accra Rehousing Scheme—2nd Report, Part I, Introduction, 1948.
34. PRAAD/CSO20/1/77, Accra Rehousing Scheme—2nd Report, Part I, Introduction, 1948.
35. PRAAD/CSO 20/1/94, E. A. Tagoe for the Tagoe Brothers to the Colonial Secretary, June 16, 1941; PRAAD/CSO/20/1/121, Odate Sakyi to the chairman of the rehousing committee, September 14, 1943; PRAAD CSO/20/1/213, West and North-West Korle Gonno New Settlement Union to the Acting Colonial Secretary, November 12, 1943. Also see Bin-Kasim, "Politics of Disaster."
36. PRAAD/RG5/1/245, Gold Coast, Report of the Accra Earthquake Rehousing Committee, 1940; PRAAD/CSO20/1/112, Accra Rehousing Scheme: Progress Report—February 1944; PRAAD/CSO20/1/77, Accra Rehousing Scheme—2nd Report, Part I, Introduction, 1948.
37. PRAAD/CSO14/1/329, Chairman of Accra Rehousing Committee to the Colonial Secretary Accra, March 20, 1940; PRAAD/CSO14/1/329, Government Sociologist, The Income of Fishermen, March 29, 1940.
38. PRAAD/CSO14/1/329, Untitled, July 14, 1942.
39. PRAAD/CSO14/1/329, Untitled, July 14, 1942.
40. *Daily Graphic*, "161 Employees"; Bin-Kasim, "Politics of Disaster."
41. Harris, "From Trusteeship to Development," 312; Wright, "Ambiguous Modernisms." 225–26.

42. PRAAD/CSO14/1/329; Government Sociologist, The Income of Fishermen, March 29, 1940; PRAAD/CSO14/1/329, Untitled, July 14, 1942.
43. PRAAD/RG5/1/245, Gold Coast, Report of the Accra Earthquake Rehousing Committee, 1940.
44. PRAAD/RG5/1/245, Gold Coast, Report of the Accra Earthquake Rehousing Committee, 1940.
45. PRAAD/RG5/1/245, Gold Coast, Report of the Accra Earthquake Rehousing Committee, 1940.
46. PRAAD/CSO20/12/14, The Secretary of States for the Colonies, August 25, 1943; PRAAD/CSO20/12/14, Secretary of State for the Colonies, September 4, 1943; PRAAD/CSO20/12/14, Mr. Maxwell Fry, Town Planning Adviser for West Africa, December 29, 1943.
47. PRAAD/CSO20/12/14, E. Maxwell Fry to the Minister, Town Planning, June 15,1944. PRAAD/CSO20/12/14, Memorandum for the 5th Meeting of the Civil Members Committee to be Held on the Appointment of Town Planning Adviser for West Africa, February 1, 1944.
48. PRAAD/CSO20/12/20, Accra Town Plan 1944–47; PRAAD/CSO14/3/489, Secretary for Social Services to the Colonial Secretary: Housing Schemes, May 23, 1944; Office of the Secretary and Executive Office Accra, "Town and Country Planning in the Gold Coast" Bulletin No. 2.
49. PRAAD/CSO20/12/20, Accra Town Plan 1944–47; Ministry of Housing, *Accra: A Plan for the Town* (Accra: Government Printer, 1958); Office of the Secretary and Executive Office Accra, "Town and Country Planning in the Gold Coast" Bulletin No. 2.
50. PRAAD/CSO20/12/20, Accra Town Plan, 1945.
51. PRAAD/CSO20/12/20, Accra Town Plan, 1945; Office of the Secretary and Executive Office Accra, "Town and Country Planning in the Gold Coast," Bulletin No. 2.
52. PRAAD/CSO20/12/14, Town Planning in the Gold Coast: Memorandum by the Secretary and Executive Officer to the Town and Country Planning Board.
53. PRAAD/CSO20/12/20, Accra Town Plan 1944–47; PRAAD/CSO14/3/489, Secretary for Social Services to the Colonial Secretary: Housing Schemes, May 23, 1944; Office of the Secretary and Executive Office Accra, "Town and Country Planning in the Gold Coast" Bulletin No. 2.
54. PRAAD/CSO20/1/160, Meeting of Accra Town Council, May 22, 1945.
55. PRAAD/CSO20/1/130, The Christiansborg Estate Council, April 7, 1945; Beeckmans, "The 'Development Syndrome.'"
56. PRAAD/CSO20/1/130, The Christiansborg Estate Council, April 7, 1945.

57. Gold Coast, *Gold Coast Review* (1950), 37–38.
58. PRAAD/ CSO20/1/160, Meeting of Accra Town Council, May 22, 1945.
59. PRAAD/CSO20/1/162, Meeting of Accra Town Council, October 16, 1945.
60. PRAAD/CSO20/1/112, Accra Rehousing Scheme: Progress Report—February 1944; PRAAD/CSO20/1/77, Accra Rehousing Scheme—2nd Report, Part I, Introduction, 1948.
61. Melville J. Herskovits Library of African Studies Northwestern University Africana Vertical Files (NUAVF), T. M. Kodwo Mercer, "The Gold Coast Development Programme," October 1955.
62. Melville J. Herskovits Library of African Studies Northwestern University Africana Vertical Files (NUAVF), T. M. Kodwo Mercer, "The Gold Coast Development Programme," October 1955.
63. Cooper, *Africa*, 59.
64. PRAAD/CSO20/1/160, Meeting of Accra Town Council, June 19, 1945.
65. PRAAD/CSO20/1/160, Meeting of Accra Town Council, May 22, 1945.
66. PRAAD/CSO20/1/160, Meeting of Accra Town Council, May 22, 1945.
67. PRAAD/CSO20/1/160, Meeting of Accra Town Council, June 26, 1945.
68. PRAAD/CSO20/1/77, Accra Rehousing Scheme—2nd Report, Part I, Introduction, 1948.
69. Acquah, *Accra Survey*, 60; *New Ghana*, "'Accra Survey' is Title of New Book," January 14, 1959.
70. PRAAD/CSO20/1/77, Accra Rehousing Scheme—2nd Report, Part I, Introduction, 1948; Acquah, *Accra Survey*, 60.
71. Acquah, *Accra Survey*, 60; PRAAD/CSO20/1/77, Accra Rehousing Scheme—2nd Report, Part I, Introduction, 1948.
72. Anderson, "Corruption," 138–40; Anderson, *Histories of the Hanged*, 138.
73. Colony and Protectorate of Kenya, *Report on African Housing*, 2; Gold Coast, *Gold Coast Review*; Harris, "From Trusteeship to Development," 327.
74. KNADS/HAK1/5/177, Oliver Stanley to Moore, January 5, 1943; Ogilvie, *Housing of Africans*, 16–62; KNADS/RN/1/96, African Locations: Nairobi City Council Housing Schemes; KNADS/RN/1/72, N. M. Deverell, Municipal African Housing Part I: Departmental Housing, 1 August 1948.
75. Ogilvie, *Housing of Africans*, 27.
76. KNADS/HAK1/5/177, Oliver Stanley to Moore, January 5, 1943; Ogilvie, *Housing of Africans*, 16–62; KNADS/RN/1/96, African Locations: Nairobi City Council Housing Schemes; KNADS/RN/1/72, N. M. Deverell, Municipal African Housing Part I: Departmental Housing, August 1, 1948.
77. KNADS/HAK1/5/177, *East African Standard*, "Mayor on Nairobi's Slum."

78. Ogilvie, *Housing of Africans*, 16–38.
79. Ogilvie, *Housing of Africans*, 19–28.
80. Parker, *Political and Social Aspects*, 90–1; Ogilvie, *Housing of Africans*, 16–26.
81. Ogilvie, *Housing of Africans*, 27–34.
82. Parker, *Political and Social Aspects*, 90–1; Ogilvie, *Housing of Africans*, 16–26; Colony and Protectorate of Kenya, *Report on African Housing*.
83. While the success of the engineering and architectural measures is not within the scope of this work, the following chapter delves into how the environmental characteristics, coupled with the inadequate or lack of municipal services, significantly worsened the already unsanitary conditions in the neighborhoods. See Ogilvie, *Housing of Africans*, 27–31; Parker, *Political and Social Aspects*, 96–7; KNAD/RN/1/96, African Locations: Nairobi City Council Housing Schemes.
84. White, Silberman, and Anderson, *Nairobi Master Plan*, 36; Ogilvie, *Housing of Africans*, 27–28, 54.
85. Colony and Protectorate of Kenya, *Report on African Housing*, 14. Ogilvie, *Housing of Africans*, 27–28, 54.
86. Colony and Protectorate of Kenya, *Report on African*, 2–3.
87. Colony and Protectorate of Kenya, *Report on African*, 2–3.
88. KNADS/RN/1/96, F. A. Passells (City African Affairs Officer): African Housing in Nairobi, July 15, 1952; KNADS/RN/1/96, African Locations: Nairobi City Council Housing Schemes.
89. Harris, "From Trusteeship to Development," 327.
90. KNADS/RN/1/96, T. C. Colchester (Chairman of Central Housing Board), Central Housing Board, January 29, 1954.
91. KNADS/RN/1/96, F. A. Passells (City African Affairs Officer): African Housing in Nairobi, July 15, 1952; KNADS/RN/1/96, African Locations: Nairobi City Council Housing Schemes.
92. KNADS/RN/1/96, F. A. Passells (City African Affairs Officer): African Housing in Nairobi, July 15, 1952; KNADS/RN/1/96, African Locations: Nairobi City Council Housing Schemes.
93. Colony and Protectorate of Kenya, *Report on African Housing*, 6.
94. Harris, "From Trusteeship to Development," 316.
95. Harris, "From Trusteeship to Development," 327–37.
96. KNADS/HAK1/5/177, Memorandum, n.d.
97. KNADS/RN/1/77, African Housing Scheme for Nairobi, May 13, 1955; KNADS/RN/1/77, Minister of Local Government Health and Housing to the Town Clerk Nairobi, May 9, 1955.

98. KNADS/HAK1/5/470, Housing for Senior African Officer of Government in Nairobi, June 30, 1960.
99. KNADS/BY/40/2, "Education and Standard of Living in Relation to African Housing" by Mr. Nahashon Mimano, 1955; KNADS/BY/40/2, Midwifery in the Home by Dr. C Rendle Short 1955.
100. KNADS/AZG1/32/9, Mayfair Housing Estate Old Racecourse Nairobi; KNADS/AZG1/32/9, Doonholm II Doonholm Road Nairobi; Walmsley, *Nairobi*, 31; Andrew Hake, was living in Nairobi during these events between 1957 and 1969. See his *African Metropolis* (*New York: St. Martin's Press, 1977*), 64–80.
101. White, Silberman, and Anderson, *Nairobi Master Plan*, 45–46.
102. Harris, "From Trusteeship to Development."
103. White, Silberman, and Anderson submitted their report in July 1946, published in 1948. See *Nairobi Master Plan*, 1–2; Hake, *African Metropolis*, 26, 43–44, 56.
104. White, Silberman, and Anderson, *Nairobi Master Plan*, 49.
105. White, Silberman, and Anderson, *Nairobi Master Plan*, 49.
106. Anderson, "Corruption," 145; Achola, "Colonial Policy and Urban Health," 122.
107. Anderson, *Histories of the Hanged.*
108. Ogilvie, *Housing of Africans.*
109. Ogilvie. *Housing of Africans*, 57.
110. KNADS/RN/1/96, T. C. Colchester (Chairman of Central Housing Board), Central Housing Board, January 29, 1954.
111. Ogilvie, *Housing of Africans*, 57–8; KNADS/RN/1/72, N. M. Deverall, Municipal African Housing Part I: Departmental Housing, August 1, 1948.
112. KNADS/RN/1/96, African Locations: Nairobi City Council Housing Schemes; Ogilvie, *Housing of Africans.*
113. KNADS/SBY/40/2, "Education and Standard of Living in Relation to African Housing" by Mr. Nahashon Mimano. 1955; KNAD/BY/40/2, Midwifery in the Home by Dr. C. Rendle Short 1955.
114. KNADS/SBY/40/2, "Education and Standard of Living in Relation to African Housing" by Mr. Nahashon Mimano. 1955; KNAD/BY/40/2, Midwifery in the Home by Dr. C. Rendle Short 1955.
115. Ogilvie, *Housing of Africans*, 27–34.
116. KNADS/AZG1/32/9, Mayfair Housing Estate Old Racecourse Nairobi; KNAD/AZG1/32/9, Doonholm II Doonholm Road Nairobi; Walmsley, *Nairobi*, 31; Andrew Hake, was living in Nairobi during these events between 1957 and 1969. See his *African Metropolis*, 64–80.

117. Cooper, *Africa*, 27.

118. Jeffrey S. Ahlman, *Living with Nkrumahism: Nation State and Pan-Africanism in Ghana* (Athens: Ohio University Press, 2017), 6–10; Jeffrey S. Ahlman, *Kwame Nkrumah: Visions of Liberation* (Athens: Ohio University Press, 2021), 14–5. For more on Gold Coast nationalism and decolonization, see Austin, *Politics in Ghana*; Nkrumah, *Ghana*; A. Adu Boahen, *African Perspectives on Colonialism* (Baltimore, MD: Johns Hopkins University Press, 1987). David Kimble, *A Political History of Ghana: The Rise of Gold Coast Nationalism, 1850–1928* (Oxford: Clarendon Press, 1963); Apter, *Ghana in Transition.*

119. Anderson, *Histories of the Hanged.*

120. Robert Home, "Transferring British Planning Law to the Colonies: The Case of the 1938 Trinidad and Regional Planning Ordinance," *Third World Planning Review* 15, no. 4 (November 1, 1993): 397–410; See also Harris, "From Trusteeship to Development"; Beeckmans, "The 'Development Syndrome.'"

121. Akyeampong, "African Socialism."

122. Cooper, *Africa.*

123. Anderson, "Corruption."

124. Marshall, *Bukom*, 91–2.

125. Decker and McMahon, *The Idea of Development*, 2–14; Ammann and Förster, *African Cities*, 3–7; Grace, *African Motors*, 11–12.

126. Rogaski, *Hygienic Modernity*, 193–224.

CHAPTER FIVE. WASTE, 1952–1963

1. *Daily Graphic*, "Improving Sanitation," August 7, 1954.
2. *Daily Graphic*, "Improving Sanitation."
3. Interview by author, Senior Citizens in Accra, August 21, 2012.
4. Interview by author, Senior Citizens in Accra, August 21, 2012.
5. *Daily Graphic*, "Improving Sanitation"; J. A. Korsah, "Help Improve Sanitation" *Daily Graphic* Readers' Forum, August 17, 1954.
6. Ahlman, *Living with Nkrumahism*, 6–10; Ahlman, *Kwame Nkrumah*, 14–5. For more on Gold Coast nationalism and decolonization, see Austin, *Politics in Ghana*; Nkrumah, *Ghana*; Boahen, *African Perspectives*; Kimble, *Political History of Ghana*; Apter, *Ghana in Transition*; Jean Marie Allman, *The Quills of the Porcupine: Asante Nationalism in an Emergent Ghana* (Madison: University of Wisconsin Press, 1993).
7. *Daily Graphic*, "Improving Sanitation"; Korsah, "Help Improve Sanitation."

8. P. D. Dorkenoo, "Plans for 'Clean the Capital' Week," *Daily Graphic,* November 27, 1954.
9. PRAAD/CSO11/14/326, J. Quist-Therson to President Accra Town Council, December 18, 1942.
10. For some of the complaints about unremoved waste in African communities in the Accra Town Council's monthly meetings, see PRAAD/CSO20/1/162, Minutes of the General Meeting of the Accra Town Council, July 16, 1946; PRAAD/CSO20/1/164, Minutes of the General Meeting of Accra Town Council 1948; PRAAD/CSO20/1/160, Meeting of Accra Town Council, June 26, 1945; PRAAD/CSO20/1/163, Minutes of the General Monthly Meeting of the Accra Town Council, January 20, 1948.
11. PRAAD/CSO20/1/61, Proceedings of Emergency Meeting of the Accra Town Council, October 23,1945; Professor Lidia La Face, "The House-Fly: The Murderer at Your Table!" *Daily Graphic*, March 23, 1956.
12. PRAAD/CSO20/1/61, Proceedings of Emergency Meeting of the Accra Town Council, October 23, 1945.
13. PRAAD/CSO11/14/326, President Accra Town Council (Norton Jones) to J. Quist-Therson, December 4, 1942; PRAAD/CSO20/1/61, Proceedings of Emergency Meeting of the Accra Town Council, October 23, 1945; Gold Coast, *Your Questions Answered by the Accra Town Council* (Accra: The Regional Information Office British West Africa, 1948), 58–64.
14. Gold Coast, *Your Questions Answered*, 40–44.
15. PRAAD/CSO20/1/160, Meeting of Accra Town Council, June 26, 1945; For more about low-ranking employees and non-employees in British colonies and their influential role in daily public health practices and policy, see the edited volume by Ryan Johnson and Amna Khalid. Khalid's and Johnson's chapters are especially instructive. *Public Health in the British Empire: Intermediaries, Subordinates, and the Practice of Public Health, 1850–1960* (New York and London: Routledge, 2012).
16. PRAAD/CSO20/1/61, Proceedings of Emergency Meeting of the Accra Town Council, October 23, 1945.
17. James C. Scott deploys the concept to explain specific techniques of evasion and resistance. See *Weapons of the Weak: Everyday Forms of Resistance* (New Haven, CT: Yale University Press, 1985).
18. PRAAD/CSO20/1/61, Proceedings of Emergency Meeting of the Accra Town Council, October 23, 1945.
19. Interview by author, Senior Citizens in Accra, August 21, 2012.
20. PRAAD/CSO20/1/160, Meeting of Accra Town Council, June 26, 1945; CSO20/1/161, Minutes of General Monthly Meeting of the Accra Town Council, January 15, 1946;

PRAAD/CSO20/1/163, Minutes of the General Meeting of the Accra Town Council, May 20, 1947; PRAAD/CSO14/3/572, President of Accra Town Council (E. W. Ellison) to the Acting Commissioner of Lands, January 7, 1947.

21. J. A. Korsah, "Help Improve Sanitation."
22. J. A. Korsah, "Help Improve Sanitation"; *Daily Graphic*, "Improving Sanitation"; *West Africa Times*, "Improvement in Method," March 24, 1931; First Name Cocroach (probably a pseudo name), "Sanitation in Labadi: 'Improving But—'" *West Africa Times*, by April 22, 1931.
23. PRAAD/CSO20/1/161, Proceedings of Emergency Meeting of the Accra Town Council, October 23, 1945.
24. PRAAD/CSO20/1/163, Minutes of the General Meeting of the Accra Town Council, May 20, 1947; PRAAD/CSO20/1/163, Minutes of the General Meeting of the Accra Town Council, July 15, 1947.
25. PRAAD/CSO20//1/164, Minutes of the General Monthly Meeting of the Accra Town Council, June 15, 1948.
26. PRAAD/CSO20/1/163, Minutes of the General Meeting of the Accra Town Council, July 15, 1947.
27. PRAAD/CSO20/1/161, Proceedings of Emergency Meeting of the Accra Town Council, October 23, 1945; PRAAD/CSO20/1/163, Minutes of the General Meeting of the Accra Town Council, July 15, 1947; PRAAD/CSO20/1/164, Minutes of the General Meeting of the Accra Town Council, June 15, 1948.
28. PRAAD/CSO20//1/164, Minutes of the General Monthly Meeting of the Accra Town Council, June 15, 1948.
29. PRAAD/CSO20//1/164, Minutes of the General Monthly Meeting of the Accra Town Council, June 15, 1948.
30. PRAAD/CSO20/1/163, General Meeting of the Accra Town Council, January 20, 1948.
31. *Daily Graphic*, "Cleaning Up Accra," December 11, 1954; Dorkenoo, "Plans for 'Clean the Capital'"; *Daily Graphic*, "Clear Accra Slums," October 27, 1956.
32. Daniel Badu, "Clean Up Accra," *Daily Graphic*, November 24, 1954; *Daily Graphic*, "Cleaning Up Accra"; Arthur Lindsay, "Accra Slum Clearance: Please Don't Shelve This Plan Again," *Daily Graphic*, September 6, 1956; *Daily Graphic*, "Clear Accra Slums."
33. Lindsay, "Accra Slum Clearance."
34. Dorkenoo, "Plans for 'Clean the Capital'"; *Daily Graphic*, "Cleaning Up Accra"; Lindsay, "Accra Slum Clearance."
35. Hart, *Making an African City*, 36–69; Addae, *Evolution of Modern Medicine*, 113–47.
36. Plageman, "'Accra Is Changing,'" 153–58.

37. *Times of West Africa,* "The Congested Area Problem"; PRAAD/CSO20/1/161, Minutes of Monthly General Meeting of the Accra Town Council, November 20, 1945; Gold Coast, *Your Questions Answered,* 58–64; S. N. Addo, "Drainage Plan £977,000 Voted for Initial Work," *Daily Graphic,* August 14, 1956.
38. PRAAD/CSO11/14/326, President Accra Town Council (Norton Jones) to J. Quist-Therson (Barrister-at Law Accra), December 4, 1942.
39. PRAAD/CSO11/14/326, J. Quist-Therson to the Governor of the Gold Coast (Sir Alan Burns), June 7, 1943; PRAAD/CSO11/14/326, J. Quist-Therson to President Accra Town Council, April 13, 1943.
40. PRAAD/CSO11/14/326, J. Quist-Therson to President Accra Town Council, December 18, 1942.
41. Acquah, *Accra Survey,* 57–62.
42. Acquah, *Accra Survey,* 57–62.
43. PRAAD/CSO20/12/20, Accra Town Planning Scheme, 1944.
44. PRAAD/CSO20/12/20, Accra Town Planning Scheme, 1944; Acquah, *Accra Survey,* 57.
45. PRAAD/CSO11/14/326, J. Quist-Therson to the Governor of the Gold Coast (Sir Alan Burns), June 7, 1943; PRAAD/CSO11/14/326, J. Quist-Therson to President Accra Town Council, April 13, 1943; CSO11/14/326, J. Quist-Therson to the Colonial Secretary, November 9, 1944.
46. PRAAD/CSO11/14/326, J. Quist-Therson to the Colonial Secretary, November 9, 1944.
47. PRAAD/CSO11/14/326, Extract of Minutes of Meeting of the Accra Town Council, Sanitary Amenities Required at Amantra Area Christiansborg, November 28, 1944; PRAAD/CSO11/14/326, Commissioner of Lands to the Colonial Secretary, December 9, 1944.
48. Discussions during the monthly meetings of the Accra Town Council were filled with complaints about unremoved waste in African residential locations. For instance, see PRAAD/CSO20/1/162, Minutes of the General Meeting of the Accra Town Council, July 16, 1946; PRAAD/CSO20/1/164, Minutes of the General Meeting of Accra Town Council 1948.
49. PRAAD/CSO20/1/164, Minutes of Monthly General Meeting of the Accra Town Council, April 26, 1949; PRAAD/CSO20/1/164, Minutes of Monthly General Meeting of the Accra Town Council, May 17, 1949.
50. PRAAD/CSO20/1/164, Minutes of Monthly General Meeting of the Accra Town Council, February 15, 1949.
51. PRAAD/CSO20/1/160, Meeting of Accra Town Council, June 26, 1945; PRAAD/CSO20/1/161, Minutes of General Monthly Meeting of the Accra Town Council, January

15, 1946; PRAAD/CSO20/1/163, Minutes of the General Meeting of the Accra Town Council, May 20, 1947; PRAAD/CSO14/3/572, President of Accra Town Council (E. W. Ellison) to the Acting Commissioner of Lands, January 7, 1947.

52. PRAAD/CSO20/1/61, Proceedings of Emergency Meeting of the Accra Town Council, October 23, 1945; PRAAD/CSO20/1/61, Minutes of General Monthly Meeting of the Accra Town Council, July 16, 1946.
53. Gold Coast, *Your Questions Answered*, 40–44.
54. PRAAD/CSO20/12/20, Accra Town Planning Scheme, 1944; PRAAD/RG5/1/156, The Medical Officer of Health (N. S. Turbull) to the Permanent Secretary Ministry of Works, June 8, 1956; Town and Country Planning Division of the Ministry of Housing, *Accra: A Plan for the Town* (Accra: Government Printer, 1958), 79–80.
55. PRAAD/CSO20/12/20, Accra Town Planning Scheme, 1944.
56. PRAAD/RG5/1/156, The Medical Officer of Health (N. S. Turbull) to the Permanent Secretary Ministry of Works, June 8, 1956; Town and Country Panning Division of the Ministry of Housing, *Accra: A Plan*.
57. PRAAD/RG5/1/443, Development Commission to the Ministry of Works and Housing, Supplementary Report on Accra Sewerage, February 12, 1960.
58. PRAAD/RG5/1/443, Memorandum for Standing Finance and Development Committee by the Minister of Works and Housing, Accra Sewerage Scheme; Addo, "Drainage Plan"; PRAAD/RG5/1/443, Development Commission to the Ministry of Works and Housing, Supplementary Report on Accra Sewerage, February 12, 1960.
59. PRAAD/RG5/1/443, Memorandum for Standing Finance and Development Committee by the Minister of Works and Housing, Accra Sewerage Scheme, 1950s.
60. PRAAD/CSO11/14/55, Acting Permanent Secretary Ministry of Local Government to the Permanent Secretary Ministry of Works, Balfour Report on Accra Sewerage, 1955.
61. PRAAD/CSO11/14/55, Acting Permanent Secretary Ministry of Local Government to the Permanent Secretary Ministry of Works, Balfour Report on Accra Sewerage, 1955.
62. PRAAD/CSO11/14/55, Acting Permanent Secretary Ministry of Local Government to the Permanent Secretary Ministry of Works, Balfour Report on Accra Sewerage, 1955.
63. To see how Europeans used science and their modern technologies to promise progress and development, see Tilley, *Africa as a Living Laboratory*; Mitchell, *Rule of Experts*.
64. PRAAD/RG5/1/443, Memorandum for Standing Finance and Development Committee by the Minister of Works and Housing, Accra Sewerage Scheme; PRAAD/RG5/1/443, Information Paper for the Standing Development Committee Progress Report by the Minister of Works and Housing, Accra Sewerage Scheme; Phase I (Survey, Investigation, and Design).

65. Addo, “Drainage Plan”; PRAAD/RG5/1/443, Memorandum for Standing Finance and Development Committee by the Minister of Works and Housing, Accra Sewerage Scheme; PRAAD/RG5/1/443, Information Paper for the Standing Development Committee Progress Report by the Minister of Works and Housing, Accra Sewerage Scheme; Phase I (Survey, Investigation, and Design).
66. Anderson, *Histories of the Hanged*, 181–229.
67. KNADS/BY/29/29, District Commissioner to the Director of Medical Services: Sanitation—African Locations Nairobi, June 15, 1954.
68. KNADS/BY/29/29, Medical Officer of Health to the Director of Medical Services, Hygiene and Sanitation in the African Locations, 1950s.
69. KNADS/RN/29/29, The Direction of Medical Service, Memorandum on Hygiene and Sanitation in the African Locations Nairobi, 1940s.
70. KNADS/BY/13/162, Senior Medical Office of Health Municipal Council of Nairobi to Commissioner for Local Government, Plague and Native Housing in Nairobi, October 2, 1941.
71. KNADS/BY/29/29, Director of Medical Services to the District Commissioner of Nairobi, Sanitation Nairobi City, July 10, 1954.
72. KNADS/BY/29/29, Director of Medical Services to the District Commissioner of Nairobi, Sanitation Nairobi City, July 10, 1954.
73. KNAD/RN/1/96, Memorandum to the Right Honourable Oliver Lyttleton M. P. Secretary of State for the Colonies, October 5, 1952.
74. *East African Standard*, “Nairobi Refuse Men Adopt Go-Slow Policy,” January 4, 1949; Nairobi Sanitary Report, 1913; City Council of Nairobi Kenya, Twenty-First Annual Report of the Medical Officer of Health, June 12, 1951; KNADS/BY/29/29, Director of Medical Services: Sanitation Nairobi City, July 10, 1954.
75. KNADS/AZG1/28/5, F. Crawford (Deputy Governor), Nairobi Sanitary Services, August 30, 1955.
76. KNADS/RN/1/96, Note on “Health” by Mrs. Michael Wood.
77. KNADS/BY/29/29, Medical Officer of Health to the Director of Medical Services, Hygiene and Sanitation in the African Locations, 1950s.
78. KNADS/RN/1/96, Note on “Health” by Mrs. Michael Wood.
79. KNAD/BY/29/29, Hygiene and Sanitation in the African Locations Nairobi.
80. KNADS/BY/29/29, Director of Medical Services to the District Commissioner of Nairobi, Sanitation Nairobi City, July 10, 1954.
81. KNADS/BY/29/29, Director of Medical Services to the District Commissioner of Nairobi, Sanitation Nairobi City, July 10, 1954.

82. Nairobi Sanitary Report, 1913; City Council of Nairobi Kenya, Twenty-First Annual Report of the Medical Officer of Health, June 12, 1951; KNADS/BY/29/29, Director of Medical Services: Sanitation Nairobi City, July 10, 1954.
83. KNADS/AZG1/28/5, Address to the Nairobi City Council by Alderman I Somen M. B. E. on the Termination of His Office as Mayor, July 2, 1957.
84. KNADS/BY/29/29, The Director of Medical Services to the District Commissioner, July 10, 1954.
85. KNADS/HAK1/17/46, Re: Memorandum from the Africa Women's League by Municipal African Affairs Officer, September 13, 1946; KNADS/BY/29/29, The Director of Medical Services to the District Commissioner, July 10, 1954.
86. KNADS//HAK1/17/47, Memorandum: African Women's League of Nairobi Municipality and Central Province to the Secretary of State for the Colonies, August 20, 1946.
87. KNADS/HAK1/17/46, Ceremonial, Visits and Visitors, General, Mr. Creech Johns, Petitions, Native, 1946; KNADS/HAK1/17/46, African Women's League, 1947.
88. KNADS/HAK1/17/46, Re: Memorandum from the Africa Women's League by Municipal African Affairs Officer, September 13, 1946.
89. KNADS/HAK1/17/46, Re: Memorandum from the Africa Women's League by Municipal African Affairs Officer, September 13, 1946.
90. PRAAD/CSO14/3/572, President of Accra Town Council to the Acting Commissioner of Lands, January 7, 1947; PRAAD/CSO20/1/163, Minutes of the General Meeting of the Accra Town Council, May 20, 1947; KNADS/RN/1/72, N. M. Deverall, Municipal African Housing Part I: Departmental Housing, August 1, 1948.
91. KNADS/BY/29/29, The Director of Medical Services to the District Commissioner, July 10, 1954.
92. Ogilvie, *Housing of Africans.* KNADS/HAK1/5/176, Acting Director of Public Works to the Acting Director, African Quarters—Sanitation, July 22, 1950; KNADS/HAK1/5/176, General Manager East African Railways & Harbours to Acting Chief Secretary, Sanitation—African Quarters, September 27, 1950.
93. City Council of Nairobi Kenya, Twenty-First Annual Report of the Medical Officer of Health, June 12, 1951.
94. KNADS/BY/29/29, Director of Medical Services: Sanitation Nairobi City, July 10, 1954; KNADS/RN/1/77, Government Proposal: For Circulation to Members of the Deputation on African Housing, 1955.
95. KNADS/HAK1/5/176, District Commission Nairobi to the Chief Secretary, Sanitation During Civil Disturbance African Quarters, June 23, 1950.
96. KNADS/HAK1/5/176, Acting Chief Secretary to the General Manager East African

Railways & Harbours, Sanitation—African Quarters, July 28, 1950.

97. KNADS/RN/1/96, Note on "Health" by Mrs. Michael Wood, 1950s.
98. KNADS/GH/26/25, The Nairobi District African Congress—Outline of Policy, May 13, 1956.
99. Gatheru, *Child of Two Worlds*, 71–46.
100. KNADS/AZG1/28/5, Entry on the London Market by the Nairobi City Council, 1954–1964; KNADS/AZG1/28/5, Deputy Governor—Nairobi Sanitary Services, August 30, 1955.
101. KNADS/AZG1/28/5, Entry on the London Market by the Nairobi City Council, 1954–1964; KNADS/AZG1/28/5, F. Crawford (Deputy Governor), Nairobi Sanitary Services, August 30, 1955.
102. KNADS/AZG1/28/5, F Crawford Nairobi Sanitary Services, August 30, 1955.
103. KNADS/AZG1/28/5, F Crawford Nairobi Sanitary Services, August 30, 1955.
104. Walmsley, *Nairobi,* 48–9; City Council of Nairobi, *Annual Report 1955* (Nairobi: Town Hall, 1956), 27–32.
105. City Council of Nairobi Kenya, *The Thirtieth Annual Report of the Medical Officer of Health*, 1959.
106. City Council of Nairobi, *The Thirty-First Annual Report of the Medical Officer of Health 1960* (Nairobi: City Hall, 1960), 48.
107. City Council of Nairobi, *The Thirty-First Annual Report*, 35.
108. Walmsley, *Nairobi*, 48–9; City Council of Nairobi, *Annual Report 1955*, 27; City Council of Nairobi, *Annual Report 1960* (Nairobi: City Hall, 1961), 5. City Council of Nairobi, *Thirty-First Annual Report*, 53.
109. City Council of Nairobi Kenya, *Thirtieth Annual Report.*
110. The actual engineering specifications are more detailed and impressive than this description. Additionally, it goes beyond the scope of this book. Colony and Protectorate of Kenya, *Report on African Housing*; City Council of Nairobi Kenya, *Thirtieth Annual Report.*
111. City Council of Nairobi Kenya, *Thirtieth Annual Report*, 51.
112. City Council of Nairobi, *Thirty-First Annual Report*, 35.
113. City Council of Nairobi, *Thirty-First Annual Report*, 35.
114. City Council of Nairobi, *Thirty-First Annual Report*, 35.
115. Johnson and Khalid, *Public Health.*
116. Rosalind Fredericks, *Garbage Citizenship: Vital Infrastructures of Labor in Dakar, Senegal* (Durham, NC: Duke University Press, 2018); Rosalind Fredericks, "Vital Infrastructure of Trash in Dakar," *Comparative Studies of South Asia, Africa and the Middle East* 34, no. 3 (2014): 532–48.

117. Brian Larkin, "The Politics and Poetics of Infrastructure," *The Annual Review of Anthropology* 42 (2013): 327–43.
118. McFarlane, "Governing the Contaminated City," 418.
119. Sophia Stamatopoulou-Robbins, *Waste Siege: The Life of Infrastructure in Palestine* (Stanford: Stanford University Press, 2020), 20–24.
120. Stephani Elizabeth Terreni Brown, "Kampala's Shitscape: Exploring Urbanity and Sanitation in Uganda" (unpublished PhD thesis, University of Edinburgh, 2013). For the various ways that waste and its infrastructures became sites for political negotiations in the Ghanaian city of Tema, Brenda Chalfin, *Waste Works: Vital Politics in Urban Ghana* (Durham, NC: Duke University Press, 2023).
121. Chalfin, *Waste Works*, 5–11.
122. Plageman, "'Accra Is Changing,'" 153–58; For infrastructure and nationalist development, see also Brian Larkin, *Signal and Noise: Media, Infrastructure, and Urban Culture in Nigeria* (Durham, NC: Duke University Press, 2008); Larkin, "The Politics and Poetics."
123. McFarlane, "Governing the Contaminated City," 425.

EPILOGUE. EVERYTHING OLD IS NEW AGAIN

1. Poor sanitation and the prevalence of "slums" are themes that scholarship uses to foreground the discourse of dysfunctionality in African cities and government. See, for example, Parker, "Urbanization and Urban Culture"; Fourchard, "Between World History," 224.
2. T. M. Kodwo Mercer, "The Gold Coast Development Programme," October 1955.
3. Appolonia City website, https://www.appolonia.com.gh.
4. "Project Details," Tatu City website, https://www.tatucity.com/project-details/.
5. "Project Details," Tatu City website, https://www.tatucity.com/project-details/.
6. Nairobi's "slums" continued to provide housing for residents in various sectors within and outside the government, including people working in offices and industries and those working as laborers and newspaper vendors. See The National Council of Churches of Kenya, *Nairobi Demolitions*, 10.
7. Paul Stacy, *State of Slum: Precarity and Informal Governance at the Margins in Accra* (London: Zed Books, 2019); Constance Smith, *Nairobi in the Making: Landscapes of Time & Urban Belonging* (Suffolk, UK: James Currey, 2019).
8. Stacy, *State of Slum*; Smith, *Nairobi in the Making*. See the volume edited by Carole Ammann and Till Förster, which also reinforces the agency and practices of African urban residents to shape their neighborhoods and cities: Ammann and Förster, *African Cities*.

9. Gale, "Official Medical Policy," 435–37.
10. Senior official of the Accra Metropolitan Assembly, Interview by the author, summer of 2016. In an earlier article, I published an incendiary comment about this person, whose identity I prefer to continue keeping anonymous. During the interview, this interlocutor emphasized "dysfunction," which seemed to regurgitate Western criticism of African central and local governments.
11. *Canberra Times*, "Accra—A Capital of Sharp Contrasts," March 25, 1964.
12. Senior official of the Accra Metropolitan Assembly, interview by the author, summer 2016; *Canberra Times*, "Accra."
13. Thuku, *Harry Thuku: An Autobiography*, 33.
14. Ngũgĩ Wa Thiong'o, *Weep not Child* (Oxford: Heinemann, 1987), 43, 50–51.
15. Fourchard, "Between World History," 223–24.
16. Fourchard, "Between World History," 223–24.
17. See, for example, Marshall, *Bukom*; Akare, *The Slums*; Ayi Kwei Armah, *The Beautyful Ones Are Not Yet Born.* (Oxford: Heinemann, 1968).
18. See Cooper, *Africa*; Freeman, "Ghana."
19. Freeman traces this to the beginning of the postcolonial period. Still, as the book has shown, they go back to when the British colonial state established Accra as the capital and gave low priority to the sanitation of the African majority in the city. See Freeman, "Ghana," 47–49.
20. Akare, *The Slums*, 67.
21. The National Council of Churches of Kenya, *Nairobi Demolitions*, 9.

Bibliography

Archives

Commonwealth and African Studies Collections (Rhodes House Collection)

MSS.EMP.BRIT s. 332 Box 47, File 2

Kenya National Archives and Document Services

Attorney General's Records

KNADS/AG/4/14

KNADS/AG/4/15

KNAD/AG/22/455

Ministry of Health Records

KNAD/BY/13/162

KNAD/BY/40/2

KNAD/BY/46/4

Records of Lands and Settlement

KNAD/BN/56/1

KNAD/BN/56/12

KNAD/BN/73/2

Records of Nairobi City Council

KNAD/RN/1/67

KNAD/RN/1/68

KNAD/RN/1/72

KNAD/RN/1/77

KNAD/RN/1/96

KNAD/RN/29/29

Records of the Chief Secretary

KNAD/HAK1/5/176

KNAD/HAK1/5/470

KNAD/HAK1/5/177

KNAD/HAK1/17/46

KNAD/HAK1/17/47

KNAD/HAK1/5/470

Records of the Governor's Office

KNAD/AZG1/28/5

KNAD/AZG1/32/9

London School of Hygiene and Tropical Medicine

Ross/46/0/27

The National Archives—London

PRO/CO96/514

PRO/CO96/517

PRO/CO96/518

PRO/CO96/520

PRO/CO96/528

PRO/CO96/533

PRO/CO96/540

PRO/CO96/752

PRO/CO96/752/12

PRO/CO96/760/13

PRO/CO533/117

PRO/CO533/192

PROCO533/196

PRO/CO533/211

Melville J. Herskovits Library of African Studies at Northwestern University

Vertical Files (NUAVF), T. M. Kodwo Mercer, "The Gold Coast Development Programme," October 1955

Public Records and Archival Administration Department (PRAAD)—Accra

Administrative Files

PRAAD/ADM11/943

PRAAD/ADM11/1/981

Colonial Secretary Office's Series

PRAAD/CSO11/1/212

PRAAD/CSO11/14/55

PRAAD/CSO11/14/326

PRAAD/CSO14/1/283

PRAAD/CSO14/1/305

PRAAD/CSO14/1/329

PRAAD/CSO14/3/489

PRAAD/CSO14/3/572

PRAAD/CSO20/1/5

PRAAD/CSO20/1/61

PRAAD/CSO20/1/77

PRAAD/CSO20/1/80

PRAAD/CSO20/1/112

PRAAD/CSO20/1/130

PRAAD/CSO20/1/160

PRAAD/CSO20/1/161

PRAAD/CSO20/1/162

PRAAD/CSO20/1/163

PRAAD/CSO20/1/164

PRAAD/CSO20/12/7

PRAAD/CSO20/12/14

PRAAD/CSO20/12/20

PRAAD/CSO 21/8/18

PRAAD/CSO21/8/42

Ministerial Record Groups

PRAAD/RG5/1/156

PRAAD/RG5/1/245

PRAAD/RG5/1/443

Publications

Abu-Lughod, Janet. *Cairo: 1001: Years of the City Victorious.* Princeton, NJ: Princeton University Press, 1971.

———. "The Legitimacy of Comparisons in Comparative Urban Studies: A Theoretical Position and an Application to North African Cities." In *The City in Comparative*

Perspective: Cross-National Research and New Directions in Theory, edited by John Walton and Louis H. Masotti, 17–39. New York: John Wiley & Sons, 1976.

———. "Tale of Two Cities: The Origins of Modern Cairo." *Comparative Studies in Society and History* 7, no. 4 (July 1965), 429–57.

Achola, Milcah Amolo. "Colonial Policy and Urban Health: The Case of Colonial Nairobi." In *The Urban Experience in Eastern Africa c. 1750–2000* Azania Special Volume XXXVI–XXXVII. Edited by Andrew Burton, 120. Nairobi: British Institute in Eastern Africa, 2002.

Acquah, Ione. *Accra Survey: A Social Survey of the Capital of Ghana, formerly called the Gold Coast, Undertaken for the West African Institute of Social and Economic Research, 1953–1956*. London: University of London Press, 1958.

Addo, S. N. "Drainage Plan £977,000 Voted for Initial Work." *Daily Graphic*. August 14, 1956.

Ahlman, Jeffrey S. *Kwame Nkrumah: Visions of Liberation*. Athens: Ohio University Press, 2021.

———. *Living with Nkrumahism: Nation State and Pan-Africanism in Ghana*. Athens: Ohio University Press, 2017.

Akare, Thomas. *The Slums*. Oxford: Heinemann, 1981.

Akurang-Parry, Kwame Opare. "Colonial Forced Labor Policies for Road Building in Southern Ghana and International Anti-Forced Labor Pressures, 1900–1940." *African Economic History* no. 28 (2000): 1–25.

Akyeampong, Emmanuel. "African Socialism; Or the Search for an Indigenous Model of Economic Development?" African Economic History Working Paper Series, 36/2017. African Economic History Network, 2017.

———. "Bukom and the Social History of Boxing in Accra: Warfare and Citizenship in Precolonial Ga Society." *International Journal of African Historical Studies* 35, no. 1 (2002), 39–60.

Akyeampong, Emmanuel, Robert H. Bates, Nathan Nunn, and James A. Robinson, eds. *Africa's Development in Historical Perspective*. New York: Cambridge University Press, 2014.

Allman, Jena Marie. "Between the Present and History: African Nationalism and Decolonization." In *The Oxford Handbook of Modern African History*, edited by John Parker and Richard Reid (Oxford: Oxford University Press, 2013), 224–40.

———. *The Quills of the Porcupine: Asante Nationalism in an Emergent Ghana*. Madison: University of Wisconsin Press, 1993.

Ammann, Carole, and Fill Förster, eds. *African Cities and the Development Conundrum*, Vol. 10. Leiden, Netherlands: Brill, 2018.

Amoah, Frank E. K. "Accra: A Study of the Development of a West African City." Unpublished MA thesis, University of Ghana, 1964.

Anderson, David. "Corruption at City Hall: African Housing and Urban Development in

Colonial Nairobi." *Azania: Archaeological Research in Africa* 36–37, no. 1 (2010): 138–54.

———. *Histories of the Hanged: The Dirty War in Kenya and the End of Empire*. New York: W. W. Norton & Company, 2005.

Apter, David E. *Ghana in Transition*. New York: Atheneum,1963.

Armah, Ayi Kwei. *The Beautyful Ones Are Not Yet Born.* Oxford: Heinemann, 1968.

Arnold, David. *Colonizing the Body: State Medicine and Epidemic Disease in Nineteenth-Century India.* Berkeley: University of California Press, 1993.

———. "Medicine and Colonialism." In *Companion Encyclopedia of the History of Medicine*, Vol. 2, edited by W. F. Bynum and Roy Porter. London: Routledge, 1993.

Austin, Dennis. *Politics in Ghana 1946–1960.* London: Oxford University Press, 1970.

Badu, Daniel. "Clean Up Accra." *Daily Graphic.* November 24, 1954.

Baker, R. A., and R. A. Bayliss. "William John Ritchie Simpson,1855–1931: Public Health and Tropical Medicine." *Medical History* 31, no. 4 (1987): 450–65.

Bickers, Robert, ed. *Settlers and Expatriates: Britons over the Seas*. Oxford: Oxford University Press, 2010.

Bigon, Liora. *French Colonial Dakar: The Morphogenesis of an African Regional Capital.* Manchester: Manchester University Press, 2016.

———. "A History of Urban Planning and Infectious Disease: Colonial Senegal in the Early Twentieth Century." *Urban Studies Research* (2012), 1–12.

———. "Urban Planning Colonial Doctrines and Street Naming in French Dakar and British Lagos c. 1850–1930." *Urban History* 36, no. 3 (December 2009): 426–48.

Bigon, Liora, and Yossi Katz, eds. *Garden Cities and Colonial Planning: Transnationality and Urban Ideas in Africa and Palestine.* Manchester: Manchester University Press, 2014.

Bin-Kasim, Waseem-Ahmed. "Politics of Disaster: Earthquake, Rehousing, and Confronting Colonial Rule in Accra (Gold Coast/Ghana), 1939–45." *The Journal of African History* 64, no. 2 (2023): 292–305.

Bissell, William Cunningham. *Urban Design, Chaos, and Colonial Power in Zanzibar.* Bloomington: Indiana University Press, 2011.

Boahen, A. Adu. *African Perspectives on Colonialism.* Baltimore, MD: Johns Hopkins University Press 1987.

Brand, Richard R. "A Geographical Interpretation of the European Influence on Accra, Ghana since 1877." (Unpublished PhD thesis, Columbia University, 1972).

———. "The Role of Cocoa in the Growth and Spatial Organization of Accra (Ghana) Prior to 1921." *African Studies Review* 15, no. 2 (September 1972): 271–82.

British East African Protectorate. *Report on the Sanitation of Nairobi*, 1913.

British East African Protectorate. *Report on the Sanitation of Nairobi, Report on the Townships of Naivasha, Nakuru, and Kisumu by George Bransby Williams.* London: Waterlow and Sons, 1907.

Brown, G. H. "Sir William John Ritchie Simpson." *Lancet* IV (1931): 414.

Brown, James W. "Increased Intercommunication and Epidemic in Early Colonial Ashanti." In *Disease in African History: An Introductory Survey and Case Studies*, edited by Gerald W. Hartwig and K. David Patterson. Durham, NC: Duke University Press, 1978.

Brown, Spencer H. "A Tool of Empire: The British Medical Establishment in Lagos, 1861–1905." *The International Journal of African Historical Studies* 37, no. 2 (2004): 309–43.

Burke, Timothy. *Lifebuoy Men, Lux Women: Commodification Consumption & Cleanliness in Modern Zimbabwe.* Durham, NC: Duke University Press, 1996.

Burton, Andrew, *African Underclass: Urbanisation Crime & Colonial Order in Dar es Salaam.* Nairobi: The British Institute on East Africa, 2005.

———. "Townsmen in the Making: Social Engineering and Citizenship in Dar es Salaam, c. 1945–1960." *The International Journal of African Historical Studies* 36, no. 2 (2003): 331–65.

Canberra Times. "Accra—A Capital of Sharp Contrasts." March 25, 1964.

Cell, John W. "Anglo-Indian Medical Theory and the Origins of Segregation in West Africa." *The American Historical Review* 91, no. 2 (April 1986): 307–35.

Chalfin, Brenda. *Waste Works: Vital Politics in Urban Ghana*. Durham, NC: Duke University Press, 2023.

City Council of Nairobi Kenya. *The Thirtieth Annual Report of the Medical Officer of Health*, 1959.

City Council of Nairobi. *Annual Report 1955.* Nairobi: Town Hall, 1956.

———. *Annual Report 1960.* Nairobi: City Hall, 1961.

———. *The Thirty-First Annual Report of the Medical Officer of Health 1960*. Nairobi: City Hall, 1960.

Colonial Office. *Report of the Commission of Enquiry into Disturbances in the Gold Coast 1948.* London: His Majesty's Stationery Office, 1948.

Colony and Protectorate of Kenya. *Report of the Local Government Commission*, vol. 1. London: The Crown Agents for the Colonies, 1927.

Colony and Protectorate of Kenya. *Report on African Housing in Townships and Trading Centers* by E. A. Vasey CMB. Nairobi: The Government Printer, 1950.

Cooper, Frederick. *Africa since 1940: The Past of the Present*, 2nd ed. New York: Cambridge University Press, 2019.

Cooper, Harold. "West African Race Rapport Supplants 'Mosquito Politics.'" *African News* 1, no. 9 (November 1954): 4.

Curtin, Philip D. "The End of the 'White Man's Grave?' Nineteen-Century Mortality in West

Africa." *Journal of Interdisciplinary History* 21, no. 1 (Summer 1990): 63–88.

———. "Medical Knowledge and Urban Planning in Tropical Africa." *The American Historical Review* 90, no. 3 (June 1985): 594–613.

———. "'The White Man's Grave:' Image and Reality, 1780–1850." *Journal of British Studies* 1 no. 1 (November 1961): 94–110.

Daily Graphic. "161 Employees of Housing Department to be Sacked." March 12, 1955.

———. "Cleaning Up Accra." December 11, 1954.

———. "Clear Accra Slums." October 27, 1956.

———. "Houses will be Ready Soon." March 12, 1955.

———. "Improving Sanitation." August 7, 1954.

Davis, Mike. *Planet of Slums*. London: Verso, 2006.

Decker, Corrie, and Elisabeth McMahon. *The Idea of Development in Africa: A History* Cambridge: Cambridge University Press, 2021.

Denoon, Donald. "Understanding Settler Societies." *Historical Studies* 18, no. 73 (1979): 511–27, 517–18.

Dorkenoo, B. D. "Plans for 'Clean the Capital' Week." *Daily Graphic*. November 27, 1954.

———. "Real Solution to Housing Problem," *Daily Graphic*, January 20, 1955.

Dumett, Raymond E. "The Campaign against Malaria and the Expansion of Scientific Medical and Sanitary Services in British West Africa 1898–1910." *African Historical Studies* 1, no. 2 (1968): 153–97.

Dyos, H. J. "The Slums of Victoria London." *Victorian Studies* 11, no. 1 (September 1967): 2–40.

Dyos, H. J., and D. A. Reeder. "Slums and Suburbs." In *The Victorian City: Images and Reality*. Vol. I. London: Routledge & Kegan Paul, 1973.

East African Standard. "Mayor on Nairobi's Slum Conditions: Council Prepared for any Project If Clear Policy is Laid Down." July 28, 1943.

———. "Nairobi to Argue with Government over Housing Burden." October 30, 1952.

———. "Nairobi Refuse Men Adopt Go-Slow Policy." January 4, 1949.

———. "Responsibility for the African's Future: New and Statesmanlike Attitude Required." November 1, 1937.

East India (Indians in East Africa). *Correspondence in Regards the Position of Indians in East Africa (Kenya and Uganda)*. London: His Majesty's Stationery Office, 1921.

Echenberg, Myron. *Plague Ports: The Global Urban Impact of Bubonic, 1894–1901*. New York: New York University Press, 2007.

Eldredge, Elizabeth A. "Drought, Famine and Disease in Nineteenth-Century Lesotho." *African Economic History*, no. 16 (1987): 61–93.

Enwezor, Okwul, ed. *The Short Century: Independence and Liberation 1945–1994*. Munich,

Germany: Prestel, 2001.

Fahmy, Khaled. "Modernizing Cairo: A Revisionist Narrative." In *Making Cairo Medieval*, edited by Nezar AlSayyad, Irene A. Bierman, and Nasser Rabbat. New York: Lexington Books, 2005.

———. "An Olfactory Tale of Two Cities." In *Historians in Cairo: Essays in Honor of George Scalon*, edited by Jill Edwards. Cairo, Egypt: The American University Press, 2002.

Field, M. J. *Religion and Medicine of the Ga People*. London: Oxford University Press, 1937.

Fourchard, Laurent. "Between World History and State Formation: New Perspectives on Africa's Cities." *The Journal of African History* 52, no. 2 (July 2011): 223–48.

Fredericks, Rosalind. *Garbage Citizenship: Vital Infrastructures of Labor in Dakar, Senegal* Durham, NC: Duke University Press, 2018.

———. "Vital Infrastructure of Trash in Dakar." *Comparative Studies of South Asia, Africa and the Middle East* 34, no. 3 (2014): 532–48.

Freeman, Frankie. "Ghana: The Waste Land." *World Policy Institute*, 2010.

Fryer, Peter. *Black People in the British Empire: An Introduction*. London: Pluto Press, 1988.

Gadsden, Fay. "The African Press in Kenya, 1945–1952." *The Journal of African History* 21, no. 4 (1980): 515–35.

Gale, Thomas S. "Lagos: The History of British Colonial Neglect of Traditional African Cities." *African Urban Studies*, no. 5 (Fall 1979): 11–24.

———. "Official Medical Policy in British West Africa, 1870–1930." Unpublished PhD thesis, University of London, 1972.

———. "Segregation in British West Africa (La Ségrégation en Afrique Occidentale Britannique)." *Cahiers d'Études Africaines* 20, no. 80 (1980): 495–507.

———. "The Struggle against Disease in the Gold Coast: Early Attempts at Urban Sanitary Reforms." *Transactions of the Historical Society of Ghana* 16, no. 2 (January 1995): 185–203.

Gaskell, S. Martin, ed. *Slums*. London: Leicester University Press, 1990.

Gatheru, R. Mugo. *Child of Two Worlds: A Kikuyu's Story*. New York: Frederick A. Praeger, 1964.

Ghana Information Services. *Ten Great Years*. Accra: Ghana Information Service, 1960.

Gilbert, Alan. "The Return of the Slum: Does Language Matter?" *International Journal of Urban and Regional Research* 31, no. 4 (December 2007): 697–713.

Gocking, Roger S. *The History of Ghana*. Westport, CT: Greenwood Press, 2005.

Goerg, Odile. "From Hill Station (Freetown) to Downtown Conakry (First Ward): Comparing French and British Approaches to Segregation in Colonial Cities at the Beginning of the Twentieth Century," *Canadian Journal of African Studies / Revue Canadienne des Études Africaines* 32, no. 1 (1998): 1–31.

Gold Coast. *The Gold Coast Review: A Review of the Events of 1920–1926 and the Prospects of*

1927–1928. Accra, 1927.

Gold Coast. *Report to the Secretary of State for the Colonies on the Outbreak of Plague in the Gold Coast Colony and Ashanti by Professor Sir William Simpsons*, 1925, 7.

Gold Coast. *Your Questions Answered by the Accra Town Council*. Accra: The Regional Information Office British West Africa, 1948.

Gold Coast Colony. *Report on the Medical Department for the Year 1938*. Accra: Government Printing Department, 1939.

Gold Coast Independence. "Mr. Jones Nelson Moves for Important Social Services." February 25, 1939.

———. "Proceedings of the Meeting between the Ga Manche and the Manchemei and the Town Council." October 7, 1922.

———. "The Public Health and Sanitation." August 26, 1922.

Gold Coast Independent. "Accra Town Council." January 27, 1940.

———. "The Accra Town Council and Demolition of Houses." January 13, 1940.

———. "Clearing Up the Areas: First Steps to Rebuild Accra, Flaws in the Scheme." January 20, 1940.

———. "Compulsory Land Acquisition: Arbitrary Taking over by Government, Ownership Privileges Seriously Affected." August 19, 1939.

———. "Fishermen Meet on Removal of Fishing industry to Chorker: Young Men Object." July 15, 1939.

———. "Fishermen Meet with Theodore Taylor on New Fishing Township." July 22, 1939.

———. "The Ga Manche Broadcasts on Earthquake Disasters." July 22, 1939.

———. "Government Housing Scheme: Plan for Repayment, Economic Condition of the Masses." January 27, 1940.

———. "Kumasi New Layout: What About Accra, The Metropolis of the Colony." May 11, 1929.

———. "Neither Government nor Council is Prepared to Advance Money to House Owners to Rebuild." December 30, 1939.

———. "The New Accra: Plans for its Building." July 8, 1939.

———. "Rebuilding Accra: Government to Launch and Subsidize, A Campaign." July 1, 1939.

———. "Sanitary and Housing Conditions." July 13, 1929.

———. "Small-Time Measure: A Good Job Once and for All." July 8, 1939.

———. "Unofficial Councilors Protests Against Indiscriminate Demolition." January 13, 1940.

Gold Coast Leader. "The Mosquito Eropaganda and Segregation." August 12–26, 1911.

Gold Coast Nation. "Notes and Comments." April 24, 1913.

———. "Notes and Comments: A New Segregation Theory, the Tables Have Turned." March 20, 1913.

———. "The Gold Coast Independent Olorun Fumi House, Station Road Accra, Saturday, August 3rd, 1918: The Accra Town Council and the Town Councils Ordinance 1891." August 3, 1918.

Good, Kenneth. "Settler Colonialism: Economic Development and Class Formation." *The Journal of Modern African Studies* 14, no. 4 (December 1976): 597–620.

Grace, Joshua. *African Motors: Technology, Gender, and the History of Development.* Durham, NC: Duke University Press, 2021.

Grant, Richard. *Globalizing City: The Urban and Economic Transformation of Accra Ghana*, Syracuse, NY: Syracuse University Press, 2009.

Hake, Andrew. *African Metropolis*. New York: St. Martin's Press, 1977.

Harris, Richard. "From Trusteeship to Development: How Class and Gender Complicated Kenya's Housing Policy, 1939–1963." *Journal of Historical Geography* 34 (2008): 314–27.

Harrison, Mark. "Disease, Diplomacy, and International Commerce: The Origins of International Sanitary Regulation in the Nineteenth Century." *Journal of Global History* 1, no. 2 (July 2006): 197–217.

Hart, Jennifer. *Making an African City: Technopolitics and the Infrastructure of Everyday Life in Colonial Accra.* Bloomington: Indiana University Press, 2024.

Harvey, David. "Labour, Capital, and Class Struggle around the Built Environment in Advanced Capitalist Society." In *Classes, Power, and Conflict: Classical and Contemporary Debates*, edited by Anthony Giddens and David Held. Basingstoke, UK: Macmillan, 1982.

———. *Paris, Capital of Modernity*. New York: Routledge, 2003.

Hayford, Casely. *Gold Coast Native Institutions: With Thoughts upon a Healthy Imperial Policy for the Gold Coast for the Gold Coast and Ashanti*. London: Sweet and Maxwell Limited, 1903.

Headrick, Daniel R. *The Tools of Empire: Technology and European Imperialism in the Nineteenth Century.* New York: Oxford University Press, 1981.

Hirst, Terry. *The Struggle for Nairobi*. Nairobi: Mazingira Institute, 1994.

Hodgkin, Thomas. *Nationalism in Colonial Africa*. London: Frederick Muller, 1956.

Home, Robert. *Of Planting and Planning: The Making of British Colonial Cities*. 2nd ed. London: Routledge, 2013.

———. "Transferring British Planning Law to the Colonies: The Case of the 1938 Trinidad Town and Regional Planning Ordinance." *Third World Planning Review* 15, no. 4 (November 1993): 397–410.

Huang, Yu-ting, and Rebecca Weaver-Hightower, eds. *Archiving Settler Colonialism: Culture Space and Race*. London: Routledge, 2019.

Hyde, Dave. "The Nairobi General Strike [1950]: From Protest to Insurgency," in *The Urban*

Experience in Eastern Africa, edited by Andrew Burton. Nairobi: British Institute in Eastern Africa, 2002.

Jackson, Iain, and Ola Uduku. "Sub-Saharan Africa." In *Architecture and Urbanism in the British Empire*, The Oxford History of the British Empire Companion Series. Oxford: Oxford University Press, 2016.

Johnson, Ryan. "'An All-white Institution:' Defending Private Practice and the Formation of the West African Medical Staff." *Medical History* 54 (2010): 237–54.

Johnson, Ryan. "Mantsemei, Interpreters, and the Successful Eradication of Plague: The 1908 Plague Epidemic in Colonial Accra." In *Public Health in the British Empire: Intermediaries, Subordinates, and the Practice of Public Health, 1850–1960*, edited by Ryan Johnson and Amna Khalid, 143. New York: Routledge, 2012.

Johnson, Ryan, and Amna Khalid, eds. *Public Health in the British Empire: Intermediaries, Subordinates, and the Practice of Public Health, 1850–1960*. New York and London: Routledge, 2012.

Kennedy, Dane. *Islands of White: Settler Society and Culture in Kenya and Southern Rhodesia, 1890–1939*. Durham, NC: Duke University Press, 1987.

Kenya Colony and Protectorate. *Annual Report of the Commissioner for Local Government, Lands, and Settlements, 1932*. Nairobi: The Government Printer, 1933.

Kenyatta, Jomo. *Facing Mount Kenya: The Tribal Life of Gikuyu*. New York: Vintage Books, 1965.

Kilson, Marion. *African Urban Kinsmen: The Ga of Central Accra*. New York: St. Martin's Press, 1974.

Kimble, David. *A Political History of Ghana: The Rise of Gold Coast Nationalism, 1850–1928*. Oxford: Clarendon Press, 1963.

King, Anthony D. *Colonial Urban Development: Culture Social Power and Environment*. London: Routledge & Paul, 1976.

———. *Urbanism, Colonialism, and the World-Economy: Cultural and Spatial Foundations of the World Urban System*. London: Routledge, 1990.

Korsah, J. A. "Help Improve Sanitation" Daily Graphic Readers' Forum, August 17, 1954.

Kwarteng, Kwasi. *Ghosts of Empire: Britain's Legacies in the Modern World*. London: Bloomsbury, 2011.

La Face, Lidia. "The House-Fly: The Murderer at Your Table!" *Daily Graphic*. March 23, 1956.

Larkin, Brian. "The Politics and Poetics of Infrastructure." *The Annual Review of Anthropology* 42 (2013): 327–43.

———. *Signal and Noise: Media, Infrastructure, and Urban Culture in Nigeria*. Durham, NC: Duke University Press, 2008.

Lindsay, Arthur. "Accra Slum Clearance: Please Don't Shelve This Plan Again." *Daily Graphic.* September 6, 1956.

Locatelli, Francesca, and Paul Nugent, eds. *African Cities: Competing Claims on Urban Spaces.* Leiden, Netherlands: Brill, 2009.

Lonsdale, John. "Kenya: Home County and African Frontier." In *Settlers and Expatriates: Britons over the Seas*, edited by Robert Bickers, 74–111. Oxford: Oxford University Press, 2010.

Lyons, Maryine. *The Colonial Disease: A Social History of Sleeping Sickness in Northern Zaire, 1900–1940*. Cambridge: Cambridge University Press, 1992.

Mamdani, Mahmood. "Beyond Settler and Native as Political Identities: Overcoming the Political Legacy of Colonialism." *Comparative Studies in Society and History* 43, no. 4 (October 2001): 651–64.

———. *Citizen and Subject: Contemporary African and the Legacy of Late Colonialism.* Princeton: Princeton University Press, 1996.

Marshall, Bill. *Bukom*. London: Longman, 1979.

Mayne, Alan. *Slums: The History of a Global Injustice.* London: Reaktion Books, 2017.

McFarlane, Colin. "Governing the Contaminated City: Infrastructure and Sanitation in Colonial and Postcolonial Bombay." *International Journal of Urban and Regional Research* 32, no. 2 (June 2008): 415–35.

Mckeown, Thomas. *The Modern Rise of Population*. London: Edward Arnold, 1977.

McVicar, Kenneth Gordon. "Twilight of an East African Slum: Pumwani and the Evolution of African Settlement in Nairobi." Unpublished PhD thesis, University of California Los Angeles, 1968.

Ministry of Housing, *Accra: A Plan for the Town.* Accra: Government Printer, 1958.

Mitchell, Timothy. *Colonizing Egypt.* Berkeley: University of California Press, 1988.

———. *Rule of Experts: Egypt, Technopolitics, and Modernity*. Berkeley: University of California Press, 2002.

Mohamed, Jama. "Epidemics and Public Health in Early Colonial Somaliland." *Social Science and Medicine* 48 (1999): 507–21.

Moradi, Alexander. "Confronting Colonial Legacies—Lessons from Human Development in Ghana and Kenya." *Journal of International Development* 20 (2008): 1107–21.

Morgan, Kenneth O. *Twentieth-Century Britain.* Oxford: Oxford University Press, 2000.

Murunga, Godwin R. "'Inherently Unhygienic Races': Plague and the Origins of Settler Dominance in Nairobi, 1899–1907." In *African Urban Spaces in Historical Perspective*, edited by Steven J. Salm and Toyin Falola, 104–9. Rochester, NY: University of Rochester Press, 2005.

Myers, Garth Andrew. *Verandahs of Power: Colonialism and Space in Urban Africa.* New York: Syracuse University Press, 2003.

Nabila, John. "Depopulation in Northern Ghana: Migration of the Frafra People." In *Interdisciplinary Approaches to Population Studies*, edited by Abrahams S. David, Ebenezer Laing, and Nelson O. Addo. Accra: University of Ghana, 1972.

Ndege, George Oduor. *Health, State, and Society in Kenya*. Rochester, NY: University of Rochester Press, 2001.

Nevanlinna, Anja Kervanto. *Interpreting Nairobi: The Cultural Study of Built* Forms. Helsinki, Finland: Bibliotheca Historica, 1996.

New Ghana. "'Accra Survey' is Title of New Book." January 14, 1959.

Newell, Stephanie. *Histories of Dirt: Media and Urban Life in Colonial and Postcolonial Lagos*. Durham, NC: Duke University Press, 2020.

———. *The Power to Name: A History of Anonymity in Colonial West Africa.* Athens: Ohio University Press, 2013.

Ngalamulume, Kalala. *Colonial Pathologies, Environment, and Western Medicine in Saint-Louis-du-Senegal 1867–1920*. New York: Peter Lang, 2012.

———. "Keeping the City Totally Clean: Yellow Fever and the Politics of Prevention in Colonial Saint-Louis-du-Sénégal 1850–1914." *The Journal of African History* 45, no. 2 (2004): 183–202.

Nightingale, Carl H. *Segregation: A Global History of Divided Cities*. Chicago: University of Chicago Press, 2012.

Nixon, Rob. *Slow Violence and the Environmentalism of the Poor.* Cambridge, MA: Harvard University Press, 2011.

Njoh, Ambe J. "Colonial Philosophies, Urban Space, and Racial Segregation in British and French Colonial Africa." *Journal of Black Studies* 38, no. 4 (March 2008): 579–99.

———. *Planning Power: Social Control and Planning in Colonial Africa*. London: UCL Press, 2007.

———. *Urban Planning and Public Health in Africa: Historical, Theoretical, and Practical Dimensions of a Continent's Water and Sanitation Problematic*. Farnham, UK: Ashgate, 2012.

Nkrumah, Kwame. *Ghana: The Autobiography of Kwame Nkrumah*. London: Panaf Books, 1957.

Odukoya, Adelaja Odutola. "Settler and Non-Settler Colonialism in Africa." In *The Palgrave Handbook of African Politics Governance and Development*, edited by Samuel Ojo Oloruntoba and Toyin Falola, 173–86. New York: Palgrave Macmillan, 2018.

Office of the Secretary and Executive Office Accra. "Town and Country Planning in the Gold Coast" Bulletin No. 2.

Ogilvie, G. C. W. *The Housing of Africans in the Urban Areas of Kenya*. Nairobi: The Kenya Information Office, 1946.

Otiso, Kefa M. "Colonial Urbanization and Urban Management in Kenya." In *African Urban Spaces in Historical Perspective*, edited by Steven J. Salm and Toyin Falola, 83. Rochester, NY: University of Rochester Press, 2005.

Packard, Randall M. *White Plague, Black Labor: Tuberculosis and the Political Economy of Health and Disease in South Africa*. Berkeley: University of California Press, 1989.

Parker, John. *In My Time of Dying: A History of Death and the Dead in West Africa.* Princeton: Princeton University Press, 2021.

———. *Making the Town: Ga State and Society in Early Colonial Accra*. Portsmouth, NH: Heinemann, 2000.

———. "Urbanization and Urban Cultures." In *The Oxford Handbook of Modern African History*, edited by John Parker and Richard Reid, 359–77. Oxford: Oxford University Press, 2013.

Parker, John, and Richard Reid, eds. *The Oxford Handbook of Modern African History*. Oxford: Oxford University Press, 2013.

Parker, Mary. *Political and Social Aspects of the Development of Municipal Government in Kenya with Special Reference to Nairobi*. Nairobi: The Government of Kenya, 1948.

Parnell, Susan. "Creating Racial Privilege: The Origins of South African Public Health and Town Planning Legislation." *Journal of Southern African Studies* 19, no. 3 (September 1993): 471–88.

Parsons, Timothy H. "Jumping Tribal Boundaries: Space, Mobility, and Identity in Kenya." In *Mapping Migration, Identity, and Space*, edited by Tebea Linhard and Timothy H. Parsons. Cham, Germany: Palgrave Macmillan, 2019.

———. "'Kibra is our Blood:' The Sudanese Military Legacy in Nairobi's Kibera Location, 1902–1968." *The International Journal of African Historical Studies* 30, no. 1 (1997): 87–122.

———. *The Second British Empire: In the Crucible of the Twentieth Century*. Lanham, MD: Rowman & Littlefield, 2014.

Patel, Zarina. *Challenge to Colonialism: The Struggle of Alibhai Mulla Jeevanjee for Equal Rights in Kenya*. Nairobi: The Standard Ltd., 1997.

Patterson, K. David. "Health in Urban Ghana: The Case of Accra 1900–1940." *Social Science and Medicine* 13B (1979): 251–68.

Pellow, Deborah. *Landlords and Lodgers: Socio-Spatial Organization in an Accra Community*. Westport, CT: Praeger, 2002.

Plageman, Nate. "'Accra Is Changing. Isn't It?': Urban Infrastructure, Independence, and Nation in the Gold Coast's 'Daily Graphic,' 1954–57." *The International Journal of African Historical*

Studies 43, no. 1 (2010): 137–59.

Plange, Nii-K. "'Opportunity Cost' and Labor Migration: A Misinterpretation of Prosletarianisation in Northern Ghana." *The Journal of Modern African Studies* 17, no. 4 (December 1979): 655–76.

Quarcoopome, Samuel S. "Political Activities in Accra: 1924–1945." Unpublished MA thesis, University of Ghana, 1980.

Quayson, Ato. *Oxford Street Accra: City Life and the Itineraries of Transnationalism.* Durham, NC: Duke University Press, 2014.

Roberts, Jonathan. "The Black Death in the Gold Coast: African and British Responses to the Bubonic Plague Epidemic of 1908." *Gateway* 3 (2001): 1–52.

———. *Sharing the Burden of Sickness: A History of Healing and Medicine in Accra* Bloomington: Indiana University Press, 2021.

Robinson, Jennifer. "A Perfect System of Control? State Power and 'Native Locations' in South Africa." *Environment and Planning* 8, no. 2 (1990): 135–62

Rogaski, Ruth. *Hygienic Modernity: Meanings of Health and Disease in Treaty-Port China* Berkeley: University of California Press, 2004.

Ross, Robert J., and Gerard J. Telkamp, eds. *Colonial Cities: Essays on Urbanism in a Colonial Context.* Dordrecht, Netherlands: Martinus Nijhoff Publishers, 1985.

Sackeyfio-Lenoch, Naaborko. *The Politics of Chieftaincy: Authority and Property in Colonial Ghana, 1920–1950.* Rochester, NY: University of Rochester Press, 2014.

———. "The Politics of Land and Urban Space in Colonial Accra," *History in Africa* 39 (2012): 293–329.

Said, Edward. *Culture and Imperialism.* New York: Knopf, 1993.

———. *Orientalism.* New York: Vintage Books, 1979.

Salm, Steven J., and Toyin Falola, eds. *African Urban Spaces in Historical Perspective.* Rochester, NY: University of Rochester Press, 2005.

Scobey, David M. *Empire City: The Making and Meaning of New York City Landscape* Philadelphia, PA: Temple University Press, 2002.

Scott, David. *Epidemic Disease in Ghana 1901–1960.* London: Oxford University Press, 1965.

Scott, James C. *Weapons of the Weak: Everyday Forms of Resistance.* New Haven, CT: Yale University Press, 1985.

Simone, AbdouMaliq. *For the City Yet to Come: Changing African Life in Four Cities.* Durham, NC: Duke University Press, 2004.

Simpson, William John R. *Report on Plague in the Gold Coast in 1908.* London: J & C Churchill, 1909.

———. *Report on Sanitary Matters in the East Africa Protectorate, Uganda, and Zanzibar.*

London: Colonial Office, 1915.

———. *Report of Sanitary Matters in Various West African Colonies and the Outbreak of Plague in the Gold Coast.* London: Darling and Sons Ltd., 1909.

Smith, Constance. *Nairobi in the Making: Landscapes of Time and Urban Belonging*. Suffolk, UK: James Currey, 2019.

Smart, James. *A Jubilee History of Nairobi.* Nairobi: East African Standard, 1950.

Stacy, Paul. *State of Slum: Precarity and Informal Governance at the Margins in Accra*. London: Zed Books, 2019.

Stamatopoulou-Robbins, Sophia. *Waste Siege: The Life of Infrastructure in Palestine*. Stanford: Stanford University Press, 2020.

Stepan, Nancy Leys. *Eradication: Ridding the World of Diseases Forever?* Ithaca, NY: Cornell University Press, 2011.

Swanson, Maynard W. "'The Asiatic Menace:' Creating Segregation in Durban 1870–1900." *The International Journal of African Historical Studies* 16, no. 3 (1983): 401–21.

———. "The Sanitation Syndrome: Bubonic Plague and Urban Native Policy 1900–1909." *The Journal of African History* 18, no. 3 (1977): 387–410.

———. "Urban Origins of Separate Development." *Race* x, no. 1 (1968): 31–40.

Talton, Benjamin. "'Kill Rats and Stop Plague': Race, Space, and Public Health in Postconquest Kumasi." *Ghana Studies* 22 (2019): 95–113.

Terreni Brown, Stephanie Elizabeth. "Kampala's Shitscape: Exploring Urbanity and Sanitation in Uganda." Unpublished PhD thesis, University of Edinburgh, 2013.

The Colonial Office. *Labor Conditions in West Africa, Reported by Major G. St. J. Orde Browne, O. B. E.* London: His Majesty's Stationary Office, 1941.

The National Council of Churches of Kenya. *Nairobi Demolitions: What Next?* Nairobi: Church House, 1991.

Thiong'o, Ngũgĩ Wa. *Weep Not Child.* Oxford: Heinemann, 1987.

Thornton White, L. W., L. Silberman, and P. R. Anderson. *Nairobi Master Plan for a Colonial Capital: A Report Prepared for the Municipal Council of Nairobi.* London: His Majesty's Stationary Office, 1948.

Thuku, Harry. *Harry Thuku: An Autobiography with the Assistance of Kenneth King*. Nairobi: Oxford University Press, 1970.

Tilley, Helen. *Africa as a Living Laboratory: Empire, Development, and the Problem of Scientific Knowledge 1870–1950*. Chicago: University of Chicago Press, 2011.

Times of West Africa. "The Congested Area Problem." February 13, 1935.

———. "Gigantic Slum Clearance Scheme at Work in England." August 13, 1934.

———. "Korle Gonno Layout Insanitary Condition of Native Area." June 25, 1934.

———. "Slum Clearance." November 22, 1934.

———. "The Square that is Bukom: Populous and Neglected Area, Muddy Streets and Stagnant Square." May 13, 1933.

Town and Country Planning Division of the Ministry of Housing. *Accra: A Plan for the Town*. Accra: Government Printer, 1958.

Turshen, Meredith. *The Political Ecology of Disease in Tanzania*. New Brunswick, NJ: Rutgers University Press, 1984.

Walmsley, R. W. *Nairobi: The Geography of a New City*. Kampala, Uganda: East African Literature Bureau, 1957.

Ward, W. E. F. *A History of Ghana*. London: George Allen and Unwin Ltd., 1958.

Webel, Mari. "Medical Auxiliaries and the Negotiation of Public Health in Colonial North-Western Tanzania." *The Journal of African History* 54, no. 3 (November 2013): 393–416.

Werlin, Herbert H. *Governing an African City: A Study of Nairobi*. New York: Africana Publishing Co., 1974.

West Africa Times. "Improvement in Method." March 24, 1931.

———. "Sanitation and Housing: The Alternatives." May 9, 1931.

Wheatley, Paul. *City as Symbol*. London: University College, 1969.

White, Luise. *The Comforts of Home: Prostitution in Colonial Nairobi*. Chicago: University of Chicago Press, 1990.

———. "Prostitution, Identity, and Class Consciousness in Nairobi during World War II." *Signs* 11, no. 2 (Winter 1986): 255–73.

Wright, Gwendolyn. "Ambiguous Modernisms of African Cities." In *The Short Century: Independence and Liberation 1945–1994*, edited by Okwul Enwezor, 225–26. Munich: Prestel, 2001.

———. *The Politics of Design in French Colonial Urbanism*. Chicago: University of Chicago Press, 1991.

Yeoh, Brenda S. A. *Contesting Space: Power Relations and the Urban Built Environment in Colonial Singapore*. Kuala Lumpur, Malaysia: Oxford University Press, 1996.

Zimring, Carl A. *Clean and White: A History of Environmental Racism in the United States*. New York: New York University Press, 2015.

Index

A

B

O

P

Q

R

S

T

U

V

W

Y

Z